PSYCHIATRIC
DIAGNOSIS

PSYCHIATRIC DIAGNOSIS

FIFTH EDITION

DONALD W. GOODWIN, M.D.
University Distinguished Professor
University of Kansas

SAMUEL B. GUZE, M.D.
Spencer T. Olin Professor of Psychiatry
and Head of the Department
Washington University School of Medicine

New York   Oxford
OXFORD UNIVERSITY PRESS
1996

Oxford University Press

Oxford   New York
Athens   Auckland   Bangkok   Bombay
Calcutta   Cape Town   Dar es Salaam   Delhi
Florence   Hong Kong   Istanbul   Karachi
Kuala Lumpur   Madras   Madrid   Melbourne
Mexico City   Nairobi   Paris   Singapore
Taipei   Tokyo   Toronto

and associated companies in
Berlin   Ibadan

Copyright © 1974, 1979, 1984, 1989, 1996 by
Oxford University Press, Inc.

Published by Oxford University Press, Inc.,
198 Madison Avenue, New York, New York 10016

Oxford is a registered trademark of Oxford University Press

Library of Congress Cataloging-in-Publication Data
Goodwin, Donald W.
Psychiatric diagnosis /
Donald W. Goodwin, Samuel B. Guze. — 5th ed.
p.   cm.   Includes bibliographical references and index.
ISBN 0–19–510421–8 (cloth). — ISBN 0–19–510422–6 (pbk.)
1. Mental illness—Classification.
2. Mental illness—Diagnosis.
I. Guze, Samuel B., 1923– . II. Title.
[DNLM: 1. Mental Disorders—diagnosis.
WM 141 G656p 1996]   RC455.2.C4G66   1996
616.89'075—dc20   DNLM/DLC   for Library of Congress   95–31245

1 3 5 7 9 8 6 4 2

Printed in the United States of America
on acid-free paper

IN MEMORIUM

ROBERT A. WOODRUFF, JR.

The inspiration for—and co-author of—
the first edition of this book

ELI ROBINS

Who, as much as any one person,
launched a new era in American psychiatry

PREFACE

TO THE

FIFTH EDITION

"The paradox of modern psychiatry is that while its practice remains uncertain, the scientific problems it poses are more interesting and exciting than those in any other branch of medicine."
—Editorial in *Lancet*,
October 17, 1987

Twenty-two years have passed since this book was first published. In that time an interesting change has occured in American psychiatry. Psychiatrists have become diagnostic-conscious.

DSM-III, the official diagnostic manual of the American Psychiatric Association, was published in 1980 and became an immediate best-seller. Previous diagnostic and statistical manuals had caused hardly a ripple. Why the change?

Possibly fatigued by unsupported theory, psychiatrists may have found some satisfaction in agreeing on what to call things. If illnesses could not be explained—and doubters were everywhere—at least they could be described. Also, with the discovery of relatively specific drug therapies, diagnosis had become *practical*. With the availability of lithium and neuroleptic drugs, distinguishing between mania and schizophrenia—once an interesting academic exercise—might now determine how a patient was treated.

With the emphasis on diagnosis, use of words like *data, reliability*, and *operational* increased. Journals brimmed over with graphs and tables; circles with arrows pointing this way and that appeared less and less. People actually stood up at meetings and asked: "Where is the evidence?"

These were real changes. We would like to think *Psychiatric Diagnosis* anticipated them. The first edition contained diagnostic criteria similar to the criteria later adopted by DSM-III. Its philosophy was described as "agnostic;" DSM-III called its approach "atheoretical." The first edition presented the features of a dozen disorders; DSM-III described 226—a difference in quantity, not kind.

That *Psychiatric Diagnosis* was a forerunner of DSM-III should not be surprising. The authors were faculty members at Washington University in St. Louis. A third of the DSM-III task force consisted of Washington University–trained psychiatrists. In the sixties and seventies Washington University's Department of Psychiatry gained the reputation of having a strong alliance with biology, taking a medical view of psychiatric illness and placing heavy reliance on reproducible data. It believed in diagnosis, and the belief caught on.

A revised edition of DSM-III was published in 1987 (DSM-III-R). Apart from the criteria for substance abuse, changes were relatively minor. Some new catergories were added. One was Late Luteal Phase Dysphoric Disorder, hormonalese for premenstrual syndrome. Some women object to premenstruel syndrome being called a psychiatric disorder. Changing the name was intended to appease them but didn't. They picketed APA headquarters and held long sessions with lawyers. The term got in anyway, but in a Needing Further Study section.

Another revision (DSM-IV) appeared in 1994. Again, changes were minor. For example, "nicotine dependence" became a disorder, while "late luteal phase dysphoric disorder" has been relegated to an appendix under its old name, "premenstrual disorder."

We have added no new catergories to the fifth edition of *Psychiatric Diagnosis*. In our view there are only about a dozen diagnostic entities in adult psychiatry that have been sufficiently studied to be useful. (For more on this heretical view, see the Preface to the First Edition.) DSM-III and its revisions introduced many new diagnostic terms. The terms used in this book were chosen because, in our judgment, they are the ones most widely used in psychiatry. Where they differ from those recommended by DSM-IV, the reason for using the older, better-known term is provided in the "Definition" section of each chapter.

The fifth edition contains much new information. This is reflected in the number of references. There are now 1,130 references, more than three times the number in the first edition. Each reference refers to somethimg in the text: if readers want to know where we got an idea, we usually can tell them. The practice of identifying sources in a psychiatry textbook has never, to our knowledge, been applied so exhaustively. In this edition we have also included more case vignettes, more neurobiology, and more information on treatment.

In general, the book hews to its original goal: to provide a concise compendium of current knowledge in psychiatry, with abundent citations, not much theory, and as little personal opinion as we could get by with.

August 1995

D.W.G.
Kansas City

S.B.G.
St. Louis

PREFACE
TO THE
FIRST EDITION

A rose is a rose is a rose
GERTRUDE STEIN

Because it remains a rose.

Classification has two functions: communication and prediction. A rose can be defined precisely. It has pinnate leaves, belongs to the rose family, and so forth. When you say "rose" to a person who knows something about the definition, communication results.

A rose also has a predictable life history: It stays a rose. If it changes into a chrysanthemum, it may not have been a rose in the first place. If roses routinely change into chrysanthemums, like caterpillars into butterflies, well and good. Natural history may include metamorphoses but they must be routine to be "natural."

Classification in medicine is called "diagnosis," and this book is about diagnosis of psychiatric conditions. Diagnostic categories—diseases, illnesses, syndromes—are included if they have been sufficiently studied to be useful. Like roses, they can be defined explicitly and have a more or less predictable course.

In choosing these categories, the guiding rule was: *Diagnosis is prognosis.* There are many diagnostic categories in psychiatry, but few are based on a clinical literature where the conditions are defined by explicit criteria and follow-up studies provide a guide to prognosis. Lacking these features, such catergories resemble what sociologists call "labeling." Two examples are "passive-aggressive personality" and "emotionally unstable personality," which, like most personality diagnoses, have been inadequatly studied for us to know whether they are useful or not.

Not every patient can be diagnosed by using the categories in this book. For them, "undiagnosed" is, we feel, more appropriate than a label incorrectly implying more knowledge than exists. Terms like "functional" and "psychogenic" and "situational reaction" are sometimes invoked by physicians to explain the unexplained. They usually mean "I don't know," and we try to avoid them.

Because classification in psychiatry is still at a primitive stage, there are reasonable grounds for questioning our choice of categories. In general, we lump rather than split. Hence we have two affective disorders—primary and secondary—rather than the half-dozen affective disorders cited in the official nomenclature. Schizophrenia is divided into "good prognosis" and "bad prognosis" schizophrenia rather than sliced more finely, as some prefer. Our justification for this is "the literature," meaning primarily follow-up studies.

"The follow-up is the great exposer of truth, the rock on which many fine theories are wrecked and upon which better ones can be built," wrote P. D. Scott. "It is to the psychiatrist what the postmortem is to the physican." Not all such studies are perfect, but we feel they are better than no studies. And inevitably there are instances where our "clinical judgment" has prevailed in evaluating the merit of individual studies. No text in psychiatry could be written today without a certain amount of this, but we have tried to limit personal opinion to a minimum. Many if not most assertions have a citation, and the reader can check the references to form his own judgment.

When the term "disease" is used, this is what is meant: A disease is a cluster of symptoms and/or signs with a more or less predictable course. Symptoms are what patients tell you; signs are what you see. The cluster may be associated with physical abnormality or may not. The essential point is that it results in consultation with a physician who specializes in recognizing, preventing, and, sometimes, curing diseases.

It is hard for many people to think of psychiatric problems as diseases. For one thing, psychiatric problems usually consist of symptons—complaints about thoughts and feelings—or behavior disturbing to others. Rarely are there signs—a fever, a rash. Almost never are there laboratory tests to confirm the diagnosis. What people say changes from time to time, as does behavior. It is usually harder to agree about symptoms than about signs. But whatever the psychiatric problems are, they have this in common with "real" diseases—they result in consultation with a physician and are associated with pain, suffering, disability, and death.

Another objection to the disease or medical "model" arises from a misconception about disease. Disease often is equated with physical abnormality. In fact, a disease is a category used by physicians, as "apples" is a catgory used by grocers. It is a useful category if precise and if the encompassed phenomena are stable over time. Diseases are conventions and may not "fit" anything in nature at all. Through the centuries, diseases have come and gone, some more useful than others, and there is no guarantee that our present "diseases"—medical or psychiatric—will represent the same clusters of symptoms and signs a hundred years from now that they do today. On the contrary, as more is learned, more useful clusters surely will emerge.

There are few explanations in this book. This is because for most psychiatric conditions there *are* no explanations. "Etiology unknown" is the hallmark of psychiatry as well as its bane. Historically, once etiogy is known, a disease stops being "psychiatric." Vitamins were discovered, whereupon vitamin-deficiency psychiatric disorders no longer were treated by psychiatrists. The spirochete was found, then penicillin, and neurosyphilis, once a major psychiatric disorder, became one more infection treated by nonpsychiatrists.

Little, however, is really known about most medical illnesses. Even infectious diseases remain puzzles in that some infected individuals have symptoms and others do not.

People continue to speculate about etiology, of course, and this is good if it produces testable hypotheses and bad if speculation is mistaken for truth. In this book, speculation largely is avoided, since it is available so plentifully elsewhere.

A final word about this approach to psychiatry. It is sometimes called "organic." This is misleading. A better term, perhaps, is "agnostic." Without evidence, we do not believe pills are better than words. Without evidence, we do not believe chemistry is more important than upbringing. Without evidence, we withhold judgment.

Advocacy is not the purpose of this book. Rather, we hope it will be useful in applying current knowledge to those vexatious problems—crudely defined and poorly understood—that come within the jurisdiction of psychiatry.

Saint Louis   D. W. G.
December 1973

CONTENTS

PSYCHIATRIC
DIAGNOSIS

1

AFFECTIVE (MOOD) DISORDERS

DEFINITION

There is a pitch of unhappiness so great that the goods of nature may be entirely forgotten, and all sentiment of their existence vanish from the mental field. For this extremity of pessimism to be reached, something more is needed than observation of life and reflection upon death. The individual must in his own person become the prey of pathological melancholy. . . . Such sensitiveness and susceptibility to mental pain is a rare occurrence where the nervous constitution is entirely normal; one seldom finds it in a healthy subject even where he is the victim of the most atrocious cruelties of outward fortune . . . it is positive and active anguish, a sort of psychical neuralgia wholly unknown to healthy life.

WILLIAM JAMES (58)

Depression and euphoria are the primary symptoms of affective disorders, but not the only ones. Associated with low moods are such symptoms as insomnia, anorexia, suicidal thoughts, and feelings of worthlessness or of being a burden to others; associated with euphoria are such symptoms as hyperactivity and flight of ideas. The extent of depression or euphoria is often inappropriate to the patient's life situation, a fact sometimes as obvious to patients as to their relatives and friends.

3

DSM-III-R renamed affective disorders, calling them "mood disorders." Mood is defined as a "prolonged emotion that colors the whole psychic life . . . generally involving depression or elation." When there is a choice between newer and older terms, this book generally opts for those most clinicians use, which in this case is the older term "affective disorders."

Whatever the name, the definition of affective (or mood) disorders remains unchanged. It refers to a group of disorders characterized by prolonged disturbances of mood, "accompanied by a full or partial manic or depressive syndrome . . . not due to any other physical or mental disorder" (*DSM-IV*).

Affective disorders have been divided and subdivided endlessly as investigators endeavor to distinguish "normal" from "abnormal" mood and to create clinical clusters with distinct natural histories, familial prevalence, course and prognoses, and response to treatment. After a century there is still no agreement about the most satisfactory classification.

Amid all this diversity, there is a common theme: Affective disorders are primarily characterized by depressed mood, elevated mood (mania), or alternations of depressed and elevated moods. The classical term for the last is "manic depressive illness"; a newer term is "bipolar disorder." The two are interchangeable. The most recent classification of affective disorders is contained in *DSM-IV*, published by the American Psychiatric Association in 1994. In this volume severe depressions are called "major depression." Criteria for major depression and mania are presented in Tables 1.1 and 1.2.

Milder forms of a depressive syndrome are called "dysthymic disorder"; milder forms of mania are called "hypomania"; and

Table 1.1 Diagnostic criteria for Major Depressive Episode (*DSM-IV*)

A. Five (or more) of the following symptoms have been present during the same 2-week period and represent a change from previous functioning; at least one of the symptoms is either (1) depressed mood or (2) loss of interest or pleasure

Table 1.1 (*Continued*)

NOTE: Do not include symptoms that are clearly due to a general medical condition, or mood-incongruent delusions or hallucinations.

(1) Depressed mood most of the day, nearly every day, as indicated by either subjective report (e.g., feels sad or empty) or observation made by others (e.g., appears tearful). NOTE: In children and adolescents, can be irritable mood

(2) Markedly diminished interest or pleasure, in all, or almost all, activities most of the day, nearly every day (as indicated by either subjective account or observation made by others)

(3) Significant weight loss when not dieting or weight gain (e.g., a change of more than 5% of body weight in a month), or decrease or increase in appetite nearly every day. NOTE: In children, consider failure to make expected weight gains

(4) Insomnia or hypersomnia nearly every day

(5) Psychomotor agitation or retardation nearly every day (observable by others, not merely subjective feelings of restlessness or being slowed down)

(6) Fatigue or loss of energy nearly every day

(7) Feelings of worthlessness or excessive or inappropriate guilt (which may be delusional) nearly every day (not merely self-reproach or guilt about being sick)

(8) Diminished ability to think or concentrate, or indecisiveness, nearly every day (either by subjective account or as observed by others)

(9) Recurrent thoughts of death (not just fear of dying), recurrent suicidal ideation without a specific plan, or a suicide attempt or a specific plan for committing suicide

B. The symptoms cause clinically significant distress or impairment in social, occupational, or other important areas of functioning

C. The symptoms are not due to the direct physiological effects of a substance (e.g., a drug of abuse, a medication) or a general medical condition (e.g., hypothyroidism)

D. The symptoms are not better accounted for by bereavement, i.e., after the loss of a loved one

All tables in this book attributed to DSM-IV were adapted from diagnostic criteria in the *Diagnostic and Statistical Manual of Mental Disorders*, Fourth Edition, American Psychiatric Association, Washington D.C. 1995.

milder expressions of bipolar disorder are called "cyclothymic disorder."

Confounding the nosologic confusion is the use of two other terms: "primary affective disorder" and "secondary affective disorder." As used in this book primary affective disorder refers to individuals who have had no previous psychiatric disorder or else only episodes of depression or mania. Secondary affective disorder refers to patients with a preexisting psychiatric illness other than depression or mania. Affective disorder is defined as bipolar when mania occurs, whether depressions occur or not. When the

Table 1.2　Diagnostic criteria for Manic Episode (*DSM-IV*)

A. A distinct period of abnormally and persistently elevated, expansive, or irritable mood, lasting at least 1 week (or any duration if hospitalization is necessary)

B. During the period of mood disturbance, three (or more) of the following symptoms have persisted (four if the mood is only irritable) and have been present to a significant degree:

(1) Inflated self-esteem or grandiosity

(2) Decreased need for sleep (e.g., feels rested after only 3 hours of sleep)

(3) More talkative than usual or pressure to keep talking

(4) Flight of ideas or subjective experience that thoughts are racing

(5) Distractibility (i.e., attention too easily drawn to unimportant or irrelevant external stimuli)

(6) Increase in goal-directed activity (either socially, at work or school, or sexually) or psychomotor agitation

(7) Excessive involvement in pleasurable activities that have a high potential for painful consequences (e.g., engaging in unrestrained buying sprees, sexual indiscretions, or foolish business investments)

C. The mood disturbance is sufficiently severe so as to cause marked impairment in occupational functioning or in usual social activities or relationships with others, or to necessitate hospitalization to prevent harm to self or others, or there are psychotic features

D. The symptoms are not due to the direct physiological effects of a substance (e.g., a drug of abuse, a medication, or other treatment) or a general medical condition (e.g., hyperthyroidism)

disorder involves solely depression, the term "unipolar" affective disorder or major depression is often used.

For all these terms, more than disturbed mood is required. There must be a syndrome, a group of characteristic clinical features that distinguish one disorder from another.

HISTORICAL BACKGROUND

Descriptions of affective disorder began with Hippocrates. The term "melancholia" is usually attributed to him, as is the notion that it results from the influence of black bile and phlegm on the brain "darkening the spirit and making it melancholy" (73).

About five hundred years later, early in the second century A.D., Aretaeus of Cappadocia recognized and recorded an association between melancholia and mania:

Those affected with melancholia are not everyone of them affected according to one particular form; they are either suspicious of poisoning or flee to the desert from misanthropy, or turn superstitious, or contract a hatred of life. If at any time a relaxation takes place, in most cases hilarity supervenes . . . the patients are dull or stern, dejected or unreasonably torpid, without any manifest cause . . . they also become peevish, dispirited, sleepless, and start up from a disturbed sleep. Unreasonable fear also seizes them, if the disease tends to increase . . . they complain of life, and desire to die" (65). Aretaeus observed that affective disorder was often episodic but also occurred in a chronic, unremitting form. Like Hippocrates, he attributed the cause to a humoral imbalance: "If it [black bile] be determined upwards to the stomach and diaphragm, it forms melancholy, for it produces flatulence and eructations of the fetid and fishy nature, and it sends rumbling wind downwards and disturbs the understanding. (73)

The nineteenth-century French physician Falret described an episodic variety of depression with remissions and attacks of increasing duration, an illness occurring more frequently among women than men, sometimes associated with precipitating events, sometimes alternating with mania (*la folie circulaire*). Falret and his contemporary Baillarger (who also described recurring attacks of mania and malancholia) probably influenced Kraepelin's later concept of manic depressive psychosis.

In 1896 Kraepelin made his major contribution to psychiatry by separating the functional psychoses into two groups, dementia praecox and manic depressive psychosis. Dementia praecox was chronic and unremitting with a generally bad prognosis. Manic depressive psychosis, on the other hand, did not usually end in chronic invalidism. After publishing the sixth edition of his textbook in 1896, Kraepelin continued to define the limits of dementia praecox narrowly, but he expanded those of manic depressive psychosis to include almost all abnormalities of mood. Patients with chronic depressions were included as well as those with episodic illness, manics as well as depressives (69, 143).

Kraepelin had insisted that manic depressive psychosis was generally independent of social and psychological forces, that the cause of the illness was "innate." Freud and the psychoanalysts assumed the opposite. Freud in *Mourning and Melancholia*, published in 1917, outlined his theories of the psychodynamic genesis of depression (43). He hypothesized that depression had in common with the process of mourning a response to the loss of a "love-object," that is, the loss of something greatly valued. Grief, a healthy response, differed from melancholia in that the latter involved *intense* expression of ambivalent, hostile feelings, formerly associated with the object. Upon loss of the loved person or thing, these unresolved, negative feelings were directed inward, resulting in despair, a sense of worthlessness, thoughts of self-harm, and other depressive symptoms.

Since early in the twentieth century there has been considerable controversy over the distinction between "endogenous" depression and "reactive" depression. This controversy had its origin partially in the differing viewpoints of the Kraepelinians and Freudians toward mental phenomena in general. Kraepelin and his followers searched for the limits of pathological behavior by describing the symptoms of syndromes in keeping with the traditions of nineteenth-century German medicine. Freud and his pupils searched for mental mechanisms that might be most obvious in pathological states but were not limited to those states. Such differences in attitude were augmented by the fact that Kraepelinian psychiatrists dealt chiefly with severely ill, hospitalized patients, whereas Freudian psychiatrists tended to treat mildly ill, nonhospitalized patients. The differences have never been fully resolved. There has been classification after classification of the affective disorders, most frequently in terms of dichotomies: endogenous opposed to reactive, psychotic opposed to neurotic, agitated opposed to retarded.

A large part of the twentieth-century literature on affective disorders assumes tacitly that two basic forms of depression do exist. (This assumption has remained remarkably stable through the centuries [107].) The terms "reactive" and "neurotic" have often been equated, as have the terms "endogenous" and "psychotic." It has been assumed that depressions of the former type are milder, that they are more often a direct result of precipitating events or unique individual responses to social and psychological stress, and more recently that they are less responsive to somatic therapy. However, controversy persists about the validity of this distinction. An alternative that avoids inference about cause is the classification of affective disorders as *primary* or *secondary* (see Definition).

Reactive and endogenous depressions may be classified as either primary or secondary affective disorders. Patients with mild or severe depressions, with or without "psychotic" symptoms such as hallucinations or delusions, with many episodes or with few, and regardless of age of onset, may be diagnosed as having either primary or secondary affective disorder.

Reports have been published in the last two decades indicating that primary affective disorder should be divided into bipolar and unipolar forms (21, 50, 89, 143). (One's initial impression of the terms "bipolar" and "unipolar" is that bipolar patients have had both mania and depression, whereas unipolar patients have had either one or the other alone. "Bipolar" actually refers to patients with mania whether or not they have also had depressions. "Unipolar" refers to patients who have had depression alone.) Patients with bipolar illness have a somewhat earlier age of onset than unipolar patients. Their histories are characterized by more frequent and shorter episodes, even when depression is considered alone. There is a greater prevalence of affective disorder among relatives of bipolar patients than among relatives of unipolar patients.

Many of the questions about affective disorders that have plagued investigators are still unresolved. At present there is no way to evaluate the importance of precipitating events in either bipolar or unipolar illness. There have been preliminary efforts to divide unipolar primary affective disorder into early-onset and late-onset forms (144), but as yet no generally accepted subclassification of unipolar illness exists. An abiding problem is the old question of how to separate the experience of bereavement from that of depression.

EPIDEMIOLOGY

Estimates of the prevalence of primary affective disorder depend on the sample or population studied and on the definition of the illness. Older studies of large groups of patients selected from isolated areas—Iceland (54) and the Danish islands of Bornholm (42) and Samsø (108)—indicated that 5 percent of men and 9 percent of women can expect to have primary affective disorder at some time during their lives. A study by the National Institute of Mental Health (NIMH) tends to confirm these findings, showing a prevalence of bipolar and unipolar disorders of about 5 percent in the general population (88). Much higher rates, however, have been reported in other studies (137); thus it is difficult to know which data are most reliable.

Problems in ascertainment may not be the only explanation for the variability. Cultural and genetic differences may be important in determining the actual prevalence of affective disorders. For example, a 1983 study of 12,500 Amish individuals in Pennsylvania yielded a prevalence rate of 1 percent for primary affective disorder (37). The Amish are a culturally and genetically homo-geneous population consisting of large extended families that live in a socially cohesive environment in which alcoholism, drug abuse, and sociopathy are virtually absent. It is conceivable that reports of higher rates of affective disorder were based on samples "contaminated" by individuals with other psychiatric disorders or possibly that the Amish have a smaller genetic propensity for affective disorders than other populations. Finally, as the Amish study was one of the first to use *DSM-III* criteria, a third explana-tion is that previous studies used looser criteria that produced inflated rates because of false positives.

In any case, private psychiatric hospitals report that primary affective disorder is the problem for which patients are most fre-quently admitted, and the same is true of many psychiatric clinics.

Furthermore, whatever the chief diagnosis, depression is a common reason for psychiatric consultation. Among patients with panic disorder in one study, for example, half presented with a secondary depression (146). Secondary depression is also fre-quently the reason for psychiatric consultation among alcoholics, hysterics, and other patients who come to a psychiatric clinic (53, 146, 147). Depression—primary and secondary—is clearly the most common diagnosis in psychiatry (55, 137).

Most studies show that primary affective disorder is more com-mon in women than men (101, 135). However, this may only apply to unipolar disorder where women, in some studies, out-number men by two to one (135). Apparently, men and women share about equally the risk of suffering bipolar disorder (9).

A link between bipolar affective disorder and above-average occupational or educational achievement has been suggested (145). Some studies raise the possibility that primary affective disorder especially affects socially striving individuals who feel great need for social success and approval (13, 29, 45, 54). The low prevalence of affective disorder among the Amish (37) may reflect their simple life style and unconcern for material success—although this explanation is just as speculative as the others.

CLINICAL PICTURE

The classification of affective disorders remains controversial. *DSM-IV*, for example, does not distinguish between "primary" and "secondary" affective disorder. We make the distinction for the following reason: Although the symptoms of primary and secondary affective disorder are similar, the two conditions have different prognostic and therapeutic implications (53, 111, 144). Primary affective disorder, which occurs in the absence of a preexisting psychiatric disorder or a chronic debilitating medical illness, consists of discrete episodes interspersed with periods of normality. In the case of secondary affective disorders, when the preexisting illness is chronic, which is usually the case, the patient is *not* well between episodes. Depressions that are indistinguishable symptomatically from primary affective disorder occur commonly in obsessive-compulsive disorder, phobic disorders, panic disorder, somatization disorder, alcohol and drug dependence, and antisocial personality. In fact, almost all psychiatric disorders, including schizophrenia and brain syndromes, are associated with an increased risk of secondary depression. (Secondary mania is much less common.)

A further advantage of the primary–secondary distinction is that some studies indicate that primary affective disorder involves a higher risk of suicide than does a secondary affective disorder (except for alcoholism, which also involves a considerable suicide risk [52]).

Finally, decisions about treatment will be influenced by distinguishing primary from secondary affective disorder; the preexisting illness as well as the depressive syndrome must be treated in the latter.

The chief complaints of patients with a depressive episode are usually psychological: feelings of worthlessness, despair, or ideas of self-harm. But it is also common for depressed patients to complain chiefly of pains, tachycardia, breathing difficulty, gastrointestinal dysfunction, headache, or other somatic disturbances (24).

The dysphoric mood eperienced by patients with depressive

illness is usually characterized as sadness or despondency, but some patients describe themselves as feeling hopeless, irritable, fearful, worried, or simply discouraged. Occasionally, patients will present with what seems to be primary affective disorder, though they report minimal feelings of dysphoria. Such patients may complain of insomnia and anorexia. They may even cry profusely while telling the examining physician that they do not feel sad. These patients are unusual, but not unknown to psychiatrists.

Other characteristic symptoms of depression are anorexia with weight loss; insomnia; early morning awakening; loss of energy, described as general tiredness or fatigability; agitation or (its opposite) psychomotor retardation; loss of interest in usual activities, including loss of interest in sex; feelings of self-reproach or guilt, which may be delusional in intensity; inability to focus one's thoughts, often with a simultaneous awareness of slowed thinking; and recurrent thought of death or suicide.

It is common for patients with primary affective disorder to say, "Something is wrong with my mind." Patients will often tell their physician that they fear they are losing their mind or have a sense of emotions out of control. It is also common for depressed patients to have a low expectancy of recovery. Such a pessimistic outlook should serve as a warning that the patient may be depressed. Medically ill patients seldom give up all hope of improvement, even if seriously ill.

In some depressed patients agitation is so overwhelming that other symptoms go almost unnoticed. These patients are brought to physicians when they are found by relatives or friends pacing, wringing their hands, bemoaning their fate, clinging to anyone who will listen. They ask for reassurance, they beg for help, yet nothing satisfies them.

In other patients retardation is prominent. Marked slowing of both thought and motor behavior occurs. Tasks that once took minutes may require hours. These patients may be so slowed that it is painful to listen to their conversation. Psychomotor retardation can be so severe that a patient becomes mute or even stuporous (68).

Paranoid symptoms can occur among patients with primary

affective disorder. There are usually exaggerated ideas of reference associated with notions of worthlessness. Characteristic delusions of patients with depression are those of a hypochondriacal
or nihilistic type. Some severely ill depressives seem to feel they
are so guilty and evil that they have become the focus of universal
abhorrence or even that the world is disintegrating because of
their terrible inadequacies and failures.

Hallucinations may also occur in primary affective disorder.
These commonly involve accusatory voices or visions of deceased
relatives associated with feelings of guilt. Delusions and hallucinations occurring in primary affective disorder are usually
"mood congruent," their content consistent with the person's
dominant mood. If a depressed person has delusions and hallucinations, the themes are commonly guilt, disease, poverty, death,
or deserved punishment. If a manic has delusions or hallucinations, they are often of inflated worth, power, or special relationship to a deity or famous person.

DSM-IV includes mood-congruence as a diagnostic feature of
affective disorders. Mood-*in*congruent psychotic features are
more often seen in schizophrenia where, for example, the patient
may seem cheerful and relaxed while describing terrifying delusional experiences. The importance of mood-congruence is based
mainly on a widespread clinical impression rather than systematic studies.

Depressed patients may or may not mention events that they
consider important in producing their illness. When a precipitating event is described, it is sometimes surprisingly trivial, difficult
for the examining physician to take seriously. Furthermore, critical evaluation of the chronology of a depressed patient's symptoms may reveal that some symptoms actually began *before* the
so-called "precipitating event" (24). This suggests that some patients who begin to feel depressed search for reasons to explain
their depression, unable or unwilling to believe they could feel as
they do for no apparent reason.

The stresful events women most frequently mention as precipi-
tants of depression are pregnancy and childbirth. In one series, 37

percent of female bipolars and 17 percent of female unipolars had their first episode of depression during pregnancy or postpatrum (59).

A change in drinking habits often accompanies depressive illness (24). Middle-aged individuals who begin to drink heavily and do not have a previous history of alcoholism may be suffering from depression. On the other hand, some individuals drink less than usual when depressed.

A physician (101) has written movingly about how it feels to have the illness:

Firstly, it is very unpleasant: depressive illness is probably more unpleasant than any disease except rabies. There is constant mental pain and often psychogenic physical pain too. If one tries to get such a patient to titrate other pains against the pain of his depression one tends to end up with a description that would raise eyebrows even in a medieval torture chamber.

Naturally, many of these patients commit suicide. They may not hope to get to heaven but they know they are leaving hell. Secondly, the patient is isolated from family and friends, because the depression itself reduces his affection for others and he may well have ideas that he is unworthy of their love or even that his friendship may harm them. Thirdly, he is rejected by others because they cannot stand the sight of his suffering.

There is a limit to sympathy. Even psychiatrists have protective mechanisms for dealing with such cases: the consultant may refer the patient to an outpatient clinic; he may allow too brief a consultation to elicit the extent of the patient's suffering; he may, on the grounds that the depression has not responded to treatment, alter his diagnosis to one of personality disorder—comforting, because of the strange but widespread belief that patients with personality disorders do not suffer.

Fourthly, and finally, the patient tends to do a great cover-up. Because of his outward depression he is socially unacceptable, and because of his inward depression he feels even more socially unacceptable than he really is. He does not, therefore, tell others how bad he feels.

Most depressives, even severe ones, can cope with routine work—initiative and leadership are what they lack. Nevertheless, many of them can continue working, functioning at a fairly low level, and their deficiencies are often covered up by colleagues. Provided some minimal degree of social and vocational functioning is present, the world leaves the depressive alone and he battles on for the sake of his god or his children, or for some reason which makes his personal torment preferable to death.

The cardinal features of mania are euphoria, hyperactivity, and flight of ideas. Not all manic patients are euphoric; some are irritable instead. Flight of ideas is a rapid digression from one idea to another. One's response to a manic patient is often that of sympathetic amusement. In fact, experienced clinicians who find themselves amused by a patient immediately consider the possibility that the patient is either manic or hypomanic (mildly manic). Flight of ideas, unlike the incoherence and tangentiality of schizophrenia, is usually understandable, even though some connections between ideas may be tenuous. (Comedians often use a well-controlled flight of ideas to amuse audiences.) Attention is often called to this symptom by a push of speech, that is, speech in which a great deal is said in a short period of time. Such speech may be accompanied by rhyming, punning, and jocular associations.

Psychotic symptoms also occur: persecutory and grandiose delusions, hallucinations, ideas of reference. They are usually mood-congruent. Some patients exhibit depression and mania simultaneously. They may cry while speaking euphorically or show other unusual combinations of symptoms.

The separation of affective states into unipolar and bipolar subtypes was first proposed by Leonhard et al. (72), and support for the separation has emerged from numerous studies in Europe and the United States. Compared to unipolars, bipolars tend to have an earlier age of onset (late twenties), cyclical depressions, a higher frequency of postpartum onsets, and a greater tendency for suicide attempts. Unipolar patients have a mean age of onset in the mid-thirties, tend to have single episodes, and find their depressions to be often confounded with anxiety (3, 35). A few studies indicate that bipolars who have had depressions respond better to lithium than unipolars (35) (Unipolar depression and major depression are synonyms.)

Among other reported differences between bipolar and unipolar disorder, bipolars are more likely to be delusional and to manifest psychomotor retardation. Unipolar patients more often have agitated depressions (14, 20, 99).

Neurochemical correlates of bipolar and unipolar affective disorder also have been reported. Schildkraut et al. (121) devised a mathematical equation that differentiates bipolar from chronic unipolar depressions; and follow-up studies by Shildkraut et al. tend to confirm the test's validity (122). The equation utilizes data on urinary catecholamines and metabolites. Italian investigators (118) reported a correlation between a urinary metabolite of norepinephrine and outcome with lithium: Bipolar patients with low excretion of the metabolite during depression responded best to lithium, supporting the theory that low levels of norepinephrine are associated with bipolar depression. The most recent evidence that bipolar and unipolar affective disorders represent two different disorders derives from positron emission tomography (PET) studies that show different group metabolism rates for discrete cerebral structures in the two disorders (124). Bipolar patients showed a reduction of glucose metabolism in structures above the tentorium, whereas unipolar depressed patients had higher values.

Some children have episodes of depression that resemble depression in adulthood: crying, social withdrawal, hypersensitivity, and behavioral problems (98). It is not clear whether such episodes are an early manifestation of primary affective disorder. Two observations suggest that they may not be: (a) As a rule, childhood depression is more common in boys, adult depression more common in women (135, 149); (b) the sleep of depressed children does not differ from that of age-matched normal children, whereas depressed adults differ from normal subjects in taking longer to fall asleep, awakening more often throughout the night, and experiencing greater early morning wakefulness (71).

Depression in adults is also associated with a reduction in slow-wave sleep (stages 3 and 4), shortened rapid eye movement (REM) latency, and increased REM density. Sleep studies of depressed children demonstrate none of these differences (149).

This suggests either that a sleep disorder makes a rather abrupt appearance within the depressive syndrome or that the depressive disorders of children and adults differ in important ways. Because human growth hormone (HGH) is excreted mostly during sleep, sleep has an additional function in children not present in adults. As a physiological state, sleep may be more protected in children than in adults. In any event, it appears that sleep measures are less useful as markers for childhood depression than for depressive illness in later years.

The dexamethasone suppression test (DST) has been called psychiatry's first laboratory test. Introduced by Carroll, it has generated both enthusiasm and criticism (23). It is only fairly *sensitive* for affective disorder: About 50 percent of patients with depression test positive, that is, resist suppression of blood cortisol levels following a dose of dexamethasone. The *specificity* of the test is higher. Only about 10 percent of *normal* control subjects are nonsuppressors. However, the specificity drops to less than 70 percent in some psychiatric conditions—including dementia and alcohol abuse—and in medical conditions that involve weight loss.

These findings were reported by an American Psychiatric Association task force (131). The report stated that positive initial DST status in depression does not add to the likelihood of antidepressant response and that a negative test is not an indication for withholding antidepressant treatment. "Although the clinical utility of the DST is limited," concluded the task force, "in certain situations its thoughtful use may aid clinical decision-making."

It has been suggested that the DST might be used to determine when antidepressant treatment should be discontinued (51). Following symptom remission in depression, there is believed to be a period of increased risk of symptom recurrence. Because there is no way to determine the length of this period, it is common practice to continue medication for at least six months after the remission of acute symptoms. Normalization of previously abnormal DST cortisol levels may indicate sufficiently diminished risk of symptom recurrence so that one can safely discontinue medication. Unfortunately, evidence that normalization of the DST predicts continued remission is mixed. Pending further evidence, most clinicians continue antidepressant drugs after remission of symptoms for several months regardless of DST results.

Another laboratory diagnostic test for depression that has been proposed involves administering thyroid-releasing hormone (TRH) to suspected depressed patients. Results vary, but in some studies half or more of unipolar patients have a "blunted" response of thyroid-stimulating hormone (TSH) secretion following a challenge with TRH. Some believe that a combination of the DST and TRH tests will identify "most" patients with unipolar depression (46), but this is debated. Even advocates of the laboratory tests do not consider them diagnostic in themselves.

NATURAL HISTORY

The natural history of primary affective disorder is variable. The age of risk extends through life. Together with the usual episodic nature of the illness, this distinguishes primary affective disorder from most other psychiatric illnesses.

The mean age of onset of primary affective disorder is approximately forty. For bipolar patients, the mean age of onset is about thirty (36). Several studies have indicated a significant correlation between family members in age of onset (59).

How often do patients experience a single episode of affective disorder without recurrence? At a conference sponsored by the NIMH (81), authorities reviewed the literature and reached these condlusions: (a) most patients who have a manic episode have multiple recurrences of depression and mania; (b) about 70 percent of patients who have a major depressive episode will have at least one subsequent episode of depression in their lifetime and about 12 percent will have subsequent manic episodes; (c) about 20 percent of patients with affective disorders develop a chronic illness difficult for physicians to manage (62).

Between episodes of illness, patients with primary affective disorder usually function well, though there are occasional residual symptoms. Bipolars may be an exception. Winokur and colleagues (142) studied remitted manic depressives and found that only 61 percent of the untreated subjects were symptom-free between acute episodes. Maintained on lithium, however, bipolars between episodes were found to be as healthy as a comparison group of nonpsychiatric patients and their episodes were much diminished in frequency and intensity.

The length of individual episodes is extremely varible, ranging from a few days to many years. In one study, 50 percent of patients recovered within one year and annual rates of recovery then declined steadily to 28 percent in the second year, 22 percent in the third year, and 18 percent in the fourth year (64).

The period for highest risk of relapse is shortly after recovery (62). About 25 percent of patients relapse within twelve weeks after recovery; 12 percent relapse within four weeks (64). The rate of relapse declines steadily thereafter. The longer the patient has remained well, the lower is his or her current risk of relapse. Increased risk of relapse is associated with (a) the presence of a chronic depression of at least two years' duration and (b) a history of at least three previous affective episodes (58). Treatment differences may account for different rates of relapse. Both lithium carbonate and antidepressant drugs prevent relapse in some patients but not others.

COMPLICATIONS

There is a clear association between primary depression and suicide: Of those who commit suicide 50 to 70 percent can be found retrospectively to have had symptoms characteristic of depression. Of those who have depression, based on a review of seventeen studies, 15 percent will eventually die by suicide (52).

Although most people who commit suicide have made previous suicide attempts, only a small percentage of attempters eventually kill themselves. Nine follow-up studies of attempters showed that no more than 2 to 4 percent are dead by suicide within five years after an attempt (96). The more medically serious the attempt, the more likely it is that a person will subsequently die by suicide—although this is a weak predictor at best—and medically trivial attempts are also sometimes followed by completed suicide.

The risk of suicide is not necessarily correlated with the severity of symptoms. An increased risk of suicide is associated with age greater than forty, with being male, and with communication of suicidal intent (112). Folklore that patients who talk of suicide do not commit suicide is untrue. Suicidal communication must be interpreted in light of the diagnosis (39). The two disorders most frequently associated with suicide are primary affective disorder and alcoholism (112).

Disregarding suicide, patients with primary affective disorder may still have an increased mortality compared with matched members of the general population. In two studies, it was found that depressed men had an increased mortality from physical disease, especially carcinoma (18, 66).

Alcoholism may be a complication of primary affective disorder. This is particularly true when a person begins to drink heavily in mid or late life because "primary" alcoholism usually begins earlier. Drug abuse may also be a complication of primary affective disorder.

Poor judgment is another complication of primary affective disorder. Manic patients often show poor judgment, going on spending sprees and making impulsive, unrealistic decisions. Depressed patients also make bad decisions. Decisions to leave a job, to move to a different city, or to separate from a spouse are sometimes the result of the restless dissatisfaction associated with depression. Many clinicians advise depressed patients not to make major life decisions until they are clearly in remission.

Studies of psychiatric illness in the postpartum period indicate that bipolar women are more likely to have episodes of depression or mania during the puerperium than at other times in their lives. Having had a postpartum episode of depression, the likelihood that a woman with bipolar illness will have another episode after subsequent pregnancy is high. Female relatives of bipolar women, if they have been affectively ill, are more likely to have had episodes of illness during the puerperium than at other times (5, 10, 19, 106).

There is a significant relationship between unipolar affective disorder and poor academic performance, including college drop-out (89, 140). In one study at a large university, students with a high number of affective symptoms received poorer grades than did others (140). Depressed students were likely to drop courses or leave college.

On psychological testing, depressed patients may show impairment in short-term but not long-term memory (127). As the clinical state improves, so does short-term memory. Depressed patients also do poorly on tests of abstract thinking, making more errors than controls on the Halstead-Reitan Category Test (120).

Sometimes the memory impairment with depression is so profound that a mistaken diagnosis of dementia is made. Memory impairment owing to depression is called "pseudodementia." Its true identity is revealed when memory returns to normal after recovery from the depression.

FAMILY STUDIES

Several studies in the 1960s reached similar conclusions about familial patterns of affective disorders: Affective disorders tend to be familial and can be subdivided into bipolar and unipolar types. In general, bipolar patients have bipolar relatives and unipolar patients have unipolar relatives (9, 94, 142).

Doubt has been cast on the validity of these reports. In a large collaborative study by the NIMH, relatives of bipolar patients had higher rates of bipolar illness than the relatives of unipolar patients, but the relatives of unipolar patients did *not* have a higher rate of unipolar illness than the relatives of bipolar patients (7).

Meanwhile, data from adoption and twin studies provide strong evidence for the role of genetic factors in affective disorders generally (63, 124). An adoption study showed that children of parents with affective disorder, when adopted out to foster parents without affective disorder, continued to have an elevated risk of affective disorder (84).

There have been numerous twin studies (4) of affective disorder, the first conducted in 1928, summarized by McGuffin, Katz and Rutherford (80). Only three dealt with unipolar affective disorder as a separate group. Of a total of 83 bipolar monozygotic probands, 72 percent had a bipolar cotwin. This contrasted with a 14 percent concordance rate in 226 dizygotic twins. The concordance rate for unipolar affective disorder was 40 percent in monozygotic twins and 11 percent in dizygotic twins. Thus, bipolar illness appears to be more strongly influenced by genetic factors than unipolar illness.

An association between unipolar affective disorder and alcoholism has been proposed by Winokur and his coworkers (133). In a series of publications they have contrasted "pure depressive illness" with "depressive spectrum disease." The latter refers to families in which there is a high prevalence of alcoholism and sociopathy among the men and a high prevalence of early onset unipolar affective disorder among the women. A study of daughters of alcoholics raised by adoptive parents compared to daughters of alcoholics raised by their own alcoholic parents revealed that the latter group did, indeed, have a high prevalence of depression but that daughters raised by adoptive parents had no more depression than did controls. This suggested that the association of depression with alcoholism in family members may be strongly influenced by environmental factors (49).

One study (87) suggests that when a patient with primary affective disorder or alcoholism has a family history of suicide attempt, the risk of suicide is increased. A family history of attempted suicide does *not* seem to predict successful suicide in patients with sociopathy, hysteria, or opiate addiction.

The mode of genetic transmission in affective disorder is non-Mendelian and almost certainly polygenic. A human leukocyte antigen (HLA) "genetic marker" for affective disorders has been reported by two groups (78, 139). Both found that pairs of siblings, when both had affective disorders, shared HLA haplotypes more often than would be expected by chance. The HLA-linked genes were on chromosome 6. Two other groups (36, 47, 140) challenged the above reports on statistical grounds and also failed to replicate the findings.

Studying a large pedigree of Amish subjects, Egland et al. (92) identified a dominant gene conferring a "strong predisposition" to manic depressive disease on the short arm of chromosome 11. However, other investigators (56) found no evidence for chromosomal linkage in three family pedigrees. They concluded that linkage in manic depression is heterogeneous and that mutations might explain the findings in the Amish sample.

DIFFERENTIAL DIAGNOSIS

Making the distinction between grief and primary affective disorder can be difficult. However, grief usually does not last as long as an episode of primary affective disorder (25–27). The majority of bereaved persons experience fewer symptoms than do patients with primary affective disorder. Furthermore, some symptoms common in primary affective disorder are relatively rare among persons experiencing bereavement, notably fear of losing one's mind and thoughts of self-harm (26, 27). If bereavement persists for more than one year, it is likely that the individual has had a preexisting psychiatric disorder.

Differential diagnosis between panic disorder and primary affective disorder can be difficult because anxiety symptoms occur frequently in primary affective disorder and depressive symptoms occur frequently in panic disorder. The distinction depends chiefly on chronology. If anxiety symptoms antedate the depressive symptoms, the diagnosis is panic disorder. If depressive symptoms appeared first, the diagnosis is primary affective disorder. Panic disorder almost always begins relatively early in life. One should be cautious about diagnosing panic disorder with secondary affective disorder when the illness begins in mid or late life (146).

Patients with primary affective disorder often report somatic symptoms; hysterics often report affective symptoms. If depressive and anxiety symptoms predominate, the diagnosis of hysteria should be made with caution, particularly if the illness did not occur until the patient was thirty or older. Though patients with primary affective disorder may report many somatic symptoms, these symptoms are seldom spread throughout the system review. Furthermore, conversion symptoms (unexplained neurological symptoms) combined with menstrual symptoms are infrequent in primary affective disorder.

Obsessions occur commonly in primary affective disorder. The distinction between obsessional illness and primary affective disorder is also made on the basis of chronology. If obsessions and compulsions antedate depressive symptoms, a diagnosis of primary affective disorder should not be made.

Distinghishing between schizophrenia and primary affective disorder is usually not a problem. Schizophrenia, a chronic illness of insidious onset, is not characterized by the remitting course found in primary affective disorder. Patients with primary affective disorder do not develop the formal thought disorder characteristically seen in schizophrenia. Occasionally, the distinction between mania and schizophrenia may be difficult. Bizarre and dramatic hallucinations, delusions, and other abnormalities of mental content like those seen in schizophrenia may occur in mania. A previous history of episodic illness with remission or the presence of euphoria, hyperactivity, or flight of ideas indicates that the diagnosis may be mania rather than schizophrenia. The physician should also be careful in making a diagnosis of schizophrenia when a patient has a family history of affective disorder. This history by itself favors the diagnosis of primary affective disorder (132).

For many years, clinicians assumed that schizophreniform illness (schizoaffective psychosis) was more closely related to schizophrenia than to primary affective disorder. Now there is increasing evidence that its relation to primary affective disorder is stronger (25, 28, 30). Family-history studies indicate that among the relatives of schizophreniform patients there is an increased prevalence of affective disorder. After remission, patients with schizophreniform illness may become ill again in episodic fashion, as do patients with primary affective disorder. Further episodes of illness may be typical of depression or mania (25).

A systematic study of eighty-eight psychiatric inpatients who were diagnosed as having either manic disorder or schizoaffective disorder revealed no differences between the two groups with regard to the clinical picture, demographic variables, individual or family history, and treatment response (2).

Organic brain syndromes are sometimes accompanied by depressive symptoms. Among patients with chronic brain syndromes, those with cerebral arteriosclerosis may be particularly likely to have episodes of secondary affective disorder (114). Pseudodementia (gross memory impairment in severely depressed patients) may lead to diagnostic confusion in deciding which is primary—the depression or the dementia (127).

Depressive or manic symptoms are side effects of certain drugs. Reserpine, alphamethyldopa, or other drugs used in the treatment of hypertension may produce depression. Steroids may produce schizophreniform illness. Some women respond to birth control pills with mild to moderate depressive symptoms (76).

CLINICAL MANAGEMENT

The management of depression in primary affective disorder always involves supportive psychotherapy (99). Many clinicians believe that *insight-directed* psychotherapy, involving examination of motives and deep feelings, is probably not wise because it tends to increase the patient's feelings of guilt. Some evidence, however, indicates that certain types of psychotherapy may be useful for mild or moderate depressions. The studies are of three types: (a) psychotherapy alone compared with control group, (b) psychotherapy compared with antidepressant drugs, and (c) combined psychotherapy and drugs compared with psychotherapy alone and drugs alone. Five types of psychotherapy have been employed in the studies: (a) cognitive therapy, (b) behavioral therapy, (c) interpersonal therapy, (d) group therapy, and (e) marital therapy.

The goal of *cognitive therapy* is to "break down existing negative cognitions and replace them with more positive functionally adaptive ones" (12). In *behavior therapy*, the patient is "trained to function effectively in interpersonal interactions so as to maximize reinforcement obtained from others" (41). "Social skills training" is one type of behavior therapy. It emphasizes assertiveness, verbal skills, and practice at making others feel more comfortable (12). *Interpersonal psychotherapy* attempts to improve the quality of the patient's social and interpersonal functioning by "enhancing ability to cope with internally and externally induced stresses, by restoring morale, and by helping the patient deal with the personal and social consequences of the disorder" (138). In *group therapy*, a psychotherapist and a group of patients attempt to effect changes in the emotional states and behavior of the patients. *Marital therapy* may be done with an individual, a couple or family, or a group of couples.

Weissman et al. (138) reviewed seventeen clinical trials that tested the efficacy of the five psychological treatments alone in comparison, and in combination, with drug therapy in samples of depressed outpatients. In all the studies, psychotherapy was more efficacious than nontreatment. The studies that compared drugs with psychotherapy were equivocal. One study found psychotherapy more efficacious than drugs; one study found both about equal; and three studies found that drugs produce relief of symptoms, whereas psychotherapy has more effect on social functioning. Four studies examined the combination of tricyclic antidepressants and psychotherapy. All found the combination more efficacious than either treatment alone or no treatment (17, 33, 115).

Based on these studies, drugs and psychotherapy combined seemed to be the treatment of choice for at least mild to moderate depressions. As Weissman et al. (138) point out, many patients will not tolerate antidepressants. Others do not wish to enter into psychotherapy. "Under either of these conditions," Weissman says, "the patient should not be denied treatment but should be offered the alternative." There are not sufficient data to say which of the psychotherapies should be used, which patients will recover quickly with no treatment, or which subtype of depressive disorder will benefit from drugs and/or psychotherapy.

There are two major somatic approaches to the management of depressive episodes: drug treatment and electrotherapy.

For many years, tricyclic antidepressants such as imipramine and amitriptyline were the most commonly used drugs for depression. They should be administered for at least three or four weeks before shifting to other drugs or to electrotherapy if there is no improvement. The side effects of tricyclic antidepressants are usually not serious. The most common are dry mouth, orthostatic hypotension, and tremor. These effects often diminish as the drug is continued. Less common, but potentially serious, are cardiac arrhythmias from tricyclics.

Individuals vary widely in their ability to metabolize tricyclic antidepressants; as much as a fortyfold difference has been reported between fast and slow metabolizers. What a physician assumes to be a therapeutic dose may actually produce toxic plasma levels or, alternatively, subtherapeutic levels of the drug. For this reason, monitoring plasma levels of tricyclics with gas liquid chromatography (available in many centers and commercial laboratories) is advised when the seemingly therapeutic dose produces either no improvement or potentially serious side effects. There is some evidence that, apart from side effects, high levels of some tricyclics are no more effective than low levels (the "therapeutic window" effect). Monitoring plasma levels may help locate the "therapeutic window."

Since the late 1980s a new class of antidepressants has become available. Called "selective serotonin-uptake inhibitors" (SSRIs), they include Prozac, Zoloft, and Paxil. They were developed because of evidence that serotonin is involved in depression (90, 91). They are as effective as tricyclic antidepressants but have fewer side effects (e.g., cardiotoxicity is nearly nonexistent). They have become very popular (99). Other SSRIs are being developed; 16 new drugs for mood disorders were scheduled for release between mid-1994 and 1997.

Lithium also relieves and possibly prevents depression, especially in bipolar depressed patients. It is less useful in unipolar depressed patients (50, 104). About 70 percent of bipolar depressions improve on lithium compared with 40 percent of unipolar depressions (67, 105). If the unipolar patient has a positive family history of bipolar disorder or hypomanic symptoms, lithium may exert a more antidepressant effect than if neither of these features exists (34, 70, 82).

The role of antidepressants in bipolar disorder is not clear. Antidepressants occasionally produce mania in depressed bipolar patients and may induce "rapid cycling" between states of mania and depression. Hence antidepressants, the treatment of choice for unipolar depression, may be deleterious in bipolar depression. A combination of lithium and antidepressants has been suggested for depressed bipolar patients to prevent a sudden onset of mania (67).

Some patients experience depression during certain times of the year, especially in the fall and early winter. *DSM-IV* includes seasonal affective disorder (SAD) as a subcategory of major depressive disorder. Criteria for SAD include a temporal relationship between the onset of bipolar disorder, or recurrent major depression, and a specific period of the year (e.g., regular appearance of depression in the fall).

Season affective disorder has been little studied, but a growing body of literature indicates that an effective treatment may exist for the condition. This involves prolonged exposure in the fall and winter months to fluorescent lighting with wavelengths similar to sunlight (113). Devices are now on the market that provide such lighting. There is disagreement about the length of exposure or the time of day when exposure is most efficacious. The effectiveness of the treatment—if definitely shown to exist—may depend on suppressing nighttime melatonin production or some other manipulation of biological rhythms (74). Investigators recommend that patients sit for as long as five hours within a few feet of the light, staring briefly at the light every minute. The possibility of resultant cataracts or retinal damage has not been fully assessed.

The drug literature is replete with warnings against combining alcohol with psychotropic drugs. In the case of alcohol and barbiturates, the combination may be lethal. There is less additive effect between alcohol and benzodiazepine tranquilizers. Combining alcohol with tricyclic antidepressants may be dangerous. Tricyclics increase the diffusion of alcohol across the blood-brain barrier, resulting in higher levels of alcohol in the brain than in the peripheral circulation (100).

Choosing the most suitable antidepressant for a particular patient is still more of an art than a science (32, 61). Often the decision is based on side effects rather than evidence of superior effectiveness. For example, amitriptyline causes sedation and is even used as a hypnotic. Imipramine has a more energizing effect and may interfere with sleep. Amitriptyline has marked anticholinergic side effects; desipramine has almost none. When dry mouth or urinary retention are bothersome, desipramine can be substituted for amitriptyline.

Monoamine oxidase inhibitors are also used for depression (110). There is no evidence they are more effective than other antidepressants, and the side effects can be more serious. Patients taking these drugs should not receive other drugs containing amphetamines or sympathomimetic substances. Foods and beverages containing tyramine (a pressor substance)—particularly cheese, some wines, and beer—should be avoided because of the danger of a hypertensive crisis.

It is not clear whether antidepressant drugs—shown in controlled studies to shorten depressive episodes, reduce the intensity of symptoms, and possibly prevent recurrence—have led to a reduction in suicide by patients with primary affective disorder

(141). The overall suicide rate has not dropped, but there is some evidence that suicide among patients with primary affective disorder has declined, whereas suicide among schizophrenics, alcoholics, and other psychiatric groups has increased (77, 116). Suicide-prevention centers, established in many cities during the 1960s, apparently have had no effect on the suicide rate.

Most psychiatrists reserve electrotherapy for patients who do not respond to antidepressants or who are so ill that they cannot be treated outside a hospital (22). Electrotherapy may be the most effective form of treatment available for depression (16, 31). When first introduced into clinical practice in the early 1940s, it frequently caused vertebral and other fractures. As advances in the drug modification of electrotherapy have been made, the procedure is less frightening and less commonly associated with complications. Patients are anesthetized briefly with a very rapid-acting barbiturate and then are given a muscle relaxant, usually succinylcholine. Electrodes are placed in the frontotemporal regions and a small, measured amount of electricity is passed between them (97, 119).

The most troublesome side effect of electrotherapy is the temporary loss of recent memory that occurs in most patients. Delivering unilateral electrotherapy to the nondominant side of the brain minimizes even this side effect (1). Electrotherapy is probably no more dangerous than treatment with drugs (60). The only absolute contraindication to this mode of therapy is increased intracranial pressure. If required, electrotherapy can be given during pregnancy or postoperatively.

Mania can be treated with phenothiazines, lithium, electrotherapy, or anticonvulsant "mood stabilizers" such as valproate (Depakote) and carbamazepine (Tegratol) (31, 79). Of these methods, electrotherapy is probably the least effective.

Lithium carbonate may be the drug of choice in the treatment of mania (102), but chlorpromazine and other sedating neuroleptics are perhaps most useful with very active manic patients. Some clinicians began to treat manics with both chlorpromazine and lithium, stopping chlorpromazine after four or five days when lithium has begun to take effect. If lithium is not effective within ten days, it probably will not be effective at all. Serum levels of lithium required for effective action are in the range of 1 meq/l (108). Generally, total doses of 1,200 to 2,400 mg of lithium per day in divided form (300 to 600 mg per dose) are required to achieve such serum levels. Because lithium is a potentially toxic drug, its use must be monitored by repeatedly checking serum levels, particularly early in treatment. Most patients experience a fine tremor of the hands at therapeutic levels of lithium (0.8 to 1.5 meq/l). At higher levels, ataxia, disorientation, somnolence, seizures, and finally circulatory collapse may occur. Long-term lithium therapy has also been associated with disturbances of thyroid and renal function, and tubular changes in the kidney have been found on autopsy. Thus, the drug should be used with caution.

The usefulness of lithium may not be limited to the treatment of acute mania. There is some evidence that the drug may reduce morbidity among bipolar patients, preventing depression as well as mania (8), and that it may also prevent depression among some unipolar patients (6, 8, 81).

Two large multicentered trials evaluating the triazolo benzodiazepine alprazolam in outpatients suffering from major depression produced encouraging results (41, 108). The antidepressant effect of alprazolam was equal to those of imipramine, amitriptyline, and doxepin. It is not known whether other benzodiazepine-type drugs are also antidepressant, but in one comparison of alprazolam and diazepam, the former was clearly a superior antidepressant (70).

REFERENCES

1. Abrams, R., Fink, M., Dornbush, R. L., Feldstein, S., Volavka, J., and Roubicek, J. Unilateral and bilateral electroconvulsive therapy. Arch. Gen. Psychiat. 27:88–91, 1972.
2. Abrams, R., and Taylor, M. A. Mania and schizo-affective disorder, manic type: a comparison. Am. J. Psychiat. 133:12, 1976.

3. Abrams, R., and Taylor, M. A. A comparison of unipolar and bipolar depressive illness. Am. J. Psychiat. *137*:9, 1084–1087, 1980.

4. Allen, M. G. Twin studies of affective illness. Arch. Gen. Psychiat. *33*:1476–1478, 1976.

5. Amsterdam, J. D., Winokur, A., Caroff, S. N., and Conn, J. The dexamethasone suppression test in outpatients with primary affective disorder and healthy control subjects. Am. J. Psychiat. *139*:3, 287–291, 1982.

6. Ananth, J. Treatment approaches to mania. Int. Pharmacopsychiat. *11*:215–231, 1976.

7. Andreasen, N. C., Rice, J., Endicott, J., Coryell, W., Grove, W. M., and Reich, T. Familial rates of affective disorder. Arch. Gen. Psychiat. *44*:461–469, 1987.

8. Angst, J., Weis, P., Grof, P., Baastrup, P. C., and Schou, J. Lithium prophylaxis in recurrent affective disorders. Brit. J. Psychiat. *116*:604–614, 1970.

9. Angst, J. Clinical typology of bipolar illness. In *Mania: An Evolving Concept*, Belmarker, R. H., and van Prang, H. M. (eds.), 61–79. Jamaica, N.Y.: SP Medical & Scientific Books, 1980.

10. Baker, M., Dorzab, J., Winokur, G., and Cadoret, R. Depressive disease: the effect of the postpartum state. Biol. Psychiat. *3*:357–365, 1971.

11. Beck, A. T. *Depression: Clinical Experimental, and Theoretical Aspects*. New York: Harper & Row, 1967.

12. Beck, A. *Cognitive Therapy and the Emotional Disorders*. New York: International Universities Press, 1976.

13. Becker, J. Achievement related to characteristics of manic-depressives. J. Abnorm. Soc. Psychol. *60*:334–339, 1960.

14. Beigel, A., and Murphy, D. L. Unipolar and bipolar affective illness. Arch. Gen. Psychiat. *24*:215–220, 1971.

15. Bellack, A. S., Hersen, M., and Himmelhoch, J. Social skills training compared with pharmacotherapy and psychotherapy in the treatment of unipolar depression. Am. J. Psychiat. *138*:1562–1567, 1981.

16. Black, D. W., Winokur, G., and Nasrallah, A. The treatment of depression: electroconvulsive therapy v antidepressants: a naturalistic evaluation of 1,495 patients. Compr. Psychiat. *28*:169–182, 1987.

17. Blackburn, I. M., Bishop, S., Glen, A. I. M., Whalley, L. J., and Christie, J. E. The efficacy of cognitive therapy in depression: a treatment trial using cognitive therapy and pharmacotherapy, each alone and in combination. Brit. J. Psychiat. *139*:181–189, 1981.

18. Bratfos, O., and Haug, J. L. The course of manic-depressive psychosis. A follow-up investigation of 215 patients. Acta Psychiat. Scand. *44*:89–112, 1968.

19. Brockington, I. F., Cernik, K. F., Schofield, E. M., Downing, A. R., Francis, A. F., and Keelan, C. Puerperal psychosis. Arch. Gen. Psychiat. *38*:829–833, 1981.

20. Brockington, I. F., Altman, E., Hillier, V. The clinical picture of bipolar affective disorder in its depressed phase. Brit. J. Psychiat. *141*:558–562, 1982.

21. Brodie, H. K., and Leff, M. J. Bipolar depression—a comparative study of patient characteristics. Am. J. Psychiat. *127*:1086–1090, 1971.

22. Buchan, H., Johnstone, E., McPherson, K., Palmer, R. L., Crow, T. J., and Brandon, S. Who benefits from electroconvulsive therapy? Combined results of the Leicester and Northwick Park Trials. Brit. J. Psychiat. *160*:355–359, 1992.

23. Carroll, B. J. The dexamethasone test for melancholia. Brit. J. Psychiat. *140*:292–304, 1982.

24. Cassidy, W. L., Flanigan, M. B., Spellman, M., and Cohen, M. E. Clinical observations in manic depressive disease. A quantitative study of 100 manic depressive patients in 50 medically sick controls. JAMA *164*:1535–1546, 1953.

25. Clayton, P. J., Rodin, L., and Winokur, G. Family history studies, III. Schizoaffective disorder, clinical and genetic factors including a one to two year follow-up. Compr. Psychiat. *9*:31–49, 1968.

26. Clayton, P. J., Halikas, J. A., and Maurice, W. L. The bereavement of the widowed. Dis. Nerv. Syst. *32*:597–604, 1971.

27. Clayton, P. J., Halikas, J. A., and Maurice, W. L. The depression of widowhood. Brit. J. Psychiat. *120*:71–78, 1972.

28. Clayton, P. J. Schizoaffective disorders. J. Nerv. Ment. Dis. *170*:646–650, 1982.

29. Cohen, M. B., Baker, G., Cohen, R. A., Fromm-Reichmann, F., and Weigert, E. V. An intensive study of 12 cases of manic depressive psychosis. Psychiatry *17*:103–137, 1954.

30. Cohen, S. M., Allen, M. G., Pollin, W., and Hrubec, Z. Relationship of schizo-affective psychosis to manic depressive psychosis and schizophrenia. Arch. Gen. Psychiat. *26*:539–546, 1972.

31. Davis, J. M. Efficacy of tranquilizing and antidepressant drugs. Arch. Gen. Psychiat. *13*:552–572, 1965.

32. de Jonghe, F., and Swinkels, J. A. The safety of antidepressants. Drugs *43*(2):40–47, 1992.

33. DiMascio, A., Weissman, M. M., Prusoff, B. A., Neu, C., Zwilling, M., and Klerman, G. L. Differential symptom reduction by drugs and psychotherapy in acute depression. Arch. Gen. Psychiat. *36*:1450–1456, 1979.

34. Dunner, D. L., Stallone, F., and Fieve, R. R. Lithium carbonate and affective disorders. Arch. Gen. Psychiat. *33*:117–120, 1976.

35. Dunner, D. L., and Fieve, R. R. The effect of lithium in depressive subtypes. In *Neuropsychopharmacology*, Deniker, A., Radouco-Thomas, B., and Villeneuve, C. (eds.), 1109–1115. New York: Pergamon Press, 1978.

36. Dunner, D. L. Unipolar and bipolar depression: recent findings from clinical and biologic studies. In *Psychobiology of Affective Disorders*, 11–24. New York: Plenum, 1980.

37. Egeland, J. A., and Hostetter, A. M. Amish study, I: affective disorders among the Amish, 1976–1980. Am. J. Psychiat. *140*:1, 56–61, 1983.

38. Egeland, J. A., Gerhard, D. S., Pauls, D. L., Sussex, J. N., Kidd, K. K., Al-

len, C. R., Hostetter, A. M., and Housman, D. E. Bipolar affective disorders linked to DNA markers on chromosome 11. Nature *325*:783, 1987.

39. Fawcett, J. Suicide risk factors in depressive disorders and in panic disorder. J. Clin. Psychiat. *53*:9–13, 1992.

40. Feighner, J. P., Aden, G. C., Fabre, L. F., Rickels, K., and Smith, W. T. Comparison of alprazolam, imipramine, and placebo in the treatment of depression. JAMA *249*:3057–3064, 1983.

41. Ferster, C. B. Behavioral approaches to depression. In *The Psychology of Depression: Contemporary Theory and Research*, Friedman, R. J., and Katz, M. M. (eds.), 29–54. New York: John Wiley & Sons, 1974.

42. Fremming, K. The expectation of mental infirmity in the sample of the Danish population. In *Occasional Papers of Eugenics*, no. 7. London: Cassell, 1951.

43. Freud, S. *Mourning and Melancholia*. In *The Complete Psychological Works of Sigmund Freud*, *14*:243–258. London: Hogarth Press, 1957.

44. Gerner, R. H., and Stanton, A. Algorithm for patient management of acute manic states: Lithium, Valproate, or Carbamazepine? J. Clin. Psychopharmacol. *12*:57S–63S, 1992.

45. Gibson, R. W. The family background and early life experience of the manic depressive patient. Psychiatry *21*:71–90, 1968.

46. Gold, M. S., Pottash, A. L. C., Extein, I., and Sweeney, D. R. Diagnosis of depression in the 1980's. JAMA *245*:1562–1564, 1981.

47. Goldin, L. R., Clerget-Darpoux, F., and Gershon, E. S. Relationship of HLA to major affective disorder not supported. Psychiat. Res. 7:29–45, 1982.

48. Goodwin, F. K., Murphy, D. L., and Dunner, D. L. Lithium response in unipolar versus bipolar depression. Am. J. Psychiat. *129*:44–47, 1974.

49. Goodwin, D. W., Schulsinger, F., Knop, J., Mednick, S., and Guze, S. B. Psychopathology in adopted and nonadopted daughters of alcoholics. Arch. Gen. Psychiat. *34*:751–755, 1977.

50. Goodwin, F. K., Murphy, D. L., Dunner, D. L., and Bunney, W. E. Lithium response in unipolar vs. bipolar depression. Am. J. Psychiat. *129*:44–47, 1972.

51. Greden, J. F., Albala, A. A., Haskett, R. F., et al. Normalization of dexamethasone suppression test: a laboratory index of recovery from endogenous depression. Biol. Psychiat. *15*:449–458, 1980.

52. Guze, S. B., and Robins, E. Suicide and primary affective disorders. Brit. J. Psychiat. *117*:437–438, 1970.

53. Guze, S. B., Woodruff, R. A., and Clayton, P. J. Secondary affective disorder: a study of 95 cases. Psychol. Med. *1*:426–428, 1971.

54. Helgason, T. Epidemiology of mental disorders in Iceland. A psychiatric and demographic investigation of 5395 Icelanders. Acta Psychiat. Scand. (Suppl.) 40:173, 1964.

55. Hirschfeld, R. M. A., and Cross, C. K. Epidemiology of affective disorders. Arch. Gen. Psychiat. *39*:35–46, 1982.

56. Hodgkinson, S., Sherrington, R., Gurling, H., Marchbanks, R., Reeders, S., Mallet, J., McInnis, M., Petursson, H., and Brynjolfsson, J. Molecular ge-

netic evidence for heterogeneity in manic depression. Nature *325*:805, 1987.

57. Hollister, L. E., Davis, K. L., and Berger, P. A. Subtypes of depression based on excretion of MHPG and response to nortriptyline. Arch. Gen. Psychiat. *37*:1107–1110, 1980.

58. James, W. *The Varieties of Religious Experience*. In *The Epidemiology of Depression*, Silverman, C. (ed.). Baltimore: Johns Hopkins Univ. Press, 1968.

59. Johnson, G. F. S., and Leeman, M. M. Onset of illness in bipolar manic-depressives and their affectively ill first-degree relatives. Biol. Psychiat. *12*:733–741, 1977.

60. Kalinowsky, L. B., and Hippius, H. *Pharmacological, Convulsive and Other Somatic Treatments in Psychiatry*. New York: Grune & Stratton, 1969.

61. Kasper, S., Fuger, J., and Möller, H.-J. Comparative efficacy of antidepressants. Drugs *43(2)*:11–23, 1992.

62. Keller, M. B., Lavori, P. W., Mueller, T. I., Endicott, J., Coryell, W., Hirschfeld, R. M., and Shea, T. Time to recovery, chronicity, and levels of psychopathology in major depression. A 5-year prospective follow-up of 431 subjects. Arch Gen. Psychiat. *49(10)*:809–816, 1992.

63. Kendler, K. S., Neale, M. C., Kessler, R. C., Heath, A. C., and Lindon, J. E. A population-based twin study of major depression in women. Arch. Gen. Psychiat. *49*:257–266, 1992.

64. Keller, M. B., Shapiro, R. W., Lavori, P. W., and Wolfe, N. Relapse in major depressive disorder. Arch. Gen. Psychiat. *39*:911–915, 1982.

65. Kendell, R. E. *The Classification of Depressive Illnesses*, Maudsley Monogr. no. 18. London: Oxford Univ. Press, 1968.

66. Kerr, T. A., Schapira, K., and Roth, M. The relationship between premature death and affective disorders. Brit. J. Psychiat. *115*:1277–1282, 1969.

67. Klein, D. F., Gittelman, R., and Quitkin, F. Review of the literature on mood-stabilizing drugs. In *Diagnosis and Drug Treatment of Psychiatric Disorders: Adults and Children*, 268–408. Baltimore: Williams & Wilkins, 1980.

68. Klerman, G. L., and Weissman, M. M. The course, morbidity, and costs of depression. Arch. Gen. Psychiat. *49*:831–834, 1992.

69. Kraepelin, E. *Manic Depressive Insanity and Paranoia*. Edinburgh: E. S. Livingstone, 1921.

70. Kupfer, D. J., Pikar, D., and Himmelhoch, J. M. Are there two types of unipolar depression? Arch. Gen. Psychiat. *32*:866–871, 1975.

71. Kupfer, D. J., and Foster, F. G. EEG sleep and depression. In *Sleep Disorders: Diagnosis and Treatment*, Williams, R. L., and Karacan, I. (eds.), 163–204. New York: John Wiley & Sons, 1978.

72. Leonhard, K., Korff, I., and Shulz, H. Die Temperamente in den Familien der monopolaren und bipolaren phasichen Psychosen. Psychiat. Neurol. *143*:416–434, 1962.

73. Lewis, A. Melancholia: a historical review. In *The State of Psychiatry: Essays and Addresses*. New York: Science House, 1967.

74. Lewy, A., Sack, R., and Singer, C. Antidepressant and circadian phase shifting effects of light. Science *235*:352–354, 1987.

75. Lundquist, G. Prognosis and course in manic depressive psychosis. A follow-up study of 319 first admissions. Acta Psychiat. Neurol (Suppl.) *35*, 1945.

76. Marcotte, D. B., Kane, F. G., Obrist, P., and Lipton, M. A. Psychophysiologic changes accompanying oral contraceptive use. Brit. J. Psychiat. *116*:165–167, 1970.

77. Martin, R. L., Cloninger, C. R., Guze, S. B., and Clayton, P. J. Mortality in 500 psychiatric outpatients. Arch. Gen. Psychiat., 1983.

78. Matthysse, S., and Kidd, K. K. Evidence of HLA linkage in depressive disorders. N. Engl. J. Med. *305*:1340–1341, 1981.

79. McElroy, S. L., Keck, Jr., P. E., Pope, Jr., H. G., and Hudson, J. I. Valproate in the treatment of bipolar disorder: literature review and clinical guidelines. J. Clin. Psychopharmacol. *12(1)*:42S–52S, 1992.

80. McGuffin, P., Katz, R., and Rutherford, J. Nature, nurture and depression: a twin study. Psychol. Med. *21(2)*:329–335, 1991.

81. Mendels, J., Secunda, S. K., and Dyson, W. L. The controlled study of the antidepressant effects of lithium carbonate. Arch. Gen. Psychiat. *26*:154–157, 1972.

82. Mendels, J., Ramsey, A., and Dyson, W. L. Lithium as an antidepressant. Arch. Gen. Psychiat. *36*:845–846, 1979.

83. Mendlewicz, J., Leboyer, M., DeBruyn, A., Malafosse, A., Sevy, S., Hirsch, D., VanBroeckhoven, C., and Mallet, J. Absence of linkage between chromosome 11p15 markers and manic-depressive illness in a Belgian pedigree. Am. J. Psychiat. *148(12)*:1683–1687, 1991.

84. Mendlewicz, J., and Rainer, J. D. Adoption study supporting genetic transmission in manic-depressive illness. Nature *268*:327–329, 1977.

85. Mendelwicz, J., Simon, P., Sevy, S., Charon, F., Brocas, H., Legros, S., and Vassart, G. Polymorphic DNA marker on X chromosome and manic depression. Lancet, 1230, May 30, 1987.

86. *Mood Disorders: Pharmacologic Prevention of Recurrences.* Public Health Service Monogr., vol. 5, no. 4, 1986.

87. Murphy, G. E., and Wetzel, R. D. Family history of suicidal behavior among suicide attempters. J. Nerv. Ment. Dis. *170*:2, 86–90, 1982.

88. Myers, J. K., Weissman, M. M., and Tischler, G. C. Six-month prevalence of psychiatric disorders in three communities. Arch. Gen. Psychiat. *41*:959–967, 1984.

89. Nicholi, A. M. Harvard dropouts: some psychiatric findings. Am. J. Psychiat. *124*:651–658, 1967.

90. Ohmori, T., Arora, R. C., and Meltzer, H. Y. Serotonergic measures in suicide brain: the concentration of 5-HIAA, HVA, and Tryptophan in frontal cortex of suicide victims. Biol. Psychiat. *32*:57–71, 1992.

91. Overstreet, D. H., Rezvani, A. H., and Janowsky, D. S. Genetic animal models of depression and ethanol preference provide support for cholinergic and serotonergic involvement in depression and alcoholism. Biol. Psychiat. *31*:919–936, 1992.

92. Pauls, D. L., Morton, L. A., and Egeland, J. A. Risks of affective illness

among first-degree relatives of bipolar I old-order Amish probands. Arch. Gen. Psychiat. *49*:703–708, 1992.

93. Perris, C. A study of bipolar (manic-depressive) and unipolar recurrent depressive psychoses. Acta Psychiat. Scand. (Suppl.) 194, 1966.

94. Perris, C. The distinction between bipolar and unipolar affective disorders. In *Handbook of Affective Disorders*, Paykel, E. S. (ed.), 45–48. New York: Guilford Press, 1982.

95. Peselow, E. D., Goldring, N., Fieve, R. R., and Wright, R. The dexamethasone suppression test in depressed outpatients and normal control subjects. Am. J. Psychiat. *140*:2, 1983.

96. Pierce, D. W. The predictive validation of a suicide intent scale: a five year follow-up. Brit. J. Psychiat. *139*:391–396, 1981.

97. Potter, W. Z., and Rudorfer, M. V. Electroconvulsive therapy—a modern medical procedure. N. Engl. J. Med. *328(12)*:882–883, 1993.

98. Poznaski, E., and Zrull, J. P. Childhood depression. Clinical characteristics of overtly depressed children. Arch. Gen. Psychiat. *23*:8–15, 1970.

99. *Practice Guidelines for Major Depressive Disorder in Adults*. American Psychiatric Association, 1993.

100. Preskorn, S. H., Irwin, G. H., Simpson, S., Friesen, D., Rinne, J., and Jerkovich, G. Medical therapies for mood disorders alter the blood–barrier. Science *213*:469–471, 1981.

101. Price, J. S. Chronic depressive illness. Brit. Med. J. *1*:1200–1201, 1978.

102. Prien, R. F., Caffey, E. M., and Klett, C. J. Comparison of lithium carbonate and chlorpromazine in the treatment of mania. Arch. Gen. Psychiat. *26*:146–153, 1972.

103. Prien, R. F., Caffey, E. M., and Klett, C. J. Relationship between serum lithium level and clinical response in acute mania treated with lithium. Brit. J. Psychiat. *120*:409–414, 1972.

104. Prien, R. F., Kupfer, D. J., and Mansky, P. A. Drug therapy in the prevention of recurrences in unipolar and bipolar affective disorders. Arch. Gen. Psychiat. *41*:1096–1104, 1984.

105. Ramsey, T. A., and Mendels, J. Lithium in the acute treatment of depression. In *Handbook of Lithium Therapy*, Johnson, F. N. (ed.), 17–25. Lancaster, England: MTP Press, 1980.

106. Reich, T., and Winokur, G. Postpartum psychoses in patients with manic depressive disease. J. Nerv. Ment. Dis. *151*:60–68, 1970.

107. Rice, J. P., Rochberg, N., Endicott, J., Lavori, P. W., and Miller, C. Stability of psychiatric diagnoses: An application to the affective disorders. Arch. Gen. Psychiat. *49*:824–830, 1992.

108. Rickels, K., Feighner, J. P., and Smith, W. T. Alprazolam, amitriptyline, doxepin, and placebo in the treatment of depression. Arch. Gen. Psychiat. *42*:134–141, 1985.

109. Rickels, K., Chung, H. R., Csanalosi, I. B., Hurowitz, A. M., London, J., Wiseman, K., Kaplan, M., and Amsterdam, J. D. Alprazolam, diazepam, imipramine, and placebo in outpatients with major depression. Arch. Gen. Psychiat. *44*:862–866, 1987.

110. Rudorfer, M. V. Monoamine oxidase inhibitors: reversible and irreversible. Psychopharmacol. Bull. *28(1)*:45–57, 1992.

111. Robins, E., and Guze, S. B. Classification of affective disorders: the primary-secondary, the endogeneous-reactive, and the neurotic-psychotic concepts. In *Recent Advances in Psychobiology of the Depressive Illnesses*, Proceedings of a workshop sponsored by the NIMH, Williams, T. A., Katz, M. M., and Shield, J. A. (eds.), Washington, D.C.: U.S. GPO, 1972.

112. Robins, E., Murphy, G. E., Wilkinson, R. H., Gassner, S., and Kayes, J. Some clinical considerations in the prevention of suicide based on a study of 134 successful suicides. Am. J. Public Health *49*:888–899, 1959.

113. Rosenthal, N., Sack, D., and Gillin, J. Seasonal affective disorder: a description of the syndrome and preliminary findings with light therapy. Arch. Gen. Psychiat. *41*:72–80, 1985.

114. Roth, M. Natural history of mental disorder in old age. J. Ment. Sci. *101*:281–301, 1955.

115. Rounsaville, B. J., Klerman, G. L., and Weissman, M. M. Do psychotherapy and pharmacotherapy for depression conflict? Arch. Gen. Psychiat. *38*:24–29, 1981.

116. Roy, A. Risk factors for suicide in psychiatric patients. Arch. Gen. Psychiat. *39*:1089–1095, 1982.

117. Sabelli, H. C., Fawcett, J., Javaid, J. I., and Bagri, S. The methylphenidate test for differentiating desipramine-responsive from nortriptyline-responsive depression. Am. J. Psychiat. *140*:212–217, 1983.

118. Saccetti, E., Vita, A., and Conte, G. Lithium prophylaxis in major affective disorders: on the specificity and sensitivity of some "new" predictors of treatment outcome. In *Current Trends in Lithium and Rubidium Therapy*, Corsini, G. V. (ed.), 165–187. Lancaster, England: MTP Press, 1984.

119. Sackeim, H. A., Prudic, J., Devanand, D. P., Kiersky, J. E., Fitzsimons, L., Moody, B. J., McElhiney, M. C., Coleman, E. A., and Settembrino, J. M. Effects of stimulus intensity and electrode placement on the efficacy and cognitive effects of electroconvulsive therapy. N. Engl. J. Med. *328*:839–846, 1993.

120. Savard, R. J., Rey, A. C., and Post, R. M. Halstead-Reitan Category Test in bipolar and unipolar affective disorders. J. Nerv. Ment. Dis. *168*:297–304, 1980.

121. Schildkraut, J. J., Orsulak, P. J., and Schatzberg, A. F. Toward a biochemical classification of depressive disorders: I. Differences in urinary excretion of MHPG and other catecholamine metabolites in clinically defined subtypes of depressions. Arch. Gen. Psychiat. *35*:1427–1433, 1978.

122. Schildkraut, J. J., Orsulak, P. J., and LaBrie, R. A. Toward a biochemical classification of depressive disorders: II. Application of multivariate discriminant function analysis to data on urinary catecholamines and metabolites. Arch. Gen. Psychiat. *35*:1436–1439, 1978.

123. Schildkraut, J. J., Schatzberg, A. F., and Orsulak, P. J. Biological discrimination of subtypes of depression. In *The Affective Disorders*, Davis, J. M.,

and Maas, J. W. (eds.), 31–51. Washington, D.C.: American Psychiatric Press, 1983.

124. Schwartz, J. M., Baxter, L. R., Mazziotta, J. C., Gerner, R. H., and Phelps, M. E. The differential diagnosis of depression. Relevance of positron emission tomography studies of cerebral glucose metabolism to the bipolar-unipolar dichotomy. JAMA *258*:1368–1374, 1987.

125. Shobe, F. O., and Brione, P. Long-term prognosis in manic-depressive illness. A follow-up investigation of 111 patients. Arch. Gen. Psychiat. *24*:334–337, 1971.

126. Silverman, C. (ed.). *The Epidemiology of Depression.* Baltimore: Johns Hopkins Univ. Press, 1968.

127. Sternberg, D. E., and Jarvik, M. E. Memory functions in depression. Arch. Gen. Psychiat. *33*:219–224, 1976.

128. Strömgren, E. *Contributions to Psychiatric Epidemiology and Genetics.* Acta Jutlandica Med. Series 16, vol. 40, 1968.

129. Suarez, B. K., and Croughan, J. Is the major histocompatibility complex linked to genes that increase susceptibility to affective disorder? A critical appraisal. Psychiat. Res. *7*:19–27, 1982.

130. Taylor, F. G., and Marshall, W. L. Experimental analysis of a cognitive-behavioral therapy for depression. Cognitive Therapy Res. *1*:59–72, 1977.

131. APA Task Force on Laboratory Tests in Psychiatry. The dexamethasone suppression test: an overview of its current status in psychiatry. Am. J. Psychiat. *144*:10, 1987.

132. Vaillant, G. E. Manic-depressive heredity and remission in schizophrenia. Brit. J. Psychiat. *109*:746–749, 1963.

133. VanValkenburg, C., Lowry, M., Winokur, G., and Cadoret, R. Depression spectrum disease versus pure depressive disease. J. Nerv. Ment. Dis. *165*:341–347, 1977.

134. Weissman, M. M., Klerman, G. L., Paykel, E. S., Prusoff, B., and Hanson, B. Treatment effects on the social adjustment of depressed patients. Arch. Gen. Psychiat. *30*:771–778, 1974.

135. Weissman, M. M., and Klerman, G. L. Sex differences and the epidemiology of depression. Arch. Gen. Psychiat. *34*:98–111, 1977.

136. Weissman, M. M., and Myers, J. K. Affective disorders in a U.S. urban community. Arch. Gen. Psychiat. *35*:1304–1311, 1978.

137. Weissman, M. M., Myers, J. K., and Harding, P. S. Psychiatric disorders in a U.S. urban community: 1975–76. Am. J. Psychiat. *135*:459–462, 1978.

138. Weissman, M. M. The psychological treatment of depression. Arch. Gen. Psychiat. *36*:1261–1269, 1979.

139. Weitkamp, L. R., Stancer, H. C., Persad, E., Flood, C., and Guttormsen, S. Depressive disorders and HLA: a gene on chromosome 6 that can affect behavior. N. Engl. J. Med. *305*:1301–1306, 1981.

140. Whitney, W., Cadoret, R. J., and McClure, J. N. Depressive symptoms and academic performance in college students. Am. J. Psychiat. *128*:766–770, 1971.

141. Winokur, G., and Black, D. W. Suicide—what can be done: N. Engl. J. Med. *327*(7):490–491, 1992.
142. Winokur, G., and Pitts, F. N. Affective disorder: VI. A family history study of prevalences, sex differences, and possible genetic factors. J. Psychiat. Res. *3*:113–123, 1965.
143. Winokur, G. Types of depressive illness. Brit. J. Psychiat. *120*:265–266, 1972.
144. Woodruff, R. A., Murphy, G. E., and Herjanic, M. The natural history of affective disorders: I. Symptoms of 72 patients at the time of index hospital admission. J. Psychiat. Res. *5*:255–263, 1967.
145. Woodruff, R. A., Robins, L. N., Winokur, G., and Reich, T. Manic depressive illness and social achievement. Acta Psychiat. Scand. *47*:237–249, 1971.
146. Woodruff, R. A., Guze, S. B., and Clayton, P. J. Anxiety neurosis among psychiatric outpatients. Compr. Psychiat. *13*:165–170, 1972.
147. Woodruff, R. A., Guze, S. B., Clayton, P. J., and Carr, D. Alcoholism and depression. Arch. Gen. Psychiat. *28*:97–100, 1973.
148. Woodruff, R. A., Guze, S. B., and Clayton, P. J. Alcoholics who see a psychiatrist compared with those who do not. Q. J. Stud. Alcohol *34*:1162–1171, 1973.
149. Young, W., Knowles, J. B., MacLean, A. W., Boag, L., and McConville, B. J. The sleep of childhood depressives: comparison with age-matched controls. Biol. Psychiat. *17*:10, 1163–1168, 1982.

2

SCHIZOPHRENIC DISORDERS

DEFINITION

Hallucinations and delusions are widely considered to be hallmarks of mental disorder and thus are of great interest to psychiatrists. These symptoms may be seen in a wide variety of illnesses, including primary affective disorders, organic mental disorders, alcoholism, drug dependence, and a group of conditions that may be called the "schizophrenic disorders." Many investigators believe that schizophrenic disorders comprise a number of different conditions, but efforts to divide them into valid subgroups have not been entirely successful, and inconsistent usage has made nomenclature confusing. Extensive work, however, has indicated that the schizophrenic disorders may be divided into two major categories: one with a relatively poor prognosis, the other with a relatively good prognosis.

When this differentiation is attempted, such labels as schizophrenia, chronic schizophrenia, process schizophrenia, nuclear schizophrenia, and nonremitting schizophrenia are used to refer to the poor-prognosis cases, whereas schizophreniform, acute schizophrenia, reactive schizophrenia, schizoaffective, and remitting schizophrenia are used for the good-prognosis cases (135).

The schizophrenic disorders are characterized, at least intermittently, by delusions and hallucinations in a clear sensorium. Other noteworthy features are a blunted, shallow, or strikingly inappropriate affect; odd, sometimes bizarre, motor behavior (termed "catatonic"); and disordered thinking in which goal-directedness and normal associations between ideas are markedly distorted (loosening of associations and tangential thinking).

Although the schizophrenic disorders are generally chronic, some cases present as episodic or single illnesses that remit and may develop in individuals whose previous general adjustment has been good. Such patients are likely to show striking affective symptoms during the acute psychotic illness. They may seem perplexed and bewildered and may be mildly disoriented. Though recovery from the psychotic episode is usual, repeated episodes are common. Subsequent episodes may be less pronounced and may sometimes resemble affective disorders (174, 175).

HISTORICAL BACKGROUND

In now-classic studies, Emil Kraepelin (1856–1926), a German psychiatrist, built upon the work of his countrymen K. L. Kahlbaum (1828–1899) and E. Hecker (1843–1909), who described "catatonia" and "hebephrenia," respectively, to lay the groundwork for present views of schizophrenia (91). After careful followup of hospitalized patients, he separated "manic depressive psychosis" from "dementia praecox." The latter term referred to the disorder now called chronic schizophrenia.

Even though Kraepelin believed dementia praecox to be a chronic disorder that frequently ended in marked deterioration of the personality, he recognized that a small number of patients recovered completely. His "narrow" view of schizophrenia has been followed by most European psychiatrists, particularly those in the Scandinavian countries and Great Britain.

A broader approach to schizophrenia (and the name itself) was offered by Eugene Bleuler (1857–1939), a Swiss psychiatrist, who realized that he might be dealing with a group of disorders (20).

His diagnostic criteria were not based on their ability to predict course and outcome, but on conformance to his hypothesis concerning the basic defect, namely, the "splitting" of psychic functions. By this he meant inconsistency, inappropriateness, and disorganization of affect, thought, and action, in the absence of obvious brain disease. Despite his less-strict approach to diagnosis and the variable course that his patients experienced, Bleuler believed that patients with schizophrenia never recovered completely, never returned to their premorbid state (*restituo ad integrum*). Because his "fundamental" symptoms included autistic thinking (defined by Bleuler as "divorce from reality"), blunted or inappropriate affect, ambivalence, and disturbed association of thought—all often difficult to define and specify— Bleuler's work set the stage for the very broad concepts of schizophrenia developed by psychoanalysts and adopted for many years by many American psychiatrists.

Psychoanalysts viewed schizophrenia primarily as a manifestation of a "weak ego." Unable to cope with the problems of life and unable to use effectively the "defenses of the ego" to handle instinctual forces and anxiety, patients "regress" to a primitive level of functioning ("primary process") manifested by thought disorder, affective poverty, disorganization, and inability to conform to the demands of "reality" (27). In this psychoanalytic view of schizophrenia, all evidence of weak ego (including a wide range of personality handicaps and abnormalities) or of "primary process" (such as hallucinations, delusions, poor reality-testing, tangential thinking, and ambivalence) may be a manifestation of schizophrenia. It is not surprising, therefore, that the diagnosis was used in a wide range of clinical situations.

In the late 1930s a number of European and American investigators began again to approach the problem of the schizophrenias in terms of predicting course, response to treatment, and long-term outcome. They were influenced first by the advent of electroconvulsive therapy (ECT—electrotherapy) and later by the introduction of the phenothiazines. Langfeldt (94), Astrup (9, 10), Retterstöl (128, 129), Leonhard (97), Ey (51), Stephens (157,

158, 159), and Vaillant (174, 175) have been leaders in these efforts.

Proper evaluation of treatment requires a knowledge of the natural history of the disorder being treated, especially the factors associated with different clinical courses and outcomes. Such factors can only be identified by follow-up studies such as those carried out by the above investigators. Thus, current clinical and research approaches to the schizophrenic disorders are based on extensive follow-up studies that are supplemented by family studies (135).

The differences in conceptualizing schizophrenic disorders between European and American psychiatrists now have largely been resolved. With the introduction of *DSM-III, DSM-III-R*, and *DSM-IV*, most psychiatrists around the world came to accept the narrower approach to schizophrenia. To a considerable degree, this consensus is based on empirical and systematic studies indicating that the narrower approach produces more consistent findings with regard to course, response to treatment, long-term outcome, and familial illness patterns. Many of these studies are discussed below.

EPIDEMIOLOGY

Chronic schizophrenia occurs in somewhat less than 1 percent of the population, but because of its early onset, chronicity, and associated disability, it is one of the most important psychiatric illnesses. A significant percentage of all hospitalized psychiatric patients suffer from this condition. The distinction between good- and poor-prognosis forms of schizophrenia has not been made consistently in epidemiologic surveys, nor is the possibility regularly raised that some of the good-prognosis cases may be other disorders, though available evidence suggests that the good-prognosis cases may be more common than the poor-prognosis ones (129). The combined prevalence of both good- and poor-prognosis disorders is probably between 1 and 2 percent.

Schizophrenic disorders are found in all cultures. A number of studies have indicated that they are more prevalent among people from lower socioeconomic backgrounds. For some investigators, this has meant that poverty, limited education, and associated handicaps predispose to schizophrenic illness. Studies have shown, however, that the association between schizophrenic illness and low socioeconomic status can be explained by "downward drift," a term that refers to the effect of an illness on the patient's socioeconomic status. If a disorder interferes with education and work performance, so that individuals are not able to complete advanced schooling or hold positions of responsibility, their socioeconomic status—characteristically defined by income, educational achievement, and job prestige—cannot be high.

Studies in England (58), Denmark (181), Finland (141), and the United States (43) have shown that the distribution of socioeconomic class among the fathers of schizophrenics is the same as in the general population, indicating that the lower socioeconomic status of patients with schizophrenic illness is at least partially the result of downward drift.

Another interesting observation concerning the epidemiology of schizophrenia is the reported tendency of schizophrenics in Europe and the United States to be born during the late winter and early spring months of the year (72, 73, 172, 178). Though most schizophrenics are not born during these months, the data suggest that something associated with such births predisposes to schizophrenic illness. One report suggests that the season of birth effect may be especially pertinent to cases arising in families without serious mental disorders (115). Other work suggests a similar association with bipolar affective disorder (26), raising the likelihood that the seasonal effect may be nonspecific. These reports do not distinguish between good-prognosis and poor-prognosis cases, so they leave the reader uncertain as to whether the observation is equally applicable to both forms of the disorder.

Recent work has suggested fairly strongly that there are significant gender differences in schizophrenia with regard to age of onset and severity of course. Male patients seem to experience earlier onset and more severe clinical manifestations and course (69, 134).

CLINICAL PICTURE

Common delusions in schizophrenia are those of persecution and control in which patients believe others are spying on them, spreading false rumors about them, planning to harm them, trying to control their thoughts or actions, or reading their minds (Table 2.1).

Table 2.1   Diagnostic criteria for Schizophrenia (*DSM-IV*)

A. *Characteristic symptoms:* Two (or more) of the following, each present for a significant portion of time during a 1-month period (or less if successfully treated):

   (1) Delusions
   (2) Hallucinations
   (3) Disorganized speech (e.g., frequent derailment or incoherence)
   (4) Grossly disorganized or catatonic behavior
   (5) Negative symptoms, i.e., affective flattening, alogia, or avolition

NOTE: Only one Criterion A symptom is required if delusions are bizarre or hallucinations consist of a voice keeping up a running commentary on the person's behavior or thoughts, or two or more voices conversing with each other.

B. *Social/occupational dysfunction:* For a significant portion of the time since the onset of the disturbance, one or more major areas of functioning such as work, interpersonal relations, or self-care are markedly below the level achieved prior to the onset (or when the onset is in childhood or adolescence, failure to achieve expected level of interpersonal, academic, or occupational achievement)

C. *Duration:* Continuous signs of the disturbance persist for at least 6 months. This 6-month period must include at least 1 month of symptoms (or less if successfully treated) that meet Criterion A (i.e., active-phase symptoms) and may include periods of prodromal or residual symptoms. During these prodromal or residual periods, the signs of the disturbance may be manifested by only negative symptoms or two or more symptoms listed in Criterion A present in an attenuated form (e.g., odd beliefs, unusual perceptual experiences)

Table 2.1   Diagnostic criteria for Schizophrenia (*DSM-IV*) (*Continued*)

D. *Schizoaffective and Mood Disorder exclusion:* Schizoaffective Disorder and Mood Disorder With Psychotic Features have been ruled out because either (1) no Major Depressive, Manic, or Mixed Episodes have occurred concurrently with the active-phase symptoms; or (2) if mood episodes have occurred during active-phase symptoms, their total duration has been brief relative to the duration of the active and residual periods.

E. *Substance/general medical condition exclusion:* The disturbance is not due to the direct physiological effects of a substance (e.g., a drug of abuse, a medication) or a general medical condition

F. *Relationship to a Pervasive Developmental Disorder:* If there is a history of Autistic Disorder or another Pervasive Developmental Disorder, the additional diagnosis of Schizophrenia is made only if prominent delusions or hallucinations are also present for at least a month (or less if successfully treated)

A young woman complained bitterly that her brother was sending special mysterious messages to her by means of television in order to make her do things that would call attention to her and lead to trouble with the police. A young man was convinced that he was being followed and observed on the streets and in various buildings, but he concluded that this was being directed by his psychiatrist as a way to monitor the patient's progress. Patients may express the belief that they are the victims of conspiracies by Catholics, neighbors, Martians, the FBI, and so on. Delusions of depersonalization are also common. These may be feelings that bizarre bodily changes are taking place, sometimes as a result of the deliberate but obscure actions of others. "My insides are rotting because they are poisoning my food. It's because they know I'm wise to them and have reported them to the police."

The most common hallucinations are auditory. They may involve solitary or multiple voices. The patient may or may not recognize the voices or talk back to them. The voices may seem to come from within the patient's body or from outside sources such as radios or walls. The voices may criticize, ridicule, or threaten;

often they urge the patient to do something she or he believes is wrong.

Visual hallucinations are also frequent (60). These may vary from frightening vague forms to images of dead or absent relatives to scenes of violence or hell. Olfactory hallucinations, which are infrequent, usually consist of unpleasant smells arising from the patient's own body. Tactile (haptic) hallucinations, also infrequent, may consist of feelings that one's genitals are being manipulated, that there are animals inside one's body, or that there are insects crawling over one's skin.

Though the so-called "typical" flat schizophrenic affect is highly characteristic when it is severe, its diagnostic value is limited because it frequently is subtle, leading to disagreement about its presence. Even when clearly present, it is not easy to describe. Patients seem emotionally unresponsive, without warmth or empathy. They can talk about frightening or shocking thoughts without seeming to experience their usual emotional impact ("inappropriate" affect). It is often difficult to feel compassion and sympathy for the patient or to believe that he can empathize with others.

Recurrent posturing, grimacing, prolonged immobility, and "wary flexibility" are dramatic examples of catatonic behavior. These may be independent symptoms or responses to auditory hallucinations.

The impaired goal-directedness of schizophrenic thought and speech may take various forms, all likely to occur in the same patient: blocking, in which the patient's thought and speech stop for periods of time only to begin again with an apparently different subject; tangential associations, in which connections between thoughts are difficult or impossible to follow; neologisms, in which the patient makes up new words; or "word salad," in which the patient's speech consists of words without any understandable sequence or meaning.

Following Kraepelin and Bleuler (20, 91), many psychiatrists group schizophrenics into paranoid, catatonic, hebephrenic, and simple types, depending on whether the predominant symptoms are delusions, bizarre motor behavior, disturbances in affect and associations, or social withdrawal and inadequacy. In practice, however, symptoms vary with time, so a patient may seem to fit several of the subclassifications during the course of his or her illness (28, 87). Attempts to identify delusions or hallucinations characteristic of good- or poor-prognosis cases have not been consistently successful (60).

Patients with schizophrenic disorders may display prominent alterations of mood, usually depression but sometimes euphoria, during the course of illness (125). Other affective symptoms— such as insomnia, anorexia, weight loss, alterations in interest and energy, impairment of mental concentration, guilt, and suicidal preoccupation—may also be present. Often, particularly early in the course of good-prognosis cases, the patients may appear confused, perplexed, somewhat disoriented. In fact, a substantial proportion of schizophrenic patients experience episodes of depression that symptomatically resemble those seen in primary major depression (67, 147). Because the first-degree relatives of such patients do not appear to have an increased prevalence of affective disorders, their depression may be regarded as symptomatic of schizophrenia rather than the manifestation of a second illness.

The introduction of a variety of brain-imaging techniques, including computerized tomography (CT), magnetic resonance (MRI), and positron emission tomography (PET), renewed interest in the possibility of identifying structural abnormalities in the brains of schizophrenic patients. A number of studies suggest that some patients have an increased cerebral-ventricle–to–brain-tissue ratio and that this may be correlated in these patients with evidence of cognitive impairment on standard neuropsychological tests. The reported percentage of such abnormalities has varied greatly in different studies and some authors have been unable to find any significant differences between schizophrenics and controls, but the findings seem important and further investigations are underway (5, 6, 40, 102, 112, 113, 130, 131, 164). A perhaps-related observation from postmortem and CT studies is that some schizophrenic patients have a smaller cerebellar vermis than control subjects (101, 180). Finally, a number of reports indicate that schizophrenic patients may have specific abnormalities in structure and function of other brain regions, including the cerebral hemispheres, the corpus callosum, and the basal ganglia (3, 4, 7, 17, 18, 22–24, 30, 39, 64–66, 75, 107, 111, 184). An especially interesting finding, because it circumvents concerns about the long-term effects of antipsychotic drugs, suggests that in young, never-medicated schizophrenics there is an abnormally high blood flow in the left globus pallidus (44). Another finding of elevated D2 dopamine receptors in drug-naive subjects may be related to this (183). The validity and significance of these findings must await further research, but recent work suggests that many schizophrenic patients have unusual or abnormal brain structure or function.

Nonetheless, one study based on measurements of the size and volume of different brain regions at autopsy found little difference between the brains of schizophrenics and controls with regard to the amygdala and the hippocampus, and only small, nonsignificant differences with regard to the volume of the ventricles (76).

It has also been reported that some schizophrenic patients have lowered platelet monoamine oxidase (MAO) activity (187). This is of interest because of the many apparent similarities between platelets and brain synaptosomes, but the significance is uncertain because similar differences in brain MAO activity have not been observed at postmortem examination (132). Postmortem examination of brains of schizophrenic patients suggests a variety of subtle anatomical changes in neuronal density in different areas and layers of the cerebral cortex (13, 29). Other studies of brain function include a report of lateral asymmetry in amygdala dopamine in schizophrenics (133). This indicates that postmortem tissue can be used for such studies despite neuroleptic drug use; the asymmetry should be independent of drug use. Finally, the possibility of a viral etiology for schizophrenia, based on elevated antibody titers, has attracted interest (36).

Some schizophrenic patients, particularly those whose illness begins later in life with prominent paranoid delusions, may have a greater degree of hearing loss than controls (46). The role of such hearing loss in the pathogenesis of auditory hallucinations is not yet clear.

Eye tracking dysfunction has been reported in schizophrenics and in their relatives. In fact, some investigators believe that a single dominant gene may account for this phenomenon and that the eye dysfunction may represent an important component of the spectrum of manifestations associated with schizophrenia (98).

The possibility of microscopic pathology in the brains of schizophrenics has been investigated with modern neuropathological methods. Subtle differences in the postmortem brains of such patients have been found, especially in the entorhinal cortex, as well as "aberrant invagination" of the brain surface, "disruption of cortical layers," "heterotopic displacement of neurons," and "paucity of neurons in superficial layers" (8); a reduction in the "numbers of small neurons (interneurons) . . . of the cingulate and prefrontal cortex" (15); and a variety of differences in the hippocampus (34, 142). This area of research presents many methodological and conceptual problems, discussed by Benes (14) and Bogerts (21).

Some psychiatrists have emphasized the difference between "positive" symptoms (delusions, hallucinations, bizarre behavior) and "negative" symptoms (apathy, withdrawal, unresponsiveness); others have challenged the usefulness of such a distinction. The issue has stimulated psychiatrists to pay more attention to the full spectrum of clinical features in this condition (108), particularly because some investigators, though not all, have reported significant correlations between certain neuroimaging findings and negative symptoms.

The criteria for diagnosing schizophrenia according to *DSM-IV* are presented in Table 2.1. Other criteria have been proposed (145) that overlap *DSM-IV* in many ways but at the same time identify somewhat different populations of patients. This does not mean, however, that the situation is chaotic. Most patients identified by one set of criteria but not by another would be diagnosed as having "possible" or "suspected" schizophrenia by nearly all clinicians and investigators. Variations among different sets of criteria reflect differences in relative importance assigned to particular features with regard to differential diagnosis. In time further research should clarify these issues.

NATURAL HISTORY

As chronic schizophrenia typically begins insidiously, it is often hard to determine when the disorder started. In retrospect, the majority of patients, but clearly not all, show certain prepsychotic personality abnormalities: excessive shyness, social awkwardness, withdrawal from personal relationships, and inability to form close relationships (the so-called "schizoid personality"). A parent put it this way: "He was always afraid to make friends and felt that other people wouldn't like him. He couldn't be comfortable with girls, never knew what to say. I'd try to help him but it was very hard to change him. He'd cry and say it made him too uncomfortable to be with others." These traits may be present from early adolescence; often they are of concern to the patient's family for months or years before delusions or hallucinations become manifest.

A number of studies have revealed an increased frequency of pregnancy and birth complications in the records of individuals who later developed schizophrenia (80) as well as in the children of schizophrenic mothers (186).

In childhood and early adolescence, long before the diagnostic symptoms of schizophrenia are evident, schizophrenics tend to have more academic difficulty in school and to achieve lower scores on intelligence tests than do their siblings and other controls (1, 93). Instead of concluding that early academic difficulty and lowered intelligence may be early manifestations of schizophrenia, some investigators (82, 116) have argued that low IQ and schizophrenia are independently transmitted, but that a low IQ is one of the factors that increases the risk of clinical schizophrenia developing in those genetically predisposed. Other work indicates that antisocial and delinquent behavior may be an early manifestation of the illness (137), as may other personality disorders involving social withdrawal and disengagement (71, 122, 144, 179).

Delusions, hallucinations, and strange behavior usually start in the late teens or twenties. At first, these aberrations may be brief and vague, so the family is not certain of their significance. Gradually they become more obvious and disturbing, usually leading to psychiatric consultation.

Schizophrenia infrequently begins after forty. The illness generally has a fluctuating course. One or more psychiatric hospitalizations commonly occur. Some schizophrenics spend most of their lives in psychiatric hospitals. Even when not hospitalized, schizophrenics lead disturbed lives: they usually fail to form satisfactory personal relationships, marry less often than their contemporaries, have poor job histories, and seldom achieve positions of responsibility. They may become neighborhood eccentrics or socially isolated residents of inner cities, doing irregular unskilled work or being supported by welfare. Schizophrenia is probably overrepresented among homeless people in at least some large cities.

In recent years, clinicians and investigators have noted an increased frequency of drug abuse and dependence and of alcoholism in a significant proportion of their schizophrenic patients. Needless to say, these complications make the care of such patients much more difficult (41).

Two developments have altered the general clinical course in schizophrenic patients: the introduction of antipsychotics and the shift away from prolonged hospitalization. With antipsychotics, significant control of hallucinations, delusions, and bizarre behavior is possible in a substantial number of cases. As a result, and because of the policy of early discharge, many patients spend far less time in psychiatric hospitals than was the case in earlier years, though rehospitalization for relatively brief periods is common.

The effectiveness if the antipsychotic agents, which seem nearly always to be associated with blocking of dopamine receptors in the brain, has led to the hypothesis that many of the clinical manifestations of schizophrenia depend on certain as-yet-unidentified dopaminergic neurons. This hypothesis has stimulated much research, but it must still be regarded as speculative (32, 33, 152). Studies of postmortem schizophrenic brains have been inconsistent in their findings on the levels of various biogenic amines, including dopamine, norepinephrine, and serotonin (16, 19, 37).

On the other hand, several investigators have reported either increased binding to, or increased numbers of, dopamine receptors in postmortem schizophrenic brains. The influence of previous treatment with dopamine-receptor-blocking antipsychotic drugs on such findings is still uncertain, because animal studies show that prolonged treatment with these antipsychotic agents may lead to similar increases in brain dopamine receptors (95, 105, 153).

Good-prognosis cases generally begin more abruptly than poor-prognosis cases, without a history of long-standing personality abnormalities. Although poor- and good-prognosis cases may differ somewhat clinically, the most important difference relates to outcome (48). When patients are seen for the first time, however, it may be difficult to predict what the course and prognosis will be. Several studies have identified criteria associated with the difference in prognosis among the schizophrenic disorders. Table 2.2 summarizes the data from these studies. When most of the criteria are present, the prognosis associated with the criteria will be accurate in the majority of cases. One study (74) suggests that these criteria work better when the diagnosis of schizophrenia includes a broader range of disorders than are included in *DSM-IV*. This may only indicate that the criteria help distinguish true schizophrenics from patients with other disorders—such as psychotic affective illness and acute intoxications—that can mimic schizophrenia.

Some patients presenting with an acute schizophrenic picture lose their psychotic features during hospitalization and begin to

Table 2.2 Nomenclature and prognostic criteria for good- and poor-prognosis cases

	Good Prognosis	Poor Prognosis
Diagnostic terms	Schizophreniform illness	Schizophrenia
	Acute Schizophrenia	Process Schizophrenia
	Schizoaffective Schizophrenia	Nuclear Schizophrenia
	Reactive Schizophrenia	Chronic Schizophrenia
	Remitting Schizophrenia	Nonremitting Schizophrenia
Prognostic criteria		
Mode of onset	Acute	Insidious
Precipitating events	Frequently reported	Usually not reported
Prepsychotic history	Good	Poor; frequent history of "schizoid" traits (aloofness, social isolation)
Confusion	Often present	Usually absent
Affective symptoms	Often present and prominent	Often absent or minimal; affective responses usually "blunted" or "flat"
Marital status	Usually married	Often single, especially males
Family history of Affective Disorder	Often present	May be present but less likely
Family history of Schizophrenia	Absent or rare	Increased

56

look like depressives (78, 109, 140). Others recover from the psychotic episode and then after a prolonged remission present with typical depression (146). These observations are of great theoretical interest. Some have interpreted them to suggest that the distinction between schizophrenic and affective disorders may be too arbitrary (146); others, emphasizing the familial prevalence of affective illness in the overlapping cases, have argued that such cases are more appropriately classified as affective disorders (173).

In the past, an apparent absence of rheumatoid arthritis in patients suffering from schizophrenia has been noted. This observation was based on long psychiatric hospitalizations and clinical records often extending over many decades. Recently, this question has received renewed attention in the hope that it may lead to new ideas about the etiology or pathogenesis of schizophrenia (45, 177).

COMPLICATIONS

In no illness is it more difficult to distinguish between the typical clinical picture and the complications than in chronic schizophrenia. For example, difficulties in school or at work are common features of schizophrenia. Yet it is usually hard to tell whether these problems arise because of the patient's disordered thinking or loss of motivation or whether they result from the reactions to the patient's abnormal behavior of teachers, fellow students and workers, or supervisors.

A suspicious, fearful, and deluded individual may not perform well in school or at work because of preoccupation with abnormal thoughts; at the same time, the withdrawn, preoccupied, and unresponsive student may draw criticism and other adverse responses from teachers and supervisors. These, in turn, will reinforce the individual's pathological responses. The definition of the disorder encompasses its natural history and at the same time specifies the complications. These include impaired education, poor work history and job achievement, celibacy, and prolonged psychiatric hospitalization. An increased risk of suicide among young patients also appears to be a complication.

Because chronic schizophrenia typically begins early in life and is characterized by recurrent or persistent manifestations, the patient's schooling and education suffer. Early school difficulties have been noted, but even among those who do well in elementary school, difficulties may arise in high school or college. Social withdrawal and loss of interest in studies may become evident. These changes coupled with the need to leave school at the onset of more dramatic symptoms eventually lead to dropping out of school in many cases. If the illness peaks after the completion of formal education, the same clinical features may lead to marked reduction of effectiveness at work, demotions, being fired, frequent job changes, and financial dependency.

Schizophrenic men are less likely to marry, presumably because male initiative is more important than female initiative in getting married. Thus a schizophrenic man would be less successful in courtship, whereas a schizophrenic woman might attract a suitor despite her illness. With the advent of modern drug treatment and the reduction in prolonged psychiatric hospitalization, marriage and childbearing rates of schizophrenics have approached those of the general population, though the sex difference persists (49, 161).

Despite the great reduction in chronic psychiatric hospitalization, no group of patients spends more time in psychiatric hospitals than schizophrenics. The majority are hospitalized for repeated, relatively brief periods, but a substantial minority of patients, perhaps one-quarter or one-third, spend many years in hospitals.

A common fear regarding deluded schizophrenic patients is that they are likely to act on their delusions and commit crimes. Available data suggest, however, that there is only a modestly increased risk of significant crimes committed by schizophrenics (68, 99). They may be arrested for vagrancy, disturbing the peace, or similar misdemeanors, but only rarely are they involved in serious or violent felonies. It needs to be emphasized, however, that many such patients are shunted away from the legal system without trial as soon as their psychiatric disorder is recognized. Thus, we may have significant underestimations about the rates of serious crimes among schizophrenics. Most experts agree, however, that serious crimes by schizophrenics represent a small percentage of all serious crimes.

Some authors have reported an increased suicide risk among young schizophrenics (42), which might represent misdiagnosis of primary affective disorder. Unfortunately, these reports did not regularly attempt to distinguish between poor- and good-prognosis cases. It may be that some of the increased suicide risk is a function of the latter state; if so, this would suggest a link between at least some cases of good-prognosis illness and primary affective disorders (135). At the same time, however, it has gradually become evident that there is a significantly increased risk of suicide in definite schizophrenic patients as well (31).

FAMILY STUDIES

All investigators have found an increased prevalence of schizophrenia among the close relatives of schizophrenics (57, 63, 67, 84, 88, 89). Most studies have indicated a prevalence of about 5 to 10 percent among first-degree relatives of index cases compared with a general population figure of just under 1 percent.

All but one of a series of twin studies reported through 1972 (Table 2.3) showed significantly higher concordance rates for schizophrenia among monozygotic twins than among dizygotic twins of the same sex (2, 50, 53, 62, 63, 79, 83, 92, 104, 138, 148, 168). The prevalence of schizophrenia among the latter was similar to the prevalence among ordinary siblings of the same sex. Although the actual concordance rates varied from study to study, probably depending on methods of ascertainment (62, 63, 86), the rate for monozygotic twins was generally three to six times that of dizygotic twins.

Table 2.3 Schizophrenia concordance rates in twins

Investigator	MZ Twins		DZ Twins (Same Sex)	
	"Strict" Schizophrenia (%)	Including "Borderline" Cases (%)	"Strict" Schizophrenia (%)	Including "Borderline" Cases (%)
Luxemberger, 1928 (Germany)	50	71	0	0
Rosanoff et al., 1934 (USA)	44	61	9	13
Essen-Möller, 1941 (Sweden)	14	71	8	17
Kallmann, 1946 (USA)		69		17
Slater, 1953 (UK)		65		14
Inouye, 1963 (Japan)		60		18
Tienari, 1963 (Finland)	6	31	5	5
Kringlen, 1966 (Norway)	28	38	6	14
Gottesman and Shields, 1966 (UK)	42	54	9	18
Fischer et al., 1969 (Denmark)	24	48	10	19
Allen et al., 1972 (USA)		27		5

Adapted from Fischer et al. (53) and Allen et al. (2)

It is worth noting that the center reporting the single failure to find a significant difference in concordance between monozygotic and dizygotic twins subsequently found just such a difference (118). In addition, an adoption study at this center showed a statistically significant effect of the biological parent's illness on the adopted-away child's risk for developing schizophrenia (169).

The failure to find complete concordance in monozygotic twins has naturally led to the conclusion that there must be important environmental factors in the etiology of schizophrenia. Often such environmental factors are assumed to be of a social or psychological nature. One report (25), however, suggested that the discordance may be related to certain "brain development deviations" to which monozygotic twins may be "specially prone." The report indicated that concordance for schizophrenia in monozygotic twins was close to 100 percent when both twins were right-handed but that it fell markedly when one or both of the twins was not clearly right-handed, suggesting that the risk of schizophrenia is somehow associated with the process of brain lateralization. Other reports have been contradictory (103, 165).

In addition, it should be noted that as discordant monozygotic twins are followed, many pairs become concordant (12), suggesting that the age of onset may be affected by nongenetic factors in some cases.

In an American study of children separated early in life from schizophrenic parents and raised by unrelated adoptive parents, schizophrenia was found in five of forty-seven children of hospitalized schizophrenic mothers and no cases were found in fifty control children (77). All five schizophrenic children had been hospitalized, three chronically; the other two were taking antipsychotic drugs. In a second study, carried out in Denmark, about 32 percent of the children of schizophrenic parents received a diagnosis in the "schizophrenia spectrum," compared to about 18 percent of controls (139); none, however, had yet been hospitalized for schizophrenia. It is unclear how many would be considered schizophrenic in the "narrow" sense. "Schizophrenia spectrum" refers to a range of disorders, including schizophrenia and personality disorders, that appear to cluster in certain families.

Another Danish study approached the problem of hereditary predisposition to schizophrenia in a different way. Monozygotic twin pairs were identified in which one twin was schizophrenic, whereas the other was not. The children of these discordant twins were studied. It was found that the frequency of schizophrenia was the same in children of nonaffected discordant schizophrenic twins as in children of affected members of discordant twin pairs (52). The prevalence of schizophrenia in all these children was about 10 percent, which is similar to the general figure for children of schizophrenic parents (62, 83). The results of all these investigations point to the likelihood of a hereditary predisposition to at least some schizophrenic illnesses.

Good- and poor-prognosis cases generally have not been distinguished in studies of the familial transmission of schizophrenia. Available evidence suggests, however, that the prevalence of affective disorders is increased in close relatives of good-prognosis cases. One interpretation given these data is that at least some good-prognosis cases are atypical forms of affective illness (135).

The recognition that schizophrenic disorders are familial and that they probably result in part from hereditary factors has focused attention on identifying at an early age those individuals within a vulnerable family who are at greatest risk of developing the clinical disorders. Such "high-risk" studies are under way in many countries (114, 144, 163). One of the first studies, conducted in Denmark (144), indicates that the risk of schizophrenia during a ten-year follow-up of ten- to twenty-year-old children of schizophrenic mothers is about eight times greater than in matched control children.

Certain measurements of autonomic nervous system function may help identify those high-risk children who will develop the clinical disorder. So may clinical measures since in at least one study childhood thought disorder correlated positively with thought disorder in adulthood (123).

A frequent problem in studies of the familial distribution of psychiatric disorders is the failure to examine both parents of index cases. As a result puzzling familial associations between different disorders may be observed. For example, in the adoption studies of schizophrenia described earlier, antisocial personality disorders have been found to be associated with schizophrenia. This may indicate that antisocial behavior can be one of the manifestations of schizophrenia, but an equally likely explanation is the tendency of some schizophrenics to mate with individuals manifesting other psychiatric disorders, especially antisocial personality (54–56, 121, 156).

Several studies have also shown a familial and even a genetic relationship between schizophrenia and schizotypal personality, thus supporting the validity of the schizophrenia-spectrum concept (88, 89, 167, 170, 171). The risks of psychiatric hospitalization and suicide are much greater in the children of schizophrenic mothers than in controls (119), though not all findings are consistent (155). In addition, close relatives of individuals with schizotypal personality disorders have an increased frequency of schizophrenia (11, 166). Schizotypal personality, described in *DSM-IV*, includes many of the chronic personality features seen in schizophrenia but does not include delusions or hallucinations.

From time to time, case reports of both schizophrenia and bipolar affective disorder in the same family have been published (126, 166). The significance of these observations is uncertain because of the possibility of the two conditions occurring together by chance alone.

DIFFERENTIAL DIAGNOSIS

The differential diagnosis between poor- and good-prognosis cases has already been discussed. Most studies indicate that when patients fulfill the criteria of either good-prognosis or poor-prognosis illness, in the majority of cases the clinical course and long-term prognosis will be consistent with the classification. Certain data suggest that the improved outcome in some series of poor-prognosis schizophrenics may be the result of improved treatment (129). A major element in the differentiation between good- and poor-prognosis cases is "premorbid adjustment." Inconsistent findings may reflect difficulties in defining and measuring such adjustment (150, 162, 163), and additional studies are needed in which patients are clearly separated on the basis of how long they have been sick before psychiatric evaluation.

A small number of patients hospitalized for depression will, at follow-up, turn out to be suffering from chronic schizophrenia (136). This is much more likely to be the case when the depression is characterized by striking delusions or hallucinations. Some patients who present with the symptoms of somatization disorder will show at follow-up the full clinical picture of chronic schizophrenia (185), but this too is infrequent.

Obsessional disorder, early in its course, occasionally is difficult to distinguish from schizophrenia. If the obsessions are bizarre or if the patient clearly does not have insight into the abnormal nature of his thoughts and impulses, it may not be possible to make a confident diagnosis. The risk of schizophrenia in patients with obsessional disorder is small after the first year or two of illness and when the obsessions are classical (61).

A clinical picture resembling schizophrenia has been described in association with temporal lobe epilepsy (38, 117, 149). Patients presenting this clinical picture cannot be distinguished from typical schizophrenics, but the absence of an increased prevalence of schizophrenia in their close relatives suggests that one is dealing with a separate entity.

Although many good-prognosis cases are probably manifestations of affective illness, the question of differential diagnosis is often one of diagnostic conventions or style. Certain delusions (those of poverty, sinfulness, disease) are common in depressions, and others (those of overconfidence and unusual powers) in mania. Different delusions (those of control, persecution, depersonalization) are more likely to lead to a diagnosis of schizophrenia.

The differential diagnosis of good-prognosis illness and organic brain syndrome may also at times be a matter of convention. If disorientation and memory impairment are transient and less striking than the delusions, hallucinations, and bizarre behavior, a diagnosis of schizophrenia may be made. Patients with systemic medical illnesses affecting the brain such as lupus erythematosus may develop psychiatric symptoms that vary over time from those of depression to those of a brain syndrome, with a schizophrenic picture in between. Most patients with brain syndromes, however, present no problem in differential diagnois. Even with striking delusions and hallucinations are present, the persistent disorientation and memory impairment point to the correct diagnosis.

Persistent alcoholic hallucinosis is a syndrome of striking hallucinations, chiefly auditory, with a clear sensorium, that follows alcohol withdrawal. It may occur either after other withdrawal symptoms have subsided or in the absence of other manifestations of withdrawal. Alcoholic hallucinosis usually subsides within a couple of weeks. Occasionally, it persists and becomes chronic, thus resembling schizophrenia. Family studies have been undertaken to determine whether there is an increased prevalence of schizophrenia in close relatives (thus suggesting that the alcoholism precipitated or was superimposed on typical schizophrenia) or whether there is no increased prevalence (suggesting that, like epilepsy, alcoholism may produce a "symptomatic schizophrenia"). The findings are contradictory and the issue cannot yet be resolved (143, 145).

Amphetamines, taken chronically in large quantities, can cause a schizophrenia-like illness (35). This psychotic state will almost always subside within ten to fourteen days after the drug is discontinued. In rare chronic cases, the situation is similar to that seen in chronic alcoholic hallucinosis, where it is uncertain which came first—the drug abuse or the schizophrenic disorder. Cocaine abuse can also bring about a schizophrenia-like condition very similar to that seen in association with amphetamines.

Other psychotomimetic drugs such as LSD and PCP are responsible for a substantial percentage of cases of acute psychosis seen in emergency rooms or admitted to psychiatric hospitals. When first seen, it is not possible to distinguish such cases from naturally occurring acute schizophrenia, and sometimes one finds that a patient with chronic schizophrenia is suffering an acute intensification of the illness as the result of using these drugs.

CLINICAL MANAGEMENT

Antipsychotic medication, coupled with a policy of early discharge from psychiatric hospitals, made possible in part by the antipsychotics, has become the keystone of standard treatment. Occasionally, the combination of antipsychotics and electroconvulsive treatments may produce better results than antipsychotics alone (151). Delusions, hallucinations, and bizarre behavior may be at least partially controlled by adequate doses of antipsychotics, though these drugs probably do not affect as much the emotional blunting and social withdrawal associated with schizophrenia. Larger doses are usually needed during acute exacerbations but may be reduced as the patient's symptoms abate.

The prolonged use of antipsychotics may lead to certain undesirable consequences. Even at moderate dosage levels, parasympatholytic, or atropine-like, effects and Parkinsonism are common. At higher doses, lenticular opacities (47, 59, 127) and, more important, tardive dyskinesia (81, 85) have been described in many long-term patients. Patients receiving large doses of thioridazine may develop a condition resembling retinitis pigmentosa that causes visual impairment and blindness (70). A variety of skin rashes (188), a form of intrahepatic obstructive jaundice (which may rarely lead to chronic biliary cirrhosis) (90), and bone marrow toxicity may occur (110, 124), all probably as a result of special hypersensitivity. Despite these and other untoward reactions, the introduction of the antipsychotics represents a major advance in the treatment of schizophrenia.

The so-called "atypical neuroleptics," of which clozapine is a widely used example, appear to offer much better results in a significant minority of schizophrenic patients who have proven resistant to standard antipsychotic drugs. A number of new neuroleptics are being developed and there is hope that these will reduce side effects and improve patient compliance. Some patients may also benefit from the use of benzodiazepines in addition to neuroleptics (100, 182).

Antipsychotic drugs do not control all schizophrenic symptoms. Patients continue to suffer from intermittent delusions and hallucinations, personality changes, and general social impairment. Many experienced clinicians believe, though, that the reduction in chronic hospitalization and the greater efforts at rehabilitation resulting from an increased optimism about more effective treatment prevent some personality deterioration.

The return of chronic schizophrenic patients to the community is not without problems. Many patients are severe burdens to their families. Although they may be better following drug treatment, they are not well. They continue to experience symptoms and their adjustment to family life is difficult and stressful. Also, most chronic schizophrenic patients are not able to support themselves financially and require family or community help. Recent work (120, 160) continues to support previous reports (96, 106, 154, 176) suggesting that some schizophrenic patients do better and require fewer hospitalizations if their family members show less "expressed emotion," referring to overt criticism and pressure on the ill relative. In some cases, efforts to help the family with these reactions seem to result in milder symptoms in the patient and fewer hospitalizations.

Good-prognosis cases are generally episodic. As in chronic schizophrenia, antipsychotics may help. In many cases, electrotherapy produces remission.

REFERENCES

1. Albee, G., Lane, E., and Reuter, J. M. Childhood intelligence of future schizophrenics and neighborhood peers. J. Psychol. *58*:141–144, 1964.
2. Allen, M. G., Cohen, S., and Pollin, W. Schizophrenia in veteran twins: a diagnostic review. Am. J. Psychiat. *128*:939–945, 1972.
3. Andreasen, N. C., Dennert, J. W., Olsen, S. A., and Damasio, A. R. Hemispheric asymmetries and schizophrenia. Am. J. Psychiat. *139*:427–430, 1982.
4. Andreasen, N., Nasrallah, H. A., Dunn, V., Olson, S. C., Grove, W. M., Ehrhardt, J. C., Coffman, J. A., and Crossett, J. H. W. Structural abnormalities in the frontal system in schizophrenia. Arch. Gen. Psychiat. *43*:136–144, 1986.
5. Andreasen, N. C., Olsen, S. A., Dennert, J. W., and Smith, M. R. Ventricular enlargement in schizophrenia: relationship to positive and negative symptoms. Am. J. Psychiat. *139*:297–302, 1982.
6. Andreasen, N. C., Smith, M. R., Jacoby, C. G., Dennert, J. W., and Olsen, S. A. Ventricular enlargement in schizophrenia: definition and prevalence. Am. J. Psychiat. *139*:292–296, 1982.
7. Andreasen, N. C., Rezai, K., Alliger, R., Swayze, V. M., Flaum, M., Kirch-

ner, P., Cohen, G., and O'Leary, D. S. Hypofrontality in neuroleptic-naive patients and in patients with chronic schizophrenia. Arch. Gen Psychiat. *49*:943–958, 1992.

8. Arnold, S. E., Hyman, B. T., Van Hoesen, G. W., and Damascio, A. R. Some cytoarchitectural abnormalities of the entorhinal cortex in schizophrenia. Arch. Gen. Psychiat. *48*:625–632, 1991.

9. Astrup, C., Fossum, A., and Holmboe, R. *Prognosis in Functional Psychoses.* Springfield, Ill.: C. C. Thomas, 1962.

10. Astrup, C., and Noreik, K. *Functional Psychoses: Diagnostic and Prognostic Models.* Springfield, Ill.: C. C. Thomas, 1966.

11. Battaglia, M., Gasperini, M., Sciuto, G., Diaferia, G., and Bellodi, L. Psychiatric disorders in the families of schizophrenic subjects. Schizophr. Bull. *17*:659–668, 1991.

12. Belmaker, R., Pollin, W., Wyatt, R. J., and Cohen, S. A follow-up of monozygotic twins discordant for schizophrenia. Arch. Gen. Psychiat. *30*:219–222, 1974.

13. Benes, F. M., Davidson, J., and Bird, E. D. Quantitative cytoarchitectural studies of the cerebral cortex of schizophrenics. Arch. Gen. Psychiat. *43*:31–35, 1986.

14. Benes, F. M. Post-mortem structural analysis of schizophrenic brain: study designs and the interpretation of data. Psychiat. Dev. *3*:213–226, 1988.

15. Benes, F. M., McSparren, J., Bird, E. D., Sangiovanni, J. P., and Vincent, S. L. Deficits in small interneurons in prefrontal and cingulate cortices of schizophrenic and schizoaffective patients. Arch. Gen. Psychiat. *48*:996–1001, 1991.

16. Bennett, Jr., J. P., Enna, S. J., Bylund, D. B., Gillin, J. C., Wyatt, R. J., and Snyder, S. H. Neurotransmitter receptors in frontal cortex of schizophrenics. Arch. Gen. Psychiat. *36*:927–934, 1979.

17. Berman, K. F., Zec, R. F., and Weinberger, D. R. Physiologic dysfunction of dorsolateral prefrontal cortex in schizophrenia. Arch. Gen. Psychiat. *43*:126–135, 1986.

18. Bigelow, L. B., Nasrallah, H. A., and Rauscher, F. P. Corpus callosum thickness in chronic schizophrenia. Brit. J. Psychiat. *142*:284–287, 1983.

19. Bird, E. D., Spokes, E. G. S., and Iversen, L. L. Increased dopamine concentration in limbic areas of brain from patients dying with schizophrenia. Brain *102*:347–360, 1979.

20. Bleuler, E. *Dementia Praecox or the Group of Schizophrenias*, Zinkin J., trans. New York: International Universities Press, 1950.

21. Bogerts, B. Recent advances in the neuropathology of schizophrenia. Schizophr. Bull. *19*:431–445, 1993.

22. Bogerts, B., Meertz, E., and Schonfeldt-Bausch, R. Basal ganglia and limbic system pathology in schizophrenia. Arch. Gen. Psychiat. *42*:784–791, 1985.

23. Bogerts, B., Ashtari, M., Degreef, G., Alvir, J. MaJ., Bilder, R. M., and Lieberman, J. A. Reduced temporal limbic structure volumes on magnetic reso-

nance images in first episode schizophrenia. Psychiat. Res. Neuroimaging *35*:1–13, 1990.

24. Bogerts, B., Lieberman, J. A., Ashtari, M., Bilder, R. M., Degreef, G., Lerner, G., Johns, C., and Masiar, S. Hippocampus-amygdala volumes and psychopathology in chronic schizophrenia. Biol. Psychiat. *33*:236–246, 1993.

25. Boklage, C. E. Schizophrenia, brain asymmetry development, and twinning: cellular relationship with etiological and possibly prognostic implications. Biol. Psychiat. *12*:19–35, 1977.

26. Boyd, J. H., Pulver, A. E., and Stewart, W. Season of birth: schizophrenia and bipolar disorder. Schizophr. Bull. *12*:173–186, 1986.

27. Brenner, D. *Elementary Textbook of Psychoanalysis*. New York: International Universities Press, 1955.

28. Brill, N., and Glass, J. Hebephrenic schizophrenic reactions. Arch. Gen. Psychiat. *12*:545–551, 1965.

29. Brown, R., Colter, N., Corsellis, J. A. N., Crow, T. J., Frith, C. D., Jagoe, R., Johnstone, E. C., and Marsh, L. Postmortem evidence of structural brain changes in schizophrenia. Arch. Gen. Psychiat. *43*:36–42, 1986.

30. Buchsbaum, M. S., Cappelletti, J., Ball, R., Hazlett, E., King, A. C., Johnson, J., Wu, J., and DeLisi, L. E. Positron emission tomographic image measurement in schizophrenia and affective disorders. Ann. Neurol. *15*:S157–S165, 1984.

31. Caldwell, C. B., and Gottesman, I. I. Schizophrenics kill themselves too: a review of risk factors for suicide. Schizophr. Bull. *16*:571–589, 1990.

32. Carlsson, A. Does dopamine play a role in schizophrenia? Psychol. Med. *7*:583–598, 1977.

33. Carlsson, A. Antipsychotic drugs, neurotransmitters, and schizophrenia. Am. J. Psychiat. *135*:164–173, 1978.

34. Christison, G. W., Casanova, M. F., Weinberger, D. R., Rawlings, R., and Kleinman, J. E. A quantitative investigation of hippocampal pyramidal cell size, shape, and variability of orientation in schizophrenia. Arch. Gen. Psychiat. *46*:1027–1032, 1989.

35. Connell, P. H. *Amphetamine Psychosis*, Maudsley Monogr., no. 5. London: Oxford Univ. Press, 1958.

36. Crow, T. J. A re-evaluation of the viral hypothesis: is psychosis the result of retroviral integration at a site close to the cerebral dominance gene? Brit. J. Psychiat. *145*:243–253, 1984.

37. Crow, T. J., Baker, H. F., Cross, A. J., Joseph, M. H., Lofthouse, R., Longden, A., Owen, F., Riley, G. J., Glover V., and Killpack, W. S. Monoamine mechanisms in chronic schizophrenia: post-mortem neurochemical findings. Brit. J. Psychiat. *134*:249–256, 1979.

38. Davison, K. Schizophrenic-like psychoses associated with organic cerebral disorders: a review. Psychiat. Dev. *1*:1–34, 1983.

39. DeLisi, L. E., Hoff, A. L., Schwartz, J. E., Shields, G. W., Halthore, S. N., Gupta, S. M., Henn, F. A., and Azad, A. K. Brain morphology in first

episode schizophrenic-like psychotic patients: a quantitative magnetic resonance imaging study. Biol. Psychiat. *29*:159–175, 1991.

40. Dennert, J. W., and Andreasen, N. C. CT scanning and schizophrenia: a review. Psychiat. Dev. *1*:105–121, 1983.

41. Drake, R. E., Osher, F. C., Noordsy, D. L., Hurlbut, S. C., Teague, G. B., and Beaudett, M. S. Diagnosis of alcohol use disorders in schizophrenia. Schizophr. Bull. *16*:57–67, 1990.

42. Drake, R. E., Gates, C., Whitaker, A., and Cotton, P. G. Suicide among schizophrenics: a review. Compr. Psychiat. *26*:90–100, 1985.

43. Dunham, H. W. *Community and Schizophrenia*. Detroit: Wayne State Univ. Press, 1965.

44. Early, T. S., Reiman, E. M., Raichle, M. E., and Spitznagel, E. L. Left globus pallidus abnormality in never-medicated patients with schizophrenia. Proc. Natl. Acad. Sci. U.S.A. *84*:561–563, 1987.

45. Eaton, W. W., Hayward, C., and Ram, R. Schizophrenia and rheumatoid arthritis: a review. Schizophr. Res. *6*:181–192, 1992.

46. Editorial. Hearing loss and perceptual dysfunction in schizophrenia. Lancet *2*:848–849, 1981.

47. Edler, K., Gottfries, C. G., Haslund, J., and Raun, J. Eye changes in connection with neuroleptic treatment especially concerning phenothiazines and thioxanthenes. Acta Psychiat. Scand. *47*:377–385, 1971.

48. Eitlinger, L., Laane, C. V., and Langfeldt, G. The prognostic value of the clinical picture and the therapeutic value of physical treatment in schizophrenia and the schizophreniform states. Acta Psychiat. Neurol. Scand. *33*:33–53, 1958.

49. Erlenmeyer-Kimling, L., Nicol, S., Rainer, J. D., and Deming, E. Changes in fertility rates of schizophrenic patients in New York State. Am J. Psychiat. *125*:916–927, 1969.

50. Essen-Moller, E. *Psychiatrische Untersuchungen an einer Serie von Zwillingen*. Copenhagen: Ejnar Munksgaard, 1941.

51. Ey, H. Unity and diversity of schizophrenia: clinical and logical analysis of the concept of schizophrenia. Am. J. Psychiat. *115*:706–714, 1959.

52. Fischer, M. Psychoses in the offspring of schizophrenic twins and their normal co-twins. Brit. J. Psychiat. *118*:43–52, 1971.

53. Fischer, M., Harvald, B., and Hauge, M. A Danish twin study of schizophrenia. Brit. J. Psychiat. *115*:981–990, 1969.

54. Fowler, R. C., and Tsuang, M. T. Spouses of schizophrenics: a blind comparative study. Compr. Psychiat. *16*:339–342, 1975.

55. Fowler, R. C., Tsuang, M. T., and Cadoret, R. J. Parental psychiatric illness associated with schizophrenia in the siblings of schizophrenics. Compr. Psychiat. *18*:271–275, 1977.

56. Fowler, R. C., Tsuang, M. T., and Cadoret, R. J. Psychiatric illness in the offspring of schizophrenics. Compr. Psychiat. *18*:127–134, 1977.

57. Frangos, E., Athanassenas, G., Tsitourides, S., Katsanou, N., and Alexandrakou, P. Prevalance of DSM III schizophrenics among the first-degree relatives of schizophrenic probands. Acta Psychiat. Scand. *72*:382–386, 1985.

58. Goldberg, E. M., and Morrison, S. L. Schizophrenia and social class. Brit. J. Psychiat. *109*:785–802, 1963.
59. Gombos, G., and Yarden, P. E. Ocular and cutaneous side-effects after prolonged chlorpromazine treatment. Am. J. Psychiat. *123*:872–874, 1967.
60. Goodwin, D. W., Alderson, P., and Rosenthal, R. Clinical significance of hallucinations in psychiatric disorders. Arch. Gen. Psychiat. *24*:76–80, 1971.
61. Goodwin, D. W., Guze, S. B., and Rohins, E. Follow-up studies in obsessional neurosis. Arch. Gen. Psychiat. *20*:182–187, 1969.
62. Gottesman, I. I., and Shields, J. Contributions of twin studies to perspectives in schizophrenia. In *Progress in Experimental Personality Research*, vol. 3, Maher, B. A. (ed.), 1–84. New York: Academic Press, 1966.
63. Gottesman, I. I., and Shields, J. *Schizophrenia: The Epigenetic Puzzle.* Cambridge: Cambridge Univ. Press, 1982.
64. Gur, R. E., Resnick, S. M., Alavi, A., Gur, R. C., Caroff, S., Dann, R., Silver, F. L., Saykin, A. J., Chawluk, J. B., Kushner, M., and Reivich, M. Regional brain function in schizophrenia. I. A positron emission tomography study. Arch. Gen. Psychiat. *44*:119–125, 1987.
65. Gur, R. E., Resnick, S. M., Gur, R. C., Alavi, A., Caroff, S., Kushner, M., and Reivich, M. Regional brain function in schizophrenia: II. Repeated evaluation with positron emission tomography. Arch. Gen. Psychiat. *44*:126–129, 1987.
66. Gur, R. E., and Pearlson, G. D. Neuroimaging in schizophrenia research. Schizophr. Bull. *19*:337–353, 1993.
67. Guze, S. B., Cloninger, C. R., Martin, R. L., and Clayton, P. J. A follow-up and family study of schizophrenia. Arch. Gen. Psychiat. *40*:1273–1276, 1983.
68. Guze, S. B., Goodwin, D. W., and Crane, J. B. Criminality and psychiatric disorders. Arch. Gen. Psychiat. *20*:583–591, 1969.
69. Hambrecht, M., Maurer, K., and Häfner, H. Gender differences in schizophrenia in three cultures. Results of the WHO Collaborative study on psychiatric disability. Social Psychiat. Psychiat. Epidemiol. *27*:117–121, 1992.
70. Hagopian, V., Stratton, D., and Busiek, R. Five cases of pigmentary retinopathy associated with thioridazine administration. Am. J. Psychiat. *123*:97–100, 1966.
71. Hanson, D. R., Gottesman, I. I., and Heston, L. L. Some possible childhood indicators of adult schizophrenia inferred from children of schizophrenics. Brit. J. Psychiat. *129*:142–154, 1976.
72. Hare, E. H. Season of birth in schizophrenia and neurosis. Am. J. Psychiat. *132*:1168–1171, 1975.
73. Hare, E., and Moran, P. A relation between seasonal temperature and the birth rate of schizophrenic patients. Acta Psychiat. Scand. *63*:396–405, 1981.
74. Harrow, M., Westermeyer, J. F., Silverstein, M., Strauss, B. S., and Cohler, B. J. Predictors of outcome in schizophrenia: the process-reaction dimensions. Schizophr. Bull. *12*:195–207, 1986.

75. Harvey, I. H., Ron, M. A., Du Boulay, G., Wicks, D., Lewis, S. W., and Murray, R. M. Reduction of cortical volume in schizophrenia on magnetic resonance imaging. Psychol. Med. *23*:591–604, 1993.
76. Heckers, S., Heinsen, H., Heinsen, Y. C., and Beckmann, H. Limbic structure and lateral ventricle in schizophrenia. Arch. Gen. Psychiat. *47*:1016–1022, 1990.
77. Heston, L. Psychiatric disorders in foster home-reared children of schizophrenic mothers. Brit. J. Psychiat. *112*:819–825, 1966.
78. Hoedemaker, F. S. Psychotic episodes and postpsychotic depression in young adults. Am. J. Psychiat. *127*:606–610, 1970.
79. Inouye, E. Similarity and dissimilarity of schizophrenia in twins. Proceedings of the 3rd World Congress on Psychiatry, *1*:524–530. Montreal: Univ. of Toronto Press, 1963.
80. Jacobsen, B., and Kinney, D. K. Perinatal complications in adopted and non-adopted schizophrenics and their controls. Acta Psychiat. Scand. *62(Suppl. 285)*:337–346, 1980.
81. Jeste, D. V., and Wyatt, R. J. Therapeutic strategies against tardive dyskinesia. Arch. Gen. Psychiat. *39*:803–815, 1982.
82. Jones, M. B., and Offord, D. R. Independent transmission of IQ and schizophrenia. Brit. J. Psychiat. *126*:185–190, 1975.
83. Kallmann, F. J. The genetic theory of schizophrenia. An analysis of 691 twin index families. Am. J. Psychiat. *103*:309–322, 1946.
84. Karlsson, J. L. Family transmission of schizophrenia: a review and synthesis. Brit. J. Psychiat. *140*:600–606, 1982.
85. Kazamatsuri, H., Chien, C., and Cole, J. O. Therapeutic approaches to tardive dyskinesia. Arch. Gen. Psychiat. *27*:491–499, 1972.
86. Kendler, K. S. Overview: a current perspective on twin studies of schizophrenia. Am. J. Psychiat. *140*:1413–1425, 1983.
87. Kendler, K. S., Gruenberg, A. M., and Tsuang, M. T. Subtype stability in schizophrenia. Am. J. Psychiat. *142*:827–832, 1985.
88. Kendler, K. S., Gruenberg, A. M., and Tsuang, M. T. Psychiatric illness in first-degree relatives of schizophrenic and surgical control patients. Arch. Gen. Psychiat. *42*:770–779, 1985.
89. Kendler, K. S., Masterson, C. C., and Davis, K. L. Psychiatric illness in first-degree relatives of patients with paranoid psychosis, schizophrenia and medical illness. Brit. J. Psychiat. *147*:524–531, 1985.
90. Kohn, N., and Myerson, R. Xanthomatous biliary cirrhosis following chlorpormazine. Am. J. Med. *31*:665–670, 1961.
91. Kraepelin, E. *Dementia Praecox and ParaAhrenia* (Barclay R. M., trans.; Robertson, G. M., ed.). Edinburgh: E. & S. Livingstone, 1919.
92. Kringlen, E. Schizophrenia in twins. An epidemiological-clinical study. Psychiatry *29*:172–184, 1966.
93. Lane, E., and Albee, G. W. Childhood intellectual differences between schizophrenic adults and their siblings. Am. J. Orthopsychiat. *35*:747–753, 1965.
94. Langfeldt, G. The prognosis in schizophrenia. Acta Psychiat. Neurol. Scand. Suppl. *110*:7–66, 1956.

95. Lee, T., and Seeman, P. Elevation of brain neuroleptic/dopamine receptors in schizophrenia. Am. J. Psychiat. *137*:191–197, 1980.

96. Leff, J., Kuipers, L., Berkowitz, R., Vaughn, C., and Sturgeon, D. Life events, relatives' expressed emotion and maintenance neuroleptics in schizophrenic relapse. Psychol. Med. *13*:799–806, 1983.

97. Leonhard, K. *Aufteilung der endogenen Psychosen.* Berlin: Akademie-Verlag, 1966.

98. Levy, D. L., Holzman, P. S., Matthysse, S., and Mendell, N. R. Eye tracking dysfunction and schizophrenia: a critical perspective. Schizophr. Bull. *19*:461–536, 1993.

99. Lindquist, P., and Allebeck, P. Schizophrenia and crime. A longitudinal follow-up of 644 schizophrenics in Stockholm. Brit. J. Psychiat. *157*:345–350, 1990.

100. Lingjaerde, O. Benzodiazepines in the treatment of schizophrenia: an updated survey. Acta Psychiat. Scand. *84*:453–459, 1991.

101. Lippmann, S., Manshadi, M., Baldwin, H., Drasin, G., Rice, J., and Alrajeh, S. Cerebellar vermis dimensions on computerized tomographic scans of schizophrenic and bipolar patients. Am. J. Psychiat. *139*:667–668, 1982.

102. Luchins, D. Computed tomography in schizophrenia. Arch. Gen. Psychiat. *39*:859–860, 1982.

103. Luchins, D., Pollin, W., and Wyatt, R. J. Laterality in monozygotic schizophrenic twins: an alternative hypothesis. Biol. Psychiat. *15*:87–93, 1980.

104. Luxenburger, H. Vorliufiger Bericht uber psychiatrischen Serieuntersuchungen an Zwillingen. Z. Ges. Neurol. Psychiat. *176*:297–326, 1928.

105. Mackay, A. V. P., Bird, E. D., Spokes, E. G., Rossor, M., Iversen, L. L., Creese, I., and Snyder, S. H. Dopamine receptors and schizophrenia: drug effect on illness. Lancet *2*:915–916, 1980.

106. MacMillan, J. F., Gold, A., Crow, T. J., Johnson, A. L., and Johnstone, E. C. Expressed emotion and relapse. Brit. J. Psychiat. *148*:133–143, 1986.

107. Mathew, R. J., Meyer, J. S., Francis, D. J., Schoolar, J. C., Weinman, M., and Mortel, K. F. Regional cerebral blood flow in schizophrenia: a preliminary report. Am. J. Psychiat. *138*:112–113, 1981.

108. McGlashan, T. H. The positive-negative distinction in schizophrenia. Review of natural history validators. Arch. Gen. Psychiat. *49*:63–72, 1992.

109. McGlashan, T. H., and Carpenter, Jr., W. T. Postpsychotic depression in schizophrenia. Arch. Gen. Psychiat. *33*:231–239, 1976.

110. McKinney, W., and Kane, Jr., F. J. Pancytopenia due to chlorpromazine. Am. J. Psychiat. *123*:879–880, 1967.

111. Merrin, E. L. Schizophrenia and brain asymmetry. An evaluation of evidence for dominant lobe dysfunction. J. Nerv. Ment. Dis. *169*:405–416, 1981.

112. Nasrallah, H. A., Jacoby, C. G., McCalley-Whitters, M., and Kuperman, S. Cerebral ventricular enlargement in subtypes of schizophrenia. Arch. Gen. Psychiat. *39*:774–777, 1982.

113. Nasrallah, H. A., Olson, S. C., McCalley-Whitters, M., Chapman, S., and

Jacoby, C. G. Cerebral ventricular enlargement in schizophrenia. Arch. Gen. Psychiat. *43*:157–159, 1986.

114. Neuchterlein, K. H. Childhood precursors of adult schizophrenia. J. Child Psychol. Psychiat. *27*:133–144, 1986.

115. O'Callaghan, E., Gibson, T., Colohan, H. A., Walshe, D., Buckley, P., Larkin, C., and Waddington, J. L. Season of birth in schizophrenia. Evidence for confinement of an excess of winter births to parents without a family history of mental disorder. Brit. J. Psychiat. *158*:764–769, 1991.

116. Offord, D. R. School performance of adult schizophrenics, their siblings and age mates. Brit. J. Psychiat. *125*:12–19, 1974.

117. Ohman, R., and Vogel, A. (eds.) Temporal lobe epilepsy, psychotic and neurological manifestations, clinical tradition and new vistas. Acta Psychiat. Scand. Suppl. *69*:313, 1984.

118. Onstad, S., Skre, I., Torgersen, S., and Kringlen, E. Twin concordance for DSM-III-R schizophrenia. Acta Psychiat. Scand. *83*:395–401, 1991.

119. Onstad, S., Skre, I., Edvardsen, J., Torgersen, S., and Kringlen, E. Mental disorders in first-degree relatives of schizophrenics. Acta Psychiat. Scand. *83*:463–467, 1991.

120. Parker, G., and Hadzi-Pavlovic, D. Expressed emotion as a predictor of schizophrenic relapse: an analysis of aggregated data. Psychol. Med. *20*:961–965, 1990.

121. Parnas, J. Mates of schizophrenic mothers. Brit. J. Psychiat. *146*:490–497, 1985.

122. Parnas, J., Schulsinger, F., Schulsinger, H., Mednick, S. A., and Teasdale, T. T. Behavioral precursors of schizophrenia spectrum. Arch. Gen. Psychiat. *39*:658–664, 1982.

123. Parnas, J., and Schulsinger, H. Continuity of formal thought disorder from childhood to adulthood in a high-risk sample. Acta Psychiat. Scand. *74*:246–251, 1986.

124. Pisciotta, A. V. Agranulocytosis induced by certain phenothiazine derivatives. JAMA *208*:1862–1868, 1969.

125. Planansky, K., and Johnston, R. Depressive syndrome in schizophrenia. Acta Psychiat. Scand. *57*:207–218, 1978.

126. Pope, H. G., and Yurgelun-Todd, D. Schizophrenic individuals with bipolar first-degree relatives: analysis of two pedigrees. J. Clin Psychiat. *51*:97–101, 1990.

127. Prien, R. F., DeLong, S. L., Cole, J. O., and Levine, J. Ocular changes occurring with prolonged high dose chlorpromazine therapy. Arch. Gen. Psychiat. *23*:464–468, 1970.

128. Retterstol, N. *Paranoid and Paranoiac Psychoses.* Springfield, Ill.: C. C. Thomas, 1966.

129. Retterstol, N. *Prognosis and Paranoid Psychoses.* Springfield, Ill.: C. C. Thomas, 1970.

130. Reveley, A. M., Reveley, M. A., and Murray, R. M. Cerebral ventricular enlargement in non-genetic schizophrenia: a controlled twin study. Brit. J. Psychiat. *144*:89–93, 1984.

131. Reveley, M. A. Ventricular enlargement in schizophrenia. The validity of computerised tomographic findings. Brit. J. Psychiat. *147*:233–240, 1985.

132. Reveley, M. A., Glover, V., Sandler, M., and Spokes, E. G. Brain monoamine oxidse activity in schizophrenics and controls. Arch. Gen. Psychiat. *38*:663–665, 1981.

133. Reynolds, G. P. Increased concentrations of lateral asymmetry of amygdala dopamine in schizophrenia. Nature *305*:527–529, 1983.

134. Riecher, A., Maurer, K., Löffler, W., Fätkenheuer, B., Heiden, W. an der, Munk-Jørgensen, P., Strömgren, E., and Häfner, H. Gender differences in age at onset and course of schizophrenic disorders. In *Search for the Causes of Schizophrenia*, vol. II, Berlin: Springer-Verlag, 1990.

135. Robins, E., and Guze, S. B. Establishment of diagnostic validity in psychiatric illness: its application to schizophrenia. Am. J. Psychiat. *126*:983–987, 1970.

136. Robins, E., and Guze, S. B. Classification of affective disorders: the primary-secondary, the endogenous-reactive, and the neurotic-psychotic concepts, In *Recent Advances in the Psychobiology of the Depressive Illnesses*, Williams, T. A., Katz, M. M., and Shield, Jr., J. A. (eds.), 283–293. Washington, D.C.: NIMH, DHEW, 1972.

137. Robins, L. *Deviant Children Grown Up.* Baltimore: Williams and Wilkins, 1966.

138. Rosanoff, A. J., Handy, I. M., Plesset, I. R., and Brush, S. The etiology of so-called schizophrenic psychoses. With special reference to their occurrence in twins. Am. J. Psychiat. *91*:247–286, 1934.

139. Rosenthal, D., Wender, P. H., Kety, S. S., Welner, J., and Schulsinger, F. The adopted-away offspring of schizophrenics. Am. J. Psychiat. *128*:307–311, 1971.

140. Roth, S. The seemingly ubiquitous depression following acute schizophrenic episodes, a neglected area of clinical discussion. Am. J. Psychiat. *127*:51–58, 1970.

141. Aslokangas, R. R. K. Social class of the parents of schizophrenic patients. Proceedings of the 18th Nordic Psychiatric Congress. Acta Psychiat. Scand. *54(Suppl. 265)*:30, 1976.

142. Scheibel, A. B., and Conrad, A. S. Hippocampal dysgenesis in mutant mouse and schizophrenic man: is there a relationship? Schizophr. Bull. *19*:23–33, 1993.

143. Schuckit, M. A., and Winokur, G. Alcoholic hallucinosis and schizophrenia: a negative study. Brit. J. Psychiat. *119*:549–550, 1971.

144. Schulsinger, H. A ten-year follow-up of children of schizophrenic mothers. Clinical assessment. Acta Psychiat. Scand. *53*:371–386, 1976.

145. Scott, D. F. Alcoholic hallucinosis—an aetiological study. Brit. J. Addict. *62*:113–125, 1967.

146. Sheldrick, C., Jablensky, A., Sartorius, N., and Shepherd, M. Schizophrenia succeeded by affective illness: catamnestic study and statistical enquiry. Psychol. Med. 7:619–624, 1977.

147. Siris, S. G. Diagnosis of secondary depression in schizophrenia: implications for DSM-IV. Schizophr. Bull. *17*:75–98, 1991.
148. Slater, E. *Psychotic and Neurotic Illnesses in Twins.* London: HMSO, 1953.
149. Slater, E., Beard, A., and Glithero, E. The schizophrenia-like psychoses of epilepsy. Brit. J. Psychiat. *109*:95–150, 1963.
150. Small, N. E., Mohs, R. C., Halperin, R., Rosen, W. G., Masterson, C., Kendler, K. S. Horvath, T. B., and Davis, K. L. A study of the reliability of reported premorbid adjustment in schizophrenic patients. Biol. Psychiat. *19*:203–211, 1984.
151. Smith, K. ECT-chlorpromazine and chlorpromazine compared in the treatment of schizophrenia. J. Nerv. Ment. Dis. *144*:284–290, 1967.
152. Snyder, S. H. The dopamine hypothesis of schizophrenia: focus on the dopamine receptor. Am. J. Psychiat. *133*:197–202, 1976.
153. Snyder, S. G. Dopamine receptors, neuroleptics, and schizophrenia. Am. J. Psychiat. *138*:460–464, 1981.
154. Spiegel, D., and Wissler, T. Family environment as a predictor of psychiatric rehospitalization. Am. J. Psychiat. *143*:56–60, 1986.
155. Squires-Wheeler, E., Skodol, A. E., Bassett, A., and Erlenmeyer-Kimling, L. DSM-III-R schizotypal personality traits in offspring of schizophrenic disorder, affective disorder, and normal control parents. J. Psychiat. Res. *23*:229–239, 1989.
156. Stephens, D. A., Atkinson, M. W., Kay, D. W., Roth, M., and Garside, R. F. Psychiatric morbidity in parents and sibs of schizophrenics and nonschizophrenics. Brit. J. Psychiat. *127*:97–108, 1975.
157. Stephens, J. H. Long-term course and prognosis of schizophrenia. Semin. Psychiat. *2*:464–485, 1970.
158. Stephens, J. H., and Astrup, C. Prognosis in "process and non-process" schizophrenia. Am. J. Psychiat. *119*:945–953, 1963.
159. Stephens, J. H., Astrup, C., Carpenter, Jr., W. T., Shaffer, J. W., and Goldberg, J. A comparison of nine systems to diagnose schizophrenia. Psychiat. Res. *6*:127–143, 1982.
160. Stirling, J., Tantam, D., Thomas, P., Newby, D., Montague, L., Ring, N., and Rowe, S. Expressed emotion and schizophrenia: the ontogeny of EE during an 18-month follow-up. Psychol. Med. *23*:771–778, 1993.
161. Stevens, B. C. *Marriage and Fertility of Women Suffering from Schizophrenia or Affective Disorders,* Maudsley Monogr. no. 19. London: Oxford Univ. Press, 1969.
162. Strauss, J. S., and Gift, T. E. Choosing an approach for diagnosing schizophrenia. Arch. Gen. Psychiat. *34*:1248–1253, 1977.
163. Strauss, J. S., Kokes, R., Klorman, R., and Sacksteder, J. Premorbid adjustment in schizophrenia: concepts, measures, and implications. Schizophr. Bull. *3*:182–245, 1977.
164. Tanaka, Y., Hazama, H., Kawahara, R., and Kobayashi, K. Computerized tomography of the brain in schizophrenic patients. Acta Psychiat. Scand. *63*:191–197, 1981.
165. Taylor, P. J., Dalton, R., Fleminger, J. J., and Lishman, W. A. Differences

between two studies of hand preference in psychiatric patients. Brit. J. Psychiat. *140*:166–173, 1982.

166. Taylor, M. A., Berenbaum, S. A., Jampala, V. C., and Cloninger, C. R. Are schizophrenia and affective disorder related? Preliminary data from a family study. Am. J. Psychiat. *150*:278–285, 1993.

167. Thaker, G., Adami, H., Moran, M., Lahti, A., and Cassady, S. Psychiatric illnesses in families of subjects with schizophrenia-spectrum personality disorders: high morbidity risks for unspecified functional psyches and schizophrenia. Am. J. Psychiat. *150*:66–71, 1993.

168. Tienari, P. Psychiatric illnesses in identical twins. Acta Psychiat. Scand. *39(Suppl. 171)*:1–195, 1963.

169. Tienari, P. Interaction between genetic vulnerability and family environment: the Finnish adoptive family study of schizophrenia. Acta Psychiat. Scand. *84*:460–465, 1991.

170. Torgersen, S. Genetic and nosological aspects of schizotypal and borderline personality disorders. Arch. Gen. Psychiat. *41*:546–554, 1984.

171. Torgersen, S. Relationship of schizotypal personality disorder to schizophrenia: genetics. Schizophr. Bull. *11*:554–563, 1985.

172. Torrey, E. F., Torrey, B. B., and Peterson, M. R. Seasonality of schizophrenic births in the United States. Arch. Gen. Psychiat. *34*:1065–1070, 1977.

173. Tsuang, M. T., Dempsey, G. M., Dvoredsky, A., and Struss, A. A. A family history study of schizo-affective disorder. Biol. Psychiat. *12*:331–338, 1977.

174. Vaillant, G. E. Prospective prediction of schizophrenic remission. Arch. Gen. Psychiat. *11*:509–518, 1964.

175. Vaillant, G. E. The prediction of recovery in schizophrenia. J. Nerv. Ment. Dis. *135*:534–543, 1962.

176. Vaughn, C. E., Snyder, K. S., Jones, S., Freeman, W. B., and Falloon, I. R. H. Family factors in schizophrenic relapse. Arch. Gen. Psychiat. *41*:1169–1177, 1984.

177. Vinogradov, S., Gottesman, I. I., Moises, H. W., and Nicol, S. Negative association between schizophrenia and rheumatoid arthritis. Schizophr. Bull. *17*:669–678, 1991.

178. Watson, C. G. Schizophrenia birth seasonality and the age-incidence artifact. Schizophr. Bull. *16*:5–10, 1990.

179. Watt, N. F. Patterns of childhood development in adult schizophrenics. Arch. Gen. Psychiat. *35*:160–165, 1978.

180. Weinberger, D. R., Kleinman, J. E., Luchins, D. J., Bigelow, L. B., and Wyatt, R. J. Cerebellar pathology in schizophrenia: a controlled postmortem study. Am. J. Psychiat. *137*:359–361, 1980.

181. Wender, P. H., Rosenthal, D., Kety, S. S., Schulsinger, F., and Welner, J. Social class and psychopathology in adoptees. Arch. Gen. Psychiat. *2*:318–325, 1973.

182. Wolkowitz, O. M., and Pickar, D. Benzodiazepines in the treatment of schizophrenia: a review and reappraisal. Am. J. Psychiat. *148*:714–726, 1991.

183. Wong, D. F., Wagner, Jr., H. N., Tune, L. E., Dannals, R. F., Pearlson, G. D., Links, J. M., Tamminga, C. A., Broussolle, E. P., Ravert, H. T., Wilson, A. A., Toung, J. K. T., Malat, J., Williams, J. A., O'Tuama, L. A., Snyder, S. H., Kuhar, M. J., and Gjedde, A. Positron emission tomography reveals elevated D2 dopamine receptors in drug naive schizophrenics. Science *234*:1558–1563, 1986.

184. Woodruff, P. W. R., Pearlson, G. D., Geer, M. J., Barta, P. E., and Chilcoat, H. D. A computerized magnetic resonance imaging study of corpus callosum morphology in schizophrenia. Psychol. Med. *23*:45–56, 1993.

185. Woodruff, R. A., Clayton, P. J., and Guze, S. B. Hysteria: studies of diagnosis, outcome, and prevalence. JAMA *215*:425–428, 1971.

186. Wrede, G., Mednick, S. A., Huttenen, M. O., and Nilsson, C. G. Pregnancy and delivery complications in the births of an unselected series of Finnish children with schizophrenic mothers. Acta Psychiat. Scand. *62*:369–381, 1980.

187. Wyatt, R. J., Potkin, S. G., and Murphy, D. L. Platelet monoamine oxidase activity in schizophrenia: a review of the data. Am. J. Psychiat. *136*:377–385, 1979.

188. Zelickson, A. Skin changes and chlorpromazine. JAMA *198*:341–344, 1966.

3

PANIC DISORDER
(ANXIETY NEUROSIS)

DEFINITION

Panic disorder is a chronic illness characterized by recurrent, acute anxiety attacks that have a definite onset and spontaneous termination. During attacks the patient is fearful and has symptoms associated with the autonomic nervous system: palpitations, tachycardia, rapid or shallow breathing, dizziness, and tremor. Between attacks, patients may be relatively asymptomatic though some experience fatigue, headache, and individual components of anxiety attacks in a persistent fashion. Panic disorder is not synonymous with anxiousness, which is a symptom rather than a syndrome. Anxiety symptoms and attacks can be part of the course of any psychiatric illness. When they occur in the absence of other significant psychiatric symptoms, the diagnosis of panic disorder is made.

Panic disorder has been known by many names (Table 3.1). Introduced by *DSM-III*, the term "panic disorder" replaced "anxiety neurosis" as the official name for the disorder. Panic disorder and anxiety neurosis will be used interchangeably in this chapter. "Anxiety neurosis" has a century-long history and is still used by many clinicians.

DSM-III-R introduced the idea that panic disorder should be

79

subdivided into two types: panic disorder with agoraphobia and panic disorder without agoraphobia. A third category, agoraphobia without panic attacks, is described in chapter 6. The criteria for panic disorder are provided in Table 3.2. Criteria for agoraphobia are given in Table 6. 3.

Anxiety is often distinguished from ordinary fear by its lack of an appropriate stimulus to explain the emotion. To highlight the apparently unmotivated nature of anxiety, the term "free-floating anxiety" is often used.

Sometimes, however, patients do experience anxiety attacks in response to a fear-provoking situation such as facing an angry employer or giving a public speech. In these cases the clinician must decide whether the anxiety is grossly out of proportion to the fear-provoking stimulus, as well as make a diagnosis based on the over-all history.

Most anxiety neurotics report that they experience some anxiety attacks without any fear-provoking stimulus, but on other occasions they overreact to situations that would produce some degree of apprehension in individuals without the disorder.

Some clinicians separate state anxiety from trait anxiety. The

Table 3.1   Terms used to describe Anxiety Neurosis (Panic Disorder)

Neurasthenia
Neurocirculatory asthenia
Nervous exhaustion
DaCosta's syndrome
Effort syndrome
Irritable heart
Soldier's heart
Somatization psychogenic cardiovascular reaction
Somatization psychogenic asthenic reaction
Anxiety reaction
Vasomotor neurosis
Personalities with mixed psychic and physical anomalies: constitutionally labile with tendency to functional disorders of specific organ systems

From Cohen and White (15)

Table 3.2 Criteria for Panic Disorder (DSM-IV)

A. Both (1) and (2):

   (1) Recurrent unexpected Panic Attacks [manifested by 4 or more of the following symptoms]:

      (a) Palpitations, pounding heart, or accelerated heart rate
      (b) Sweating
      (c) Trembling or shaking
      (d) Sensations of shortness of breath or smothering
      (e) Feeling of choking
      (f) Chest pain or discomfort
      (g) Nausea or abdominal distress
      (h) Feeling dizzy, unsteady, lightheaded, or faint
      (i) Derealization (feelings of unreality) or depersonalization (being detached from oneself)
      (j) Fear of losing control or going crazy
      (k) Fear of dying
      (l) Paresthesias (numbness or tingling sensations)
      (m) Chills or hot flushes

   (2) At least one of the attacks has been followed by 1 month (or more) of one (or more) of the following:

      (a) Persistent concern about having additional attacks
      (b) Worry about the implications of the attack or its consequences (e.g., losing control, having a heart attack, "going crazy")
      (c) A significant change in behavior related to the attacks

B. Agoraphobia may or may not be present. Agoraphobia also may exist in the absence of panic attacks (see chapter 6)

C. The Panic Attacks are not due to the direct physiological effects of a substance (e.g., a drug of abuse, a medication) or a general medical condition (e.g., hyperthyroidism)

D. The Panic Attacks are not better accounted for by another mental disorder, such as Social Phobia (e.g., occurring on exposure to feared social situations), Specific Phobia (e.g., on exposure to a specific phobic situation), Obsessive-Compulsive Disorder (e.g., on exposure to dirt in someone with an obsession about contamination), Posttraumatic Stress Disorder (e.g., in response to stimuli associated with a severe stressor), or Separation Anxiety Disorder (e.g., in response to being away from home or close relative) former refers to anxiety at any particular moment: "I feel anxious right now." The latter refers to a tendency to be anxious over a long period: "I generally feel anxious." The two forms of anxiety commonly occur together, with increased life stresses raising the anxiety of an already-anxiety-prone individual beyond the point of tolerance (59).

HISTORICAL BACKGROUND

> O lift me from the grass!
> I die! I faint! I fall!
> . . .
> My cheek is cold and white, alas!
> My heart beats loud and fast.
>
> PERCY BYSSHE SHELLEY,
> *The Indian Serenade*

It has been suggested that Shelley was having an anxiety attack when he wrote these lines. If so, he probably would have called it something else. A good possibility is "vapors," a favorite expression in the nineteenth century for anxiety reactions that also referred to fainting. Anxiety neurotics sometimes faint—probably from hyperventilating—and in the nineteenth century fainting among women was fashionable. In Victorian times the prototype of a refined young woman was a "swooner, pale and trembling, who responded to unpleasant or unusual social situations by taking to the floor in a graceful and delicious maneuver, in no way resembling the crash of the epileptic" (22). A Jane Austen heroine found one social situation "too pathetic for the feelings of Sophie and myself. We fainted alternately on a sofa." Overtight corsets may have been responsible for some of the fainting. A nineteenth-century physician, Dr. John Brown, cured fainting by "cutting the stay laces, which ran before the knife and cracked like a bow string" (22).

One of the first medical terms for anxiety neurosis was "neurasthenia," defined by an American physician, G. M. Beard, in 1869 (5). The term was used rather broadly to include patients with hysteria and obsessional illness as well as hypochondriacs, anxiety neurotics, and swooners (10).

In 1871 DaCosta reported a syndrome among Civil War military personnel that he called "irritable heart." His concept was probably more restricted than Beard's and closer to our definition of anxiety neurosis (21). DaCosta noted that for more than a century previously there had been similar reports of cases from British and German military medical sources.

The term "anxiety neurosis" was first used by Freud in 1895 to refer to patients who probably would have been called neurasthenic by other physicians at that time.

In 1950 Wheeler et al. published a twenty-year follow-up study of 173 patients with anxiety neurosis diagnosed by specific checklist criteria (89). Later Cohen et al. reported a family study based on a similar group of anxiety neurotics (14). These studies are the basis of the clinical concept of the disorder discussed in this chapter.

In the hundred years since Beard's paper on neurasthenia was published, there have been many theories regarding the cause of the disorder, ranging from constitutional weakness of the nervous system, through social and psychological factors, to more recent biochemical hypotheses. Although the cause of anxiety neurosis remains unknown, some studies have indicated that there are physiologic differences between anxiety neurotics and normal individuals (15, 42, 46, 47). Anxiety neurotics, for instance, are more responsive to painful stimuli of various types. They also have low exercise tolerance and high blood levels of lactic acid following exercise. The latter observation has led to a theory that abnormal lactate levels may be responsible for producing anxiety symptoms.

In fact, lactate can precipitate panic attacks in predisposed individuals. Liebowitz et al. (50, 52) reviewed six studies and found that panic attacks followed lactate infusion in 70 to 100 percent of patients with panic disorder. They then found that lactate-induced panic attacks could be prevented by the antidepressant imipramine, which blocks spontaneous panic attacks (53). Pitts and McClure (69) suggested that panic was induced by direct chemical action of the lactate, but alternative explanations have been proposed (53), including the possibility that lactate functions as a conditioned stimulus producing a phobic response (50, 52). Panic disorder patients, when asleep, have greater cardiac and respiratory reactivity than healthy subjects (80).

Several studies (27, 29, 67, 85, 92) have shown that panic symptoms can also be produced in panic-disorder patients by giving them carbon dioxide by inhalation. Propranolol, a drug used to relieve anxiety, reduces the symptoms produced by carbon dioxide, as does the benzodiazepine alprozolam (Xanax) (76).

EPIDEMIOLOGY

Anxiety neurosis is one of the most common psychiatric syndromes. A Boston study indicated that approximately 5 percent of the adult population is affected (15). Many patients, however, experience the syndrome in a mild form and probably never seek medical care for their symptoms (91). Many others consult family practitioners or internists rather than psychiatrists. Anxiety neurotics who see psychiatrists may represent a small group with a high prevalence of affective disorder (91).

For these reasons, prevalence estimates of anxiety neurosis vary widely. The Framingham investigators (39) reported a rate of 11 percent in a sample of 960 persons. Weissman et al. (86), studying 1,095 households in New Haven, Connecticut, found panic disorder in only 1.5 percent of the subjects. A national survey of psychotropic drug use reported a similar prevalence rate (84).

Compounding the problem of estimating prevalence is the recent tendency to consider agoraphobia a form of panic disorder. Many agoraphobics have panic attacks, but until recently it was believed that panic disorder is considerably more common than agoraphobia. There is now some question about this. In the National Institute of Mental Health (NIMH) Environmental Catchment Area study, data were obtained from three sites totaling

9,453 persons (73). The rates for panic disorder were almost identical in the three cities (New Haven, Baltimore, and St. Louis). The overall prevalence rate was 1.4 percent. When combined with agoraphobia, the prevalence ranged from 3.7 to 9.7 percent, with a combined prevalence of 6.1 percent. A more recent national survey found that panic disorder and agoraphobia were associated in about 50% of cases (24). Conceivably, the earlier studies failed to ask whether agoraphobic symptoms were present or absent.

Women have panic disorder at least twice as often as men. In the Framingham study (39), 16 percent of women were affected compared to about 5 percent of men. In most family studies, women have outnumbered men about two to one (14, 19, 65, 71).

Some studies indicate that anxiety neurotics do not differ from the general population in educational level or socioeconomic status (85), and others associate the condition with a lower educational achievement (24). There is no evidence that any specific type of childhood experience such as bereavement or birth order predisposes to the disorder (15, 90).

CLINICAL PICTURE

Anxiety attacks are the hallmark of panic disorder. The attacks usually begin suddenly, sometimes in a public place, sometimes at home, perhaps awakening the patient from sleep. There is a sense of foreboding, fear, and apprehension; a sense that one had suddenly become seriously ill; a feeling that one's life may be threatened by such illness. Among some patients there is a disturbing sense that one's body has changed or become distorted (depersonalization). Such a feeling of alien change may extend to the surrounding world (derealization).

Symptoms of labored breathing, smothering, palpitation, blurred vision, tremulousness, and weakness usually accompany the apprehension and foreboding. If a patient is examined during such an attack, signs of distress will be present: tachycardia, sweating, tachypnea, tremor, hyperactive deep tendon reflexes, and dilated pupils. An electrocardiogram taken during such an episode usually reveals sinus tachycardia. There may be localized or diffuse areas of tenderness over the anterior chest wall, possibly related to fatigue of the muscles from exaggerated thoracic breathing and involvement of costal cartilages and costovertebral joints (4).

Anxiety attacks vary in frequency among patients. Some experience them on a daily basis; others have them only once or twice a year. Other symptoms may occur between attacks. Table 3.3 lists these symptoms and their frequency as reported in one study. Again, the symptoms can occur in practically any pattern.

Cardiorespiratory symptoms are the most frequent chief complaints that anxiety neurotics report to physicians: "I have heart spells," "I think I'll smother," or "There is no way for me to get enough air." The chief complaint is occasionally psychological, but more often it indicates that the patient considers his or her disorder medical, and frequently fears that the disturbance may be very serious.

A fifty-one-year-old electrical engineer was brought to an emergency room by ambulance complaining of severe left anterior chest pain. His breathing was labored and he complained of numbness and tingling in his lips and fingers. His pulse was 110. He was perspiring heavily and obviously frightened.

The electrocardiogram was normal. Blood enzymes were within normal limits. Nevertheless, the patient was admitted to the intensive care unit. He was observed for twenty-four hours and then discharged asymptomatic.

The history revealed that the patient had first experienced severe chest pain at the age of twenty-one while watching a movie. He had many subsequent episodes of chest pain accompanied by dyspnea and anxiety and had been taken to an emergency room on at least ten previous occasions. Although the examinations were always normal, he had undergone a variety of cardiovascular procedures, including cardiac catheterization. He had never been seen by a psychiatrist and at no time was told that he very likely suffered from a common disorder called anxiety neurosis.

Table 3.3   Symptoms of Anxiety Neurosis

Symptoms	60 Patients (%)	102 Controls* (%)
Palpitation	97	9
Tires easily	93	19
Breathlessness	90	13
Nervousness	88	27
Chest pain	85	10
Sighing	79	16
Dizziness	78	16
Faintness	70	12
Apprehensiveness	61	3
Headache	58	26
Paresthesias	58	7
Weakness	56	3
Trembling	54	17
Breathing unsatisfactory	53	4
Insomnia	53	4
Unhappiness	50	2
Shakiness	47	16
Fatigued all the time	45	6
Sweating	42	33
Fear of death	42	2
Smothering	40	3
Syncope	37	11
Nervous chill	24	0
Urinary frequency	18	2
Vomiting and diarrhea	14	0
Anorexia	12	3
Paralysis	0	0
Blindness	0	0

*Healthy controls consisted of 50 men and 11 women from a large industrial plant and 41 healthy postpartum women from the Boston Lying-In Hospital

From Cohen and White (15)

Symptoms may become associated with specific situations that patients will try to avoid. For example, they may choose aisle seats in theaters, preferably close to exits, so that if an attack occurs, they will not be confined. Or, patients may avoid social situations in which an attack would be both frightening and embarrassing.

Phobias are common in patients with anxiety neurosis. Some clinicians, in fact, do not distinguish between anxiety neurosis and phobic disorders. For our purposes, anxiety neurosis is diagnosed when anxiety symptoms predominate; phobic disorder is the diagnosis when phobias predominate.

NATURAL HISTORY

Panic disorder begins early in life. Cohen and White (15) found the mean age of onset to be twenty-five. The disorder appears in most patients between the ages of eighteen and thirty-five. This is consistent with a later study (19) in which the mean age of onset was twenty-six years with a standard deviation of ten years. Some patients may remember the exact time and circumstances of the first attack. In a study by Winokur and Holemon, thirteen of thirty-one anxiety neurotics were able to describe such circumstances (90). These researchers found that four subjects remembered specifically that they had been awakened at night by their first anxiety attack. Some patients remember having their first attack at a time of stress (e.g., while making a speech in class). Thus the disorder may begin acutely with a discrete anxiety attack, but it also may begin insidiously with feelings of tenseness, nervousness, fatigue, or dizziness for years before the first anxiety attack.

Patients' initial medical contact is not always helpful. If they come to a physician complaining of cardiorespiratory symptoms, fearful of heart disease, a physician unacquainted with the natural history of anxiety neurosis may support these patients' fears by referring them to a specialist and warning that exercise should be limited.

Although patients commonly present with cardiorespiratory symptoms, they do not do so invariably. Some patients present with symptoms of "irritable colon" (55). In fact, among patients with irritable colon, anxiety neurosis is one of the most common psychiatric illnesses found. Such patients usually consult a gastro-enterologist. Among their most common presenting symptoms are abdominal cramping, diarrhea, constipation, nausea, belching, flatus, and occasionally dysphagia. ("Irritable colon" sometimes occurs in the course of other psychiatric illnesses such as hysteria or primary affective disorder. It also occurs in the absence of psychiatric illness. One study [38], in fact, suggests that food intolerance is often a major factor in the pathogenesis of the irritable bowel syndrome.)

In one long-term study of patients meeting the criteria for anxiety neurosis, gastrointestinal and musculoskeletal symptoms were as frequent as cardiovascular ones (62). For example, abdominal pain or discomfort was not far behind chest pain or discomfort and muscular aching or tension in occurrence. And during anxiety attacks, noncardiovascular symptoms such as headache or abdominal pain often became the primary focus of concern. A shift of symptoms over the follow-up period reflected the increasing chronicity of the illness. In this series, the more acute, dramatic, and disruptive manifestations tended to drop out over time. Anxiety attacks after five years were occurring in only half of the patients, and insomnia, nausea, vomiting, lightheadedness, and fainting were greatly reduced

Anxiety neurosis can occasionally be severe, but in the majority of cases the course is mild (89). Symptoms wax and wane in an irregular pattern that may or may not be associated with events and circumstances interpreted by the patient as stressful. Despite their symptoms, most anxiety neurotics live productively without social impairment. There is evidence that patients of lower social class have more severe symptoms and greater social impairment than patients with higher incomes and more education (64). One possible explanation is that lower-class people are less likely than more affluent people to encounter a physician who takes the time to provide reassurance by explaining the nature of the illness.

Seven long-term studies of patients with anxiety neurosis conducted in Boston, Oslo, Zurich, England, and Iowa show remarkably similar findings (59). On five- to twenty-year follow-up, about 50 to 60 percent of patients had recovered or were much improved. About one in five patients continued to have moderate to severe disability (Table 3.4).

Table 3.4   Disability from Anxiety Neurosis—twenty-year follow-up

Symptoms and Disability	60 Patients (%)	22 Men (%)	38 Women (%)
Well	12	13	11
Symptoms, no disability	35	46	29
Symptoms, mild disability	38	32	42
Symptoms, moderate or severe disability	15	9	18

From Wheeler et al. (89)

A follow-up of anxiety neurotics seen by a psychiatric consultation service revealed almost identical findings, suggesting that those relatively few patients who see a psychiatrist have a prognosis as favorable as the majority who do not (62). In this study, men of age thirty or more at the time of psychiatric consultation showed the poorest outcome. As the authors note, this may reflect a tendency for men to ignore lesser degrees of stress and seek medical care only when more severely impaired.

Most studies do not associate anxiety neurosis with reduced longevity. Two recent studies from the University of Iowa, however, tend to contradict this assumption (17, 18, 26). In both, men with panic disorder were twice as likely to die as expected, largely from cardiovascular disease and suicide (16, 26). Although the risk of suicide among patients with anxiety disorder is not known, several follow-up studies have found suicides occur in such patients (43, 75, 87, 89). The finding in Iowa of excess cardiovascular deaths among panic disorder patients has not been reported before.

COMPLICATIONS

Depression is the most common complication of anxiety neurosis. Woodruff and associates (91) found that 50 percent of anxiety neurotics seen in a psychiatric clinic gave a history of depression. Of 112 patients with anxiety neurosis examined in the medical clinics of a general hospital, 44 percent reported episodes of depression compared with 7 percent of surgical controls (13). The depressions seen in anxiety neurosis are relatively mild. In one study, two-thirds of the depressive episodes were of three-month duration or less (13). An equal number were associated with precipitating life events such as the loss of a family member through death or divorce, an association less commonly seen in primary affective disorder.

Because of the frequent occurrence of depression in anxiety neurosis, there has been speculation that anxiety neurosis is a variant of primary affective disorder. Both conditions are relieved by tricyclic antidepressant medication. Recent evidence indicates that there is an overlap of depression and anxiety neurosis in the relatives of depressed patients. Arguments against the illnesses being identical are: (a) anxiety neurosis has an earlier age of onset than primary affective disorder; (b) panic attacks can usually be precipitated in people with a history of spontaneous panic attacks by the intravenous infusion of sodium lactate, and this rarely happens in depressed controls (68); (c) failure of suppression in the dexamethasone suppression test occurs in about half of primary affective disorder patients but is rare in individuals with spontaneous panic attacks (6).

Drug abuse may occur as a complication of anxiety neurosis, the occasional result of overzealous medication by well-meaning physicians.

FAMILY STUDIES

Panic disorder is a strikingly familial condition (28). Crowe (20) found that two-thirds of cases had relatives affected with the same condition and that the risk in first-degree relatives was about three to four times the rate for the general population. Although some family studies suggest an overlap in the transmission of panic disorder and depression and a common diathesis hypothesis has been proposed, depression is more frequent in the family of depressives, as is panic disorder in the family of those with panic disorder.

Twin studies of anxiety disorders document a 30 to 40 percent concordance among monozygotic twins, contrasting with a 4 percent concordance among dyzygotic twins. This of course supports a genetic predisposition (80, 82, 83).

Harris et al. (33) examined the relationship between panic disorder and agoraphobia in the family members of patients with each diagnosis. The families of panic disorder patients had a morbidity risk of 20.5 percent for panic disorder but only 1.9 percent for agoraphobia. The families of agoraphobics, by contrast, had a morbidity rate of 7.7 percent for panic disorder and 8.6 percent for agoraphobia. The rate of the two diagnoses in controls was 4 percent for each condition. This study cast some doubt on the current tendency to view most cases of agoraphobia as a subtype of panic disorder because the latter ran true to type in families, overlapping very little with agoraphobia. There is, however, general agreement that many agoraphobics experience episodes of panic early in the course of their agoraphobic illness.

Several studies (14, 69) indicate an increased frequency of alcoholism among fathers of anxiety neurotics. However, it is not clear which came first: the anxiety attacks or the alcoholism. Alcoholics commonly experience anxiety attacks, particularly when hung over. Because anxiety neurosis and alcoholism both begin in adolescence or early adulthood, it is usually not possible to tell which developed first.

DIFFERENTIAL DIAGNOSIS

Anxiety symptoms and anxiety attacks can be part of any psychiatric illness. Anxiety symptoms often appear in primary affective disorder, obsessional illness, phobic disorder, hysteria, and alcoholism. In part, the diagnosis is based on chronology. Anxiety neurosis is diagnosed only if there are no other symptoms or if anxiety symptoms antedated the others.

Medical illnesses that produce symptoms resembling those of anxiety neurosis include cardiac arrhythmias (especially paroxysmal atrial tachycardia), angina pectoris, hyperthyroidism, pheochromocytoma, parathyroid disease, and mitral valve prolapse. Of these, mitral valve prolapse has received by far the greatest attention in recent years.

Mitral valve prolapse occurs in about 5 percent of the population (23, 58). Abnormal electrocardiograms (EKGs) are usually present, together with systolic clicks and late systolic murmurs, but there are usually no symptoms. Confirmation of the diagnosis is often made with the echocardiogram. Studies have shown that a high proportion of anxiety neurotics—32 to 50 percent—have mitral valve prolapse (34, 44). According to one study (40), it was also common in agoraphobia, an illness often accompanied by panic attacks.

The relationship between mitral valve prolapse and anxiety neurosis is not clear. In one study (28), the presence or absence of a prolapsed mitral valve had no influence on the induction of a panic attack by sodium lactate. In another study (44), anxiety symptoms in patients with prolapsed mitral valves responded as well to imipramine as did anxiety symptoms in patients with a normal valve.

Leaving aside this problem, the diagnosis of anxiety neurosis obviously requires the exclusion of medical conditions that give rise to similar symptoms. Clinicians who are not familiar with anxiety neurosis as a specific diagnostic entity may mistakenly attribute the symptoms to a physical condition. Studies show that a false-positive diagnosis is made in 25 percent of patients considered to have angina pectoris, some of whom almost certainly have anxiety neurosis (3). The percentage of false positives actually may be higher because of disagreement about interpreting EKGs. In one study, three cardiologists interviewed fifty-seven patients with chest pain. If any of them diagnosed angina, there was only a

55 percent chance that his two colleagues would agree with him (74). In another study of 110 EKGs read by at least one of four cardiologists as compatible with arteriosclerotic heart disease, two of the readers agreed in 60 percent of the cases, three out of the four agreed in 40 percent, and all four agreed in less than 20 percent (36). Nearly half of patients undergoing postmortem examinations who had received a diagnosis of angina pectoris show no coronary artery narrowing (49). False positives and false negatives are even found in double-blind evaluations of the two-step exercise EKG (25).

Clearly, it is important to exclude medical illness before diagnosing anxiety neurosis, but because of disagreement among clinicians, this may not be as simple as it seems.

In any case, there appears to be no characteristic EKG abnormality associated with anxiety neurosis. This conclusion came from a Framingham study of 203 cases of anxiety neurosis and 757 control subjects free of cardiovascular disease (39).

The mistake probably made most often in the evaluation of anxiety symptoms is that of overlooking primary affective disorder. Among other factors, a family history of affective disorder should alert one to the possibility that a patient with anxiety symptoms may have primary affective disorder. Also, anxiety that begins for the first time after the age of forty is commonly part of a depressive symdrome rather than a manifestation of anxiety neurosis.

Hysteria involves a broader range of medical complaints with frequent hospitalizations and operations. Anxiety neurotics are hospitalized and operated on no more frequently than other individuals. Furthermore, anxiety neurosis is *not* characterized by dramatic and medically unexplained complaints in nearly *every* area of the review of symptoms, as is the case in hysteria. Finally, sexual and menstrual complaints and conversion symptoms (unexplained neurological symptoms), common in hysteria, do not appear frequently among patients with anxiety neurosis.

Obsessional illness and phobic disorder can be mistaken for anxiety neurosis. Phobic disorder is so similar that the distinction depends on whether or not phobias dominate the clinical picture. Obsessive compulsive disorder involves obsessive ruminations and compulsive rituals. Although these may occur in mild form among patients with anxiety neurosis, they are not characteristically severe.

Anxiety neurosis also should be distinguished from the so-called "post-traumatic stress disorder." In one series (60), patients who had experienced a life-threatening accident subsequently experienced a long period of free-floating anxiety, muscular tension, irritability, impaired concentration, repetitive nightmares reproducing the accident, and social withdrawal. These symptoms persisted for six months to three years after the accident. None of the patients had cardiorespiratory or other autonomic symptoms, the hallmark of a typical anxiety neurosis. Also, in some cases referred by courts, the possibility of monetary compensation may have been a contributing factor. Supporting this possibility are a number of studies—starting with one by Heim in 1892 of survivors of falls in the Alps (35)—reporting that most individuals do not have frightening dreams or anxiety after their accidents. In any event, there is no evidence that life-threatening events precipitate anxiety neurosis as defined in this chapter (64).

DSM-IV describes a condition called "post-traumatic stress disorder, delayed type." This has the same clinical features as the above, but the symptoms do not appear until at least six months after the trauma. In 1980 the Veterans Administration announced that post-traumatic stress disorder, delayed type, was a compensable disorder. This meant that for the first time since World War I, the Department of Veterans Benefits could consider disorders to be service connected when the symptoms appeared long after military discharge.

Many veterans responded by filing claims based on their belief that they suffered from post-traumatic stress disorder, delayed type, related to traumatic war experiences. The symptoms of the disorder were well publicized in the media and in brochures distributed by national service organizations. Rarely before had so many claimants presented themselves to psychiatric examiners having read printed symptom checklists describing the diagnostic features of the disorder for which they sought compensation. Some psychiatrists were offended by the "mechanical litany of complaints recited by a well-read claimant" (2). The decision to award compensation was made even more difficult by the almost total lack of evidence that "post-traumatic stress disorder, delayed type" exists as a clinical entity.

Anxiety attacks are occasionally accompanied by hyperventilation, which produces symptoms that aggravate those of anxiety neurosis. Such symptoms are caused by lowering of pCO_2 as well as other chemical alterations, including an elevation of lactic acid. Five deep breaths produced by yawning or sighing may be enough to alter pCO_2 and produce the characteristic symptoms (12): cerebral hypoxia, a slowing of the electroencephalogram (EEG), and respiratory alkalosis, which in turn can induce tetany.

It appears that there is a group of patients who have hyperventilation syndrome (HVS) but do not meet the criteria for anxiety neurosis. In contrast to studies of anxiety neurosis, it is not known whether HVS represents a discrete syndrome or is symptomatic of other psychiatric or medical conditions. Apparently, some individuals are more susceptible than others to the effects of hyperventilation.

In one study at the Yale–New Haven Hospital, the diagnosis of HVS was made on the basis of the patient's response to overbreathing (12). Each patient suspected of having HVS was asked to overbreathe for up to three minutes or until he or she became dizzy. If the patient's reported symptoms were reproduced in their entirety and if no other explanation for the symptoms could be adduced from physical examination, medical history, or laboratory tests, the diagnosis of HVS was considered established. However, many patients had a history of conversion reactions, hypochondriasis, or "psychosomatic" illnesses; most were young women. Others had organic diseases such as adrenal insufficiency and peptic ulcer. Thus, psychiatric conditions such as Briquet's syndrome (hysteria) or medical illness actually may have been the primary disorder, with hyperventilation occurring secondarily, as it sometimes does in anxiety neurosis. In short, whether or not HVS exists as a separate syndrome is still uncertain.

Finally, the differential diagnosis of panic disorder is not complete without considering the Chinese restaurant syndrome, apparently caused by monosodium glutamate in Chinese food. This syndrome is characterized by palpitations, numbness, paresthesias, generalized weakness, and other symptoms that can mimic a panic disorder (80).

How far to pursue a physical explanation for symptoms that may represent an anxiety neurosis depends on clinical judgment, but a good deal of money is often invested in tests and consultations. In one study (62), anxiety neurotics received an average of five laboratory tests and two consultations with specialists. As the authors explained, "This is not unusual, since most patients did not consider their illness as psychiatric but saw themselves as persons suffering from undiagnosed physical conditions. This almost inevitably led to a search for an organic basis for the complaints. Sometimes the search was conducted against the physicians' better judgment in order that the patient might accept psychiatric referral. Even at that, the patients as a group were demanding and not easily satisfied. One patient's remark typified the atttitude of many, 'I do not want to be told what I haven't got. I want the doctor to find something.' Another patient stated, 'I know I am nervous, I have always been nervous, but don't try to tell me that is what is wrong.'"

CLINICAL MANAGEMENT

Psychiatric referral is rarely necessary for anxiety neurosis if the patient's physician has diagnosed the disorder correctly, understands its natural history, and is willing to discuss the syndrome with the patient. Telling the patient that there is nothing wrong physically is usually not enough. Some patients resent the implication that their symptoms might be psychological. Others continue to believe that they have a serious illness. The physician should agree that something is wrong and should describe the syndrome in lay terms. Many patients are relieved by such an explanation and thereby become receptive to further reassurance.

As noted earlier, some patients with irritable bowel syndrome or musculoskeletal complaints meet the criteria for anxiety neurosis. In these cases, treatment should focus primarily on the basic disorder—the anxiety neurosis—so that the presenting gastrointestinal or musculoskeletal complaints are viewed in this context and treated as conservatively as possible.

Supportive psychotherapy is almost always indicated, yet there is no evidence that psychological management more extensive than reassurance has any better effect than reassurance alone (90). Prolonged and expensive forms of psychotherapy are rarely indicated.

In the 1960s, Klein and colleagues in New York (44) and Marks and colleagues in England (59) found that antidepressants prevented panic attacks (66). The New York group focused on imipramine and the British group on monoamine oxidase inhibitors (MAOIs). Both types of drugs apparently had similar efficacy in preventing panic attacks, although there was some disagreement about the relief persisting after the drugs were discontinued and about the role of supportive or behavioral therapy in augmenting the effects of the drugs. In any case, antidepressants have become standard treatment for preventing panic attacks.

Except for the atypical benzodiazepine alprazolam, none of the benzodiazepines seems to prevent panic attacks (77). However, benzodiazepines reduce anticipatory anxiety between attacks. Many patients are given both drugs: a tricyclic antidepressant, for example, at night, and benzodiazepines during the day on an as-needed basis. Of the tricyclics, imipramine has been the most widely studied, but recent reports indicate that desipramine (56) and the "new generation" antidepressants (e.g., Prozac) are also effective (61). In other studies, alprazolam, the atypical benzodiazepine, has been proven to be effective not only as an anxiolytic drug but also as an agent that prevents panic attacks (when administered in rather large amounts) (11, 78, 79). Finally, cognitive therapy has been tried with panic disorder patients and seems to help (7).

There has been much speculation about the action of these drugs in reducing anxiety and preventing panic attacks. One of the most promising leads is evidence that imipramine prevents panic attacks by decreasing norepinephrine turnover in the brain, whereas alprazolam affects both benzodiazepine receptors and noradrenergic systems (8, 9, 37). Much attention has been focused on the locus ceruleus, a nucleus that serves as a relay center for the putative alarm-fear-anxiety system. Drugs that increase the firing rate of locus ceruleus neurons increase anxiety levels, whereas drugs that block the firing of these neurons apparently have opposite effects. The septohippocampal system has also been associated with anxiety (30), although this remains conjectural. However, evidence that panic disorder involves changes in brain activity has come from studies using positron emission tomography (PET) (71, 72). Patients with panic disorder who are vulnerable to lactate-induced anxiety attacks have strikingly abnormal hemispheric asymmetries of parahippocampal blood flow, blood volume, and oxygen metabolism.

The beta-adrenergic blocking agent propranolol, a drug used for cardiac arrhythmias, also may be effective in the treatment of anxiety neurosis (30, 88). Propranolol has potentially serious side effects but not usually in the low doses effective in reducing anxiety symptoms (81). The only significant one reported has been increased wheezing in asthmatic patients. Although the efficacy of propranolol in treating anxiety neurosis has not definitely been established, there is little question that it blocks some of the physiologic symptoms.

REFERENCES

1. Agras, W. S. The diagnosis and treatment of panic disorder. Annu. Rev. Med. *44*:39–51, 1993.
2. Atkinson, R. M., Henderson, R. G., Sparr, L. F., and Deale, S. Assessment of

Viet Nam veterans for posttraumatic stress disorder in Veterans Administration disability claims. Am. J. Psychiat. *139*:1118–1121, 1982.

3. Banks, T., and Shugoll, G. Confirmatory physical findings in angina pectoris. JAMA *200*:107–112, 1967.

4. Bass, C., Wade, C., Gardner, W. N., Cawley, R., Ryan, K. C., Hutchison, D. C. S., and Jackson, G. Lancet, March 19, 1983.

5. Beard, G. M. Neurasthenia or nervous exhaustion. Boston Med. Surg. J. *3*:217, 1869.

6. Carroll, B. J. The dexamethasone suppression test for melancholia. Brit. J. Psychiat. *140*:292–304, 1982.

7. Chambless, D. L., and Gillis, M. M. Cognitive therapy of anxiety disorders. J. Consult. Clin. Psychol. *61*(2):248–260, 1993.

8. Charney, D. S., and Heninger, G. R. Noradrenergic function and the mechanism of action of antianxiety treatment: I. The effect of long-term alprazolam treatment. Arch. Gen. Psychiat. *42*:458–467, 1985.

9. Charney, D. S., and Heninger, G. R. Noradrenergic function and the mechanism of action of antianxiety treatment: II. The effect of long-term imipramine treatment. Arch. Gen. Psychiat. *42*:473–481, 1985.

10. Chatel, J. C., and Peele, R. A centennial review of neurasthenia. J. Psychiat. *126*:1404–1413, 1970.

11. Chouinard, G., Annable, L., Fontaine, R., and Solyom, L. Alprazolam in the treatment of generalized anxiety and panic disorders: a double-blind placebo-controlled study. Psychopharmacology 77:229–233, 1982.

12. Christensen, B. Studies on hyperventilation. II: Electrocardiographic changes in normal man during voluntary hyperventilation. J. Clin. Invest. *24*:880, 1946.

13. Clancy, J., Noyes, R., Hoenk, P. R., and Slymen, D. J. Secondary depression in anxiety neurosis. J. Nerv. Ment. Dis. *166*:846–850, 1978.

14. Cohen, M. E., Badal, D. W., Kilpatrick, A., Ried, E. W., and White, P. D. The high familial prevalence of neurocirculatory asthenia (anxiety neurosis, effort syndrome). Am. J. Human Genet. *3*:126, 1951.

15. Cohen, M., and White, P. Life situations, emotions, and neurocirculatory asthenia (anxiety neurosis, neurasthenia, effort syndrome). Ass. Res. Nerv. Dis. Proc. *29*:832–869, 1950.

16. Coryell, W. Panic disorder and mortality. Psychiat. Clin. North Am. *11*(2):433–440, 1988.

17. Coryell, W., Noyes, R., and Clancy, J. Excess mortality in panic disorder: a comparison with primary unipolar depression. Arch. Gen. Psychiat. *39*:701–703, 1982.

18. Coryell, W., Noyes, R., and House, J. D. Am. J. Psychiat. *143*:508–510, 1986.

19. Crowe, R. R., Noyes, R., Pauls, D. L., and Slymen, D. A family study of panic disorder. Arch. Gen. Psychiat. *40*:1065–1069, 1983.

20. Crowe, R. R. The genetics of panic disorder and agoraphobia. Psychiat. Dev. 2:171–185, 1985.

21. DaCosta, J. M. On irritable heart, a clinical form of functional cardiac disorder and its consequences. Am. J. Med. Sci. *61*:17, 1871.

22. Dalessio, D. J. Hyperventilation: the vapors, effort syndrome, neurasthenia. JAMA *239*:1401–1402, 1978.

23. Devereux, R. B., Perloff, J. K., Reichek, N., and Josephson, M. E. Mitral valve prolapse. Circulation *54*, 1976.

24. Eaton, W. W., Kessler, R. C., Wittchen, H. U., and Magee, W. J. Panic and panic disorder in the United States. Am. J. Psychiat. *151*:413–420, 1994.

25. Friedberg, C. K. The two step exercise electrocardiogram: a double blind evaluation of its use in the diagnosis of angina pectoris. Circulation *26*:1254–1260, 1962.

26. Friedman, S., Jones, J. C., Chernen, L., and Barlow, D. H. Suicidal ideation and suicide attempts among patients with panic disorder: a survey of two outpatient clinics. Am. J. Psychiat. *149*:680–685, 1992.

27. Fryer, M. R., Uy, J., Martinez, B. S., Goetz, R., Klein, D. F., Fryer, A., Liebowitz, M. R., and Gorman, J. CO_2 challenge of patients with panic disorder. Am. J. Psychiat. *144*:1080–1082, 1987.

28. Goldstein, R. B., Weissman, M. M., Adams, P. B., Horwath, E., Lish, J. D., Charney, D., Woods, S. W., Sobin, C., and Wickramaratne, P. J. Psychiatric disorders in relatives of probands with panic disorder and/or major depression. Arch. Gen. Psychiat. *51*:383–394, 1994.

29. Gorman, J. M., Fyer, A. F., Gliklich, J., King, D., and Klein, D. F. Effect of sodium lactate on patients with panic disorder and mitral valve prolapse. Am. J. Psychiat. *138*:247–249, 1981.

30. Gorman, J. M., Askanazi, J., Liebowwitz, M. R., Fryer, A. J., Stein, J., Kinney, J. M., and Klein, D. F. Response to hyperventilation in a group of patients with panic disorder. Am. J. Psychiat. *141*:857–861, 1984.

31. Granville-Grossman, K. L., and Turner, P. The effect of propranolol on anxiety. Lancet *1*:788–790, 1966.

32. Gray, J. A. *The Neuropsychology of Anxiety.* Oxford: Oxford Univ. Press, 1982.

33. Grosz, H. J., and Farmer, B. B. Pitts and McClure's lactate-anxiety study revisited. Brit. J. Psychiat. *120*:415–418, 1972.

34. Harris, E. L., Noyes, R., Crowe, R. R., and Chaudhry, D. R. A family study of agoraphobia: report of a pilot study. Arch. Gen. Psychiat. *40*:1061–1064, 1983.

35. Hartman, N., Kramer, R., Brown, W. T., and Devereux, R. B. Panic disorder in patients with mitral valve prolapse. Am. J. Psychiat. *139*:669–670, 1982.

36. Heim, A. Remarks on Fatal Falls. Yearbook of the Swiss Alpine Club 27:327–337, 1892. Trans. R. Noyes R. Kletti Omega *3*:45–52, 1972.

37. Higgins, I. T. Ischemic heart disease: the problem. Milbank Mem. Fund. Q. *43*:23–31, 1965.

38. Iversen, S. *Benzodiazepine Divided*, pp. 176–185. New York: John Wiley & Sons, 1983.

39. Jones, V. A., Shorthouse, M., McLaughlan, P., Workman, E., and Hunter, J. O. Food intolerance: a major factor in the pathogenesis of irritable bowel syndrome. Lancet 1982.

40. Kannel, W. B., Dawber, T. R., and Cohen, M. E. The electrocardiogram in neurocirculatory asthenia (anxiety neurosis or neurasthenia): a study of 203

neurocirculatory asthenia patients and 757 healthy controls in the Framingham study. Ann. Intern. Med. *49*:1351–1360, 1958.

41. Kantor, J. S., Zitrin, C. M., and Zeldis, S. M. Mitral valve prolapse syndrome in agoraphobic patients. Am. J. Psychiat. *137*:467–469, 1980.

42. Kelly, D., Mittchell-Heggs, N., and Sherman, D. Anxiety and the effects of sodium lactate assessed clinically and physiologically. Brit. J. Psychiat. *119*:129–141, 1971.

43. Kelly, D., and Walter, C. J. S. A clinical and physiological relationship between anxiety and depression. Brit. J. Psychiat. *115*:401–406, 1969.

44. Kerr, T. A., Schapira, K., and Roth, M. The relationship between premature death and affective disorders. Brit. J. Psychiat. *115*:1277–1282, 1969.

45. Klein, D. F. Importance of psychiatric diagnosis in prediction of clinical drug effects. Arch. Gen. Psychiat. *37*:63–72, 1980.

46. Koenigsberg, H. W., Pollak, C. P., Fine, J., Kakuma, T. Cardiac and respiratory activity in panic disorder: Effects of sleep and sleep lactate infusions. Am. J. Psychiat. *151(8)*:1148–1152, 1994.

47. Levander-Lindgren, M. Studies in neurocirculatory asthenia (DaCosta's syndrome). Acta Med. Scand. *172*:665–683, 1962.

48. Levander-Lindgren, M. Studies in neurocirculatory asthenia (DaCosta's syndrome). Acta Med. Scand. *173*:631–637, 1963.

49. Liberthson, R., Sheehan, D. V., King, M. E., and Weyman, A. E. The prevalence of mitral valve prolapse in patients with panic disorders. Am. J. Psychiat. *142*:511–515, 1986.

50. Liebow, I. M., and Oseasohn, R. Relationship between selected clinical and electrocardiographic findings and post mortem lesions associated with ischemic heart disease. J. Chronic Dis. *17*:609–617, 1964.

51. Liebowitz, M. R., Fryer, A. J., Gorman, J. M., Dillon, D., Appleby, I. L., Levy, G., Anderson, S., Levitt, M., Palij, M., Davies, S. O., and Klein, D. F. Lactate provocation of panic attacks. Arch. Gen. Psychiat. *41*:764–770, 1984.

52. Liebowitz, M. R., Fryer, A. J., Gorman, J. M., Dillon, D., Davies, S., Stein, J. M., Cohen, B. S., and Klein, D. F. Specificity of lactate infusions in social phobia versus panic disorders. Am. J. Psychiat. *142*:947–950, 1985.

53. Liebowitz, M. R., Gorman, J. M., Fryer, A. J., Levitt, M., Dillon, D., Levy, G., Appleby, I. L., Anderson, S., Palij, M., Davies, S. O., and Klein, D. F. Lactate provocation of panic attacks. II. Biochemical and physiological findings. Arch. Gen. Psychiat. *42*:709–719, 1985.

54. Liebowitz, M. R., Gorman, J. M., Fyer, A., Dillon, D., Levitt, M., and Klein, D. F. Possible mechanisms for lactate's induction of panic. Am. J. Psychiat. *143(4)*:495–502, 1986.

55. Liebowitz, M. R., Gorman, J. M., Fyer, A. J., Levitt, M., Dillon, D., Levy, G., Appleby, I. L., Anderson, S., Palij, M., Davies, S. O., and Klein, D. F. Lactate provocation of panic attacks. Arch. Gen. Psychiat. *42*:709–719, 1985.

56. Liss, J., Alpers, D., and Woodruff, R. A. The "irritable colon" syndrome and psychiatric illness. Dis. Nerv. Syst. *34*:151–157, 1973.

57. Lydiard, R. B. Preliminary results of an open, fixed-dose study of desipramine in panic disorder. Psychopharmacol. Bull. *23*:139–140, 1987.
58. Margraf, J., Eilers, A., and Roth, W. T. Sodium lactate infusions and panic attacks: a review and critique. Psychosom. Med. *48*:23–51, 1986.
59. Markiewicz, W., Stoner, J., London, E., Hunt, S. A., and Popp, R. L. Mitral valve prolapse in one hundred presumably healthy young females. Circulation *53*:464, 1976.
60. Marks, I., and Lader, M. Anxiety states (anxiety neurosis): a review. J. Nerv. Ment. Dis. *156*:3–18, 1973.
61. Modlin, H. C. Postaccident anxiety syndrome: psychosocial aspects. Am. J. Psychiat. *123*:1008–1012, 1967.
62. Mavissakalian, M., Perel, J., Bowler, K., and Dealy, R. Trazodone in the treatment of panic disorder and agoraphobia with panic attacks. Am. J. Psychiat. *144*:785–787, 1987.
63. Noyes, R., and Clancy, J. Anxiety neurosis: a 5-year follow-up. J. Nerv. Ment. Dis. *162*:200–205, 1976.
64. Noyes, R., and Kletti, R. Depersonalization in the face of life-threatening danger: a description. Psychiatry *39*:19–27, 1976.
65. Noyes, R., Clancy, J., Crowe, R., Hoenk, P. R., and Slymen, D. J. The familial prevalence of anxiety neurosis. Arch. Gen. Psychiat. *35*:1057–1059, 1978.
66. Noyes, R., Clarkson, C., Crowe, R. R., Yates, W. R., and McChesney, C. M. A family study of generalized anxiety disorder. Am. J. Psychiat. *144*:1019–1024, 1987.
67. Noyes, R., Perry, P. Maintenance treatment with antidepressants in panic disorder. J. Clin. Psychiat. *51(A)*:24–30, 1990.
68. Papp, L. A., Klein, D. F., Gorman, J. M. Carbon dioxide hypersensitivity, hyperventilation, and panic disorder. Am. J. Psychiat. *150*:1149–1157, 1993.
69. Pitts, F. N., and McClure, J. N. Lactate metabolism in anxiety neurosis. N. Eng. J. Med. *277*:1329–1336, 1967.
70. Pitts, F. N., Meyer, J., Brooks, M., and Winokur, G. Adult psychiatric illness assessed for childhood parental loss, and psychiatric illness in family members: a study of 748 patients and 250 controls. Am. J. Psychiat. *121*(Suppl.)i–x, 1965.
71. Reich, J. The epidemiology of anxiety. J. Nerv. Ment. Dis. *174*:129–136, 1986.
72. Reiman, E. M., Raichle, M. E., Butler, F. K., Herscovitch, P., and Robins, E. A focal brain abnormality in panic disorder, a severe form of anxiety. Nature *310*:683–685, 1984.
73. Reiman, E. M. The study of panic disorder using positron emission tomography. Psychiat. Dev. *1*:63–78, 1987.
74. Robins, L. N., Helzer, G. E., and Weissman, M. M. Lifetime prevalence of specific psychiatric disorders in three sites. Arch. Gen. Psychiat. *41*:949–958, 1984.
75. Rose, G. A. Ischemic heart disease: chest pain questionnaire. Milbank Mem. Fund. Q. *43*:32–39, 1965.
76. Rosenberg, C. M. Complications of obsessional neurosis. Brit. J. Psychiat. *114*:477–478, 1968.

77. Sanderson, W. C., Wetzler, S., Asnis, G. M. Alprazolam blockade of CO_2-provoked panic in patients with panic disorder. Am. J. Psychiat. *151*:1220–1222, 1994.
78. Shader, R. I., Greenblatt, D. J. Use of benzodiazepines in anxiety disorders. N. Engl. J. Med. *328(19)*:1398–1405, 1993.
79. Sheehan, D. V., Claycomb, J. B., and Surman, O. S. The relative efficacy of alprazolam, phenelzine and imipramine in treating panic attacks and phobias. Paper presented at the 137th Annual Meeting of the American Psychiatric Association, Los Angeles, 1984.
80. Sheehan, D. V., Coleman, J. H., and Greenblatt, D. J. Some biochemical correlates of panic attacks with agoraphobia and their response to a new treatment. J. Clin. Psychopharmacol. *4*:66–75, 1984.
81. Slater, B., and Shields, J. Genetical aspects of anxiety. Brit. J. Psychiat. Special Publication no. 3: Studies of Anxiety, 62–71. Ashford, Kent: Headley Bros., 1969.
82. Tanna, V. T., Penningrowth, R. P., and Woolson, R. F. Propranolol in anxiety neurosis. Compr. Psychiat. *18*:319–326, 1977.
83. Torgersen, S. Genetics of neurosis: the effects of sampling variation upon the twin concordance ratio. Brit. J. Psychiat. *142*:126–132, 1983.
84. Torgersen, S. Genetic factors in anxiety disorders. Arch. Gen. Psychiat. *40*:1085–1089, 1983.
85. Uhlenhuth, E. H., Balter, M. B., Mellinger, G. D., Cisin, I. H., and Clinthorne, J. Symptom check list syndromes in the general population: correlations with psychotherapeutic drug use. Arch. Gen. Psychiat. *40*:1167–1173, 1983.
86. Van Den Hout, M. A., and Griez, E. Panic symptoms after inhalation of carbon dioxide. Brit. J. Psychiat. *144*:503–507, 1984.
87. Weissman, M. M., Meyers, J. K., and Harding, P. S. Psychiatric disorders in a U.S. urban community: 1975–76. Am. J. Psychiat. *135*:459–462, 1978.
88. Weissman, M. M., Klerman, G. L., Markowitz, J. S., Ouellette, R. Suicidal ideation and suicide attempts in panic disorder and attacks. N. Engl. J. Med. *321(18)*:1209–1214, 1989.
89. Wheatley, D. Comparative effects of propranolol and chlordiazepoxide in anxiety states. Brit. J. Psychiat. *115*:1411–1412, 1969.
90. Wheeler, E. O., White, P. D., Ried, E. W., and Cohen, M. E. Neurocirculatory asthenia (anxiety neurosis, effort syndrome, neuroasthenia). JAMA *142*:878–889, 1950.
91. Winokur, G., and Holemon, E. Chronic anxiety neurosis: clinical and sexual aspects. Acta Psychiat. Scand. *39*:384–412, 1963.
92. Woodruff, R. A., Jr., Guze, S. B., and Clayton, P. J. Anxiety neurosis among psychiatric outpatients. Compr. Psychiat. *13*:165–170, 1972.
93. Woods, S. W., Charney, D. S., Loke, J., Goodman, W. K., Redmond, D. E., and Heninger, G. R. Carbon dioxide sensitivity in panic anxiety. Arch. Gen. Psychiat. *43*:900–907, 1986.
94. Zautcke, J. L., Schwartz, J. A., and Mueller, E. J. Chinese restaurant syndrome: a review. Ann. Emergency Med. *15*:1210–1213, 1986.

4

SOMATIZATION DISORDER (HYSTERIA)

DEFINITION

The diagnosis of hysteria was applied to cases of unexplained physical complaints for many centuries. Building upon the earlier work of P. Briquet in France (7), Savill in England (53), and Purtell and colleagues in Boston (16, 47), investigators at Washington University in Saint Louis (1, 13–15, 23, 24, 26–32, 46) carried out a series of studies and proposed that this diagnosis be replaced by two labels: "Briquet's syndrome" (after the French psychiatrist who described a large series of such patients) and "conversion symptoms." This proposal was designed to eliminate the pejorative implications associated with the diagnosis of hysteria and to avoid the complications of inconsistent use of terminology.

Toward the same ends, *DSM-III* introduced the category of somatoform disorders in place of hysteria generally, with somatization disorder substituting for Briquet's syndrome. The place of conversion symptoms was not fully clarified.

The importance of distinguishing between Briquet's syndrome and conversion symptoms continued to be emphasized by the Washington University group. They argued that the former is typically a polysymptomatic disorder that begins early in life (usu-

105

ally in the teens, rarely after the twenties), chiefly affects women, and is characterized by recurrent, multiple somatic complaints often described dramatically. Characteristic features, all unexplained by other known clinical disorders, include varied pains, anxiety symptoms, gastrointestinal disturbances, urinary symptoms, menstrual difficulties, sexual and marital maladjustment, nervousness, mood disturbances, and "pseudoneurotical" symptoms (the last often used synonymously with the term "conversion symptoms"). Repeated visits to physicians and clinics, the use of a large number of medications—often at the same time—prescribed by different physicians, and frequent hospitalizations and operations result in a florid medical history (29, 30).

In keeping with this view, somatization disorder continues to be the term for Briquet's syndrome in *DSM-IV*. The specific diagnostic criteria are presented in Table 4.1.

It should be emphasized, however, that the diagnostic criteria for somatization disorder in *DSM-IV* are less stringent than those for Briquet's syndrome and were proposed to offer a shortcut to the diagnosis (70). As yet, we have few data about the validity of these criteria for somatization disorder from systematic, controlled follow-up and family studies. The findings thus far indicate that the two sets of criteria (for Briquet's syndrome and somatization disorder) select overlapping but somewhat different populations (15, 21).

The Saint Louis group proposed that the term "conversion symptom" be reserved for *unexlained symptoms suggesting neurological disease* such as amnesia, unconsciousness, paralysis, "spells," aphonia, urinary retention, difficulty in walking, anesthesia, and blindness—the so-called pseudoneurological or "grand hysterical" symptoms (41)."Unexplained" means only that the history, neurological examination, and diagnostic tests have failed to reveal a satisfactory explanation for the symptoms. Thus used, the term "conversion symptom" has no etiologic implication; it refers, in a descriptive way only, to a limited group of symptoms. In order to give the term greater specificity, unexplained pains and other unexplained medical symptoms that do

Table 4.1   Diagnostic criteria for 300.81 Somatization Disorder
(*DSM-IV*)

A. A history of many physical complaints beginning before age 30 years that occur over a period of several years and result in treatment being sought or significant impairment in social, occupational, or other important areas of functioning.

B. Each of the following criteria must have been met, with individual symptoms occurring at any time during the course of the disturbance:

(1) *Four pain symptoms:* a history of pain related to at least four different sites or functions (e.g., head, abdomen, back, joints, extremities, chest, rectum, during menstruation, during sexual intercourse, or during urination)

(2) *Two gastrointestinal symptoms:* a history of at least two gastrointestinal symptoms other than pain (e.g., nausea, bloating, vomiting other than during pregnancy, diarrhea, or intolerance of several different foods)

(3) *One sexual symptom:* a history of at least one sexual or reproductive symptom other than pain (e.g., sexual indifference, erectile or ejaculatory dysfunction, irregular menses, excessive menstrual bleeding, vomiting throughout pregnancy)

(4) *One Pseudoneurological symptom:* a history of at least one symptom or deficit suggesting a neurological condition not limited to pain (conversion symptoms such as impaired coordination or balance, paralysis or localized weakness, difficulty swallowing or lump in throat, aphonia, urinary retention, hallucinations, loss of touch or pain sensation, double vision, blindness, deafness, seizures; dissociative symptoms such as amnesia; or loss of consciousness other than fainting)

C. Either (1) or (2):

(1) After appropriate investigation, each of the symptoms in Criterion B cannot be fully explained by a known general medical condition or the direct effects of a substance (e.g., a drug of abuse, a medication)

(2) When there is a related general medical condition, the physical complaints or resulting social or occupational impairment are in excess of what would be expected from the history, physical examination, or laboratory findings

D. The symptoms are not intentionally produced or feigned (as in Factitious Disorder or Malingering)

not suggest neurological disease are not included in the definition. If other unexplained medical symptoms such as headaches, backaches, and abdominal pains were included, conversion symptom would mean any unexplained medical symptom and thus would lose any precision it has (29, 30).

Sometimes a related syndrome occurs as a sudden, short-lived epidemic (mass hysteria), characteristically in a school population and most frequently affecting female students (42, 57). Blackouts, dizziness, weakness, headaches, hyperventilation, nausea, and abdominal pain are the usual symptoms. Suggestion and fear are thought to be major factors in the pathogenesis of these episodes. Long-term follow-up of the affected children has not been reported, though the short-term prognosis appears to be very good.

To recapitulate: Conversion symptoms comprise a limited group of individual symptoms suggesting neurological disease. Somatization disorder or Briquet's syndrome refers to a polysymptomatic syndrome that typically includes conversion symptoms.

One criticism of the definition of Briquet's syndrome or somatization disorder is that everyone experiences many symptoms characteristic of the syndrome. It is true that most people have experienced headaches, fatigue, anorexia, nausea, diarrhea, vomiting, nervousness, and varied pains. But when responding to a physician, few report such symptoms. Most people interpet the physician's questions to mean significant symptoms; they report only symptoms that are recent, recurrent, or otherwise troublesome. Furthermore, the physician evaluates the patient's responses, ignoring symptoms that are not recent, recurrent, or disabling. He or she pays attention to symptoms that led the patient to consult a physician, take medicines, or alter usual routines. In addition, there are some symptoms that will be considered significant regardless of qualifying features, such as blindness and paralysis. These criteria—ones that physicians ordinarily use to evaluate symptoms—are the same as those applied in the studies of Briquet's syndrome or somatization disorder cited above. By these criteria, very few people report enough symptoms, otherwise unexplained medically, to warrant these diagnoses.

HISTORICAL BACKGROUND

The concept of hysteria, which probably originated in Egypt, is at least four thousand years old. The name "hysteria" has been in use since the time of Hippocrates. The original Egyptian approach to hysteria was perhaps the most fanciful. Believing that physical displacement of the uterus caused the varied symptoms, physicians treated the patient by trying to attract the "wandering uterus" back to its proper site. Sweet-smelling substances were placed in the region of the vagina to attract the errant organ; unpleasant materials were ingested or inhaled to drive it away from the upper body (62).

Although Egyptian and Greek physicians applied the diagnosis whenever they believed that unusual symptoms were caused by a displaced uterus, the available records do not provide explicit diagnostic criteria. This state of affairs persisted, and, although speculations about pathogenesis have changed through the centuries, few authors of any century, including our own, have provided specific diagnostic criteria of any kind (56).

Witchcraft, demonology, and sorcery were associated with hysteria in the Middle Ages (62). Mysterious symptoms, spells, and odd behavior were frequently considered manifestations of supernatural, evil influences. Hysterical patients were sometimes perceived as either the active evil spirit (witch, sorceress, or demon) or as the passive victim of such an evil being. Since the Middle Ages there have been speculations of many kinds about the cause of hysteria. Such speculations have included ideas about neurological weakness, neurological degeneration, the effects of various toxins, and disturbances of what Mesmer called "animal magnetism."

Hysteria became Freud's central concern during the early years of psychoanalysis (6). That interest had developed while Freud was working in Paris with Charcot, who was treating hysteria with hypnosis. The psychoanalytic concept of conversion as an ego defense mechanism, referring to unconscious conversion of "psychic energy" into physical symptoms, ultimately led to the identification of conversion symptoms with hysteria in psychoanalytic practice. Many psychoanalysts considered hysteria a simulation of illness designed to work out unconscious conflicts, partially through attention-getting and "secondary gain," a term that refers to possible advantages of illness such as sympathy and support, including financial support, from relatives and friends and being excused from various duties (71).

This view led easily to the attitude, widely held by physicians though seldom stated openly, that hysteria is a term of opprobrium to be applied whenever the patient's complaints are not explained or when the demands appear excessive. The most fully developed version of this view is the concept of the hysterical personality. Here, the emphasis is on immature, histrionic, manipulative, seductive, and attention-getting behavior regardless of the presenting complaint of present illness. In the absence of specific diagnostic criteria and systematic studies, however, use of the term has been inconsistent and confusing. Many clinicians believe that conversion symptoms, hysteria, and hysterical personality are different: all three may frequently be present in the same individual (35), but any combination is possible and patients may present any one without the other two (11, 12).

The syndromatic approach to the diagnosis of hysteria began in 1859 when the French physician Pierre Briquet published his monograph, *Traits clinique et thérapeutique à l'hystérie* (7, 39, 40). Similar descriptions of the syndrome were provided in 1909 by the English physician Savill (53) and in 1951 by the American psychiatrists Purtell, Cohen, and Robins (47). In recent decades a series of studies by Guze and colleagues has refined and clarified the concept of hysteria as a syndrome (27, 29, 30, 46, 68, 69), and in a systematic study of women diagnosed as "having a hysterical personality or as being hysterics," Blinder (3) confirmed the clinical description and familiar characteristics described below.

EPIDEMIOLOGY

A study in an urban community (65) indicated the prevalence of somatization disorder to be 0.4 percent. Assuming that nearly all of the cases occurred in women, and correcting for the sex distribution of the sample, the prevalence in urban women was just under 1 percent according to this report. In studies of hospitalized, postpartum women whose pregnancies and deliveries were without complication, the prevalence of the syndrome was between 1 and 2 percent (69).

A history of conversion symptoms, on the other hand, is commonly found when symtematic interviewing is done among hospitalized, normal, postpartum women (23), hospitalized medically ill women (68), and male and female psychiatric outpatients (32). On average, about one-quarter of such patients give a history of conversion symptoms.

All authors, except those describing psychiatric problems encountered in the military, report that the great majority of patients with the diagnosis of hysteria (using a variety of diagnostic criteria) were women (20, 33, 36, 49, 60). Nearly all men with symptoms resembling hysteria in women have had histories of associated compensation factors such as litigation following injuries, consideration for veterans' and other pensions, disability payments, or serious legal difficulties (52).

There is a generally held view that hysteria and conversion symptoms are more common among less sopphisticated, more primitive people. One group of investigators found that higher education (one or more years of college) was significantly less common in patients with conversion symptoms—with or without Briquet's syndrome—than in patients without conversion symptoms. This was also true for patients with Briquet's syndrome compared to other psychiatric patients as a group (32). Several investigators have reported that "hysterical neurosis, conversion type" is much more frequent in nonwhites than in whites and is highest in the lowest socioeconomic classes (60, 61).

Of interest is the work of J. C. Carothers, a British psychiatrist whose anthropological studies led to a theory that "psychopathy and hysteria" may be manifestations of the persistence in modern society of preliterate "magical" modes of thinking. On the basis of this theory, Carothers concluded that sociopathy should predominate in men, hysteria in women (see below) (10).

Indeed, although a history of conversion symptoms may be elicited from patients with any psychiatric disorder, two conditions are most often associated with such a history: Briquet's syndrome and sociopathy. A report indicates that women with Briquet's syndrome are significantly more likely to show an earlier birth order than are women with other psychiatric disorders (43).

In summary, a history of conversion symptoms can be found among psychiatric patients of either sex suffering from any psychiatric disorder. However, such a history is most likely to be associated with somatization disorder in women or sociopathy in men. Somatization disorder is much less common than conversion symptoms; it is seen less infrequently among men; and, like conversion symptoms, it is frequently associated with higher education.

CLINICAL PICTURE

When first seen by a psychiatrist, the typical patient with somatization disorder is a married woman in her thirties. Her history is often delivered in a dramatic, complicated fashion. She usually presents with multiple vague complaints to her general physician, and a straightforward history of the present illness is difficult if not impossible to elicit. Frequently, the physician has trouble deciding when the present illness began or even why the patient came. Table 4.2 presents the most common symptoms reported by patients with somatization disorder. Not only do they report large numbers of these and other symptoms, but the symptoms are distributed widely throughout all or nearly all organ systems. It is this range of symptoms in addition to their number that defines the condition.

The dramatic, colorful, exaggerated description of symptoms is best conveyed by quoting patients, though it should be noted that not all patients show this trait to the same degree. The following quotations are from Purtell et al. (47):

Table 4.2 The frequency of symptoms in Hysteria

Symptom	%	Symptom	%	Symptom	%
Dyspnea	72	Weight loss	28	Joint pain	84
Palpitation	60	Sudden fluctuations in weight	16	Extremity pain	84
Chest pain	72	Anorexia	60	Burning pains in rectum, vagina, mouth	28
Dizziness	84	Nausea	80	Other bodily pain	36
Headache	80	Vomiting	32	Depressed feelings	64
Anxiety attacks	64	Abdominal pain	80	Phobias	48
Fatigue	84	Abdominal bloating	68	Vomiting all nine months of pregnancy	20
Blindness	20	Food intolerances	48	Nervous	92
Paralysis	12	Diarrhea	20	Had to quit working because felt bad	44
Anesthesia	32	Constipation	64	Trouble doing anything because felt bad	72
Aphonia	44	Dysuria	44	Cried a lot	60
Lump in throat	28	Urinary retention	8	Felt life was hopeless	28
Fits or convulsions	20	Dysmenorrhea (premarital only)	4	Always sickly (most of life)	40
Faints	56	Dysmenorrhea (prepregnancy only)	8	Thought of dying	48
Unconsciousness	16	Dysmenorrhea (other)	48	Wanted to die	36
Amnesia	8	Menstrual irregularity	48	Thought of suicide	28
Visual blurring	64	Excessive menstrual bleeding	48	Attempted Suicide	12
Visual hallucination	12	Sexual indifference	44		
Deafness	4	Frigidity (absence of orgasm)	24		
Olfactory hallucination	16	Dyspareunia	52		
Weakness	84	Back pain	88		

From M. Perley and S. B. Guze (43)

Vomiting: "I vomit every ten minutes. Sometimes it lasts for two to three weeks at a time. I can't even take liquids. I even vomit water. I can't stand the smell of food."

Food intolerance: "I can't eat pastries. Always pay for it. I can't eat steak now. I throw up whole milk. I always throw up the skins of tomatoes. Pudding made with canned milk makes me sick. I have to use fresh milk."

A trance: "I passed out on the bathroom floor during my period and was still on the floor when they found me the next morning."

Weight change: "I can lose weight just walking down the street. I can hold my breath and lose weight. I was down to 65 pounds at one time."

Dysmenorrhea: "I can't work. Every month I am in bed for several days. I have had to have morphine hypos. There is a throbbing pain in the legs as if the blood doesn't circulate. Can't go to the bathroom as I faint. It's murder! I want to die. It affects my nervous system."

Sexual indifference: "Have never been interested." "It's not a normal thing to me. Disgusting. My husband has never bothered me." "It's just a part of my married life. I have to do it." "I was only disappointed. Never really enjoyed it, but I had to please my husband." "I have no feelings. It's just a duty."

Dyspareunia: "Every time I had intercourse I swelled up on one side. It's sore and burns, and afterwards is very painful." "I hate it. I have a severe pain on the right side and have to go to bed for a day."

Presenting complaints: "I am sore all over. I can't explain it. I have been sick all my life. Now I am alone since my husband died, and the doctor said I must come for help. It has taken $10,000 to keep me alive. This is my 76th hospitalization." "I have been taking care of my invalid mother and I get very little rest or sleep." "My father came here for a checkup on his diabetes and insisted that I come along. I had a nervous breakdown in 1943 and have never gotten around to being really well."

The gynecologist, the neurologist, and the psychiatrist are likely to see somatization-disorder patients with more focused complaints: the gynecologist because of menstrual pain, irregularity, lapses, or because of dyspareunia; the neurologist because of headaches, "spells," or other conversion symptoms; the psychiatrist because of suicide attempts, depression, or marital discord. But even these specialists find it difficult to obtain straightforward histories from patients with somatization disorder.

Among the characteristic recurrent or chronic symptoms in hysteria, pains are very prominent: headaches, chest pain, abdominal pain, back pain, joint pain. Abdominal, pelvic, and back pain in association with menstrual or sexual difficulties account for frequent gynecologic surgery: dilatation and curettage, uterine suspension, and salpingo-oophorectomy. Abdominal pain, back pain, dysuria, and dyspareunia account for frequent catheterization and cystoscopy. Abdominal pain, indigestion, bowel difficulties, and vomiting are associated with frequent gastrointestinal X-ray examinations and rectal and gallbladder surgery.

Repeated hospitalization and surgery are characteristic of these conditions (16). Because of the dramatic and persistent symptoms, patients are hospitalized for observation, tests, X-rays, and treatment of a wide variety of medical and surgical conditions that may be mimicked by somatization disorder.

Nervousness and anxiety symptoms (palpitation, dyspnea, chest pain, dizziness, fatigue, tremulousness) are frequent. When chest pain is prominent, it often leads to a diagnosis of heart disease, too often supported only by nonspecific deviations in the EKG. The same nervousness and anxiety symptoms, especially when associated with globus (lump in throat) or weight loss, frequently lead to thyroid studies and the diagnosis of thyroid abnormalities. Before the advent of modern laboratory methods for evaluating thyroid function, thyroidectomy was performed for suspected hyperthyroidism, particularly in older patients. Moodiness, irritability, depression, suicidal ideation, and suicide attempts are common and lead to psychiatric hospitalization (18). Hysteria accounts for a significant minority of suicide attempts (54) but rarely leads to suicide (50).

Menstrual symptoms and sexual indifference or frigidity are so characteristic that a diagnosis of Briquet's syndrome or somatization disorder should be made with care if the menstrual and sexual histories are normal. Marital discord related to sexual indifference and frigidity frequently leads to separation and divorce (27).

Recent studies emphasize a point recognized in the past—that somatization disorder is a "psychoform" condition as much as a "somatoform" one (55, 66). Patients are as prone to report a wide range of psychological or emotional symptoms as they are to report physical ones.

The question of malingering frequently arises in discussions about these patients. Although often suspected, malingering is difficult to prove. Nevertheless, malingering and factitious lesions are striking features in some cases (48). Factitious fever produced by heating thermometers with matches or friction, skin lesions produced by self-injections, and hemoptysis and hematuria produced by pricking fingers and adding blood to sputum or urine may take months or years to recognize. An occasional patient will confide that a given symptom or sign was produced artificially in the past but will insist that it is now real.

Multiple personality is another manifestation of these syndromes (4, 45). Though considered a rare phenomenon, multiple personality may be increasing in frequency, perhaps as a result of widespread attention in the news media (5, 25). Similarly, borderline personality disorder is often seen in patients meeting the criteria for Briquet's syndrome or somatization disorder. In fact, *evidence from a number of recent studies suggests that many cases of these two syndromes and both borderline and multiple personality disorders may all be manifestations of a single condition,* the various manifestations of which may vary in prominence and severity over time and with different circumstances (4, 25, 34, 45, 66).

The long-recognized association of antisocial personality and

Briquet's syndrome within the same individual and within families (1, 8, 9, 13–15, 28, 31, 59, 68), discussed below, may tie together a number of different clinical features, and one is reminded of the old tale of several blind men drawing different conclusions about an elephant from the different parts of the animal's body each touches.

Another characteristic feature of somatization disorder is the tendency of many patients to give inconsistent histories (26); thus, symptoms that lead to hospitalization on one occasion are denied on another. Though this inconsistency has not been studied systematically, it may be related to the patient's perception of the physician's response to her and her desire to influence his judgment about her illness.

The association between somatization disorder and sociopathy is of great interest. The familial aspect of this association will be discussed below (see Family Studies), but there is a clinical aspect as well. Many delinquent or antisocial adolescent girls develop somatization disorder as adults (51); many somatization-disorder patients give a history of delinquent or antisocial behavior earlier in life (31, 38); the medical histories of delinquent children indicate an increased prevalence of medical contacts (37); and many convicted women felons present with a mixed picture of sociopathy and somatization (13, 14). Thus school delinquency, repeated fighting, running away from home, a poor work record, a poor marital history, sexual promiscuity, heavy drinking, and police trouble are events found in the histories of many, though not all, such women (59). It may be pertinent that Eysenck has concluded from his studies of personality that both hysterics and psychopaths are "extroverted neurotics," a possible reason for associating the two conditions (22).

NATURAL HISTORY

As already noted, it is not easy to determine when the illness began. The vague and often inconsistent history makes the chronology of symptoms difficult to establish. The patient may insist that she has always been "sick" and may describe early difficulties that are hard to evaluate. These patients may also suffer from other illnesses, and, therefore, descriptions of childhood or adolescent disorders that allegedly were diagnosed as rheumatic fever, appendicitis, poliomyelitis, or typhoid fever can be most difficult to judge.

The symptoms fluctuate in severity, but the characteristic features persist: recurrent pains, conversion symptoms, nervousness and depression, sexual and marital discord, repeated hospitalization, and repeated surgery (27). Although systematic follow-up until death of a series of patients has not yet been reported, there is no indication that more than a minority of patients experience marked improvement or permanent remission. Twenty to thirty years of symptoms are typical, and patients who have had the illness for over forty years are not unusual. There is no evidence of excess mortality (19).

On the other hand, the long-term course of the patient with conversion symptoms is determined by the underlying illness rather than by the nature of the symptoms themselves. Because conversion symptoms may be seen in a wide variety of medical, neurologic, and psychiatric disorders (24, 33, 64), patients with these symptoms have a variable prognosis and course.

COMPLICATIONS

The most frequent and important complications of somatization disorder are repeated surgical operations, drug dependence, marital separation or divorce, and suicide attempts. The first two are presumably preventable if physicians learn to recognize the disorder and manage patients properly. Knowing that somatization disorder is an alternate explanation for various pains and other symptoms, surgery can be withheld or postponed in cases where objective indications are equivocal or missing. Habit-forming or addicting drugs should be avoided for recurrent or persistent pain. Whether the physician can modify marital discord through psychotherapy is uncertain, but recognizing the frequency of separation and divorce, the physician can certainly direct his or her attention to these problems. The same may be said about suicide attempts, but there the physician can approach patients with hysteria knowing that the risk of complicated suicide is low.

FAMILY STUDIES

Studies using the Briquet's syndrome criteria suggest that somatization disorder runs in families (1, 17, 67). It was found in one study that about 20 percent of first-degree (siblings, parents, children) female relatives of index cases met the criteria for the same condition, a tenfold increase over the prevalence in the general population of women, lending strong support to the validity of the concept of hysteria as an illness. A second study, using "blind" examiners, showed lower numbers and only a three-and-a-half-fold increase in first-degree female relatives compared to similar relatives of index women with a range of other psychiatric disorders (26), but it again confirmed the familial aggregation of cases.

Family studies also indicate that a significant association exists between somatization disorder and antisocial personality. First-degree male relatives of women selected by the Briquet's syndrome criteria show an increased prevalence of sociopathy and alcoholism (1, 26, 67). The first-degree female relatives of convicted male felons also show an increased prevalence of Briquet's syndrome (28). There findings, in conjunction with the observation that many female sociopaths present with, or develop, the full Briquet's syndrome or meet the criteria for somatization disorder (13), have suggested that at least some cases of somatization disorder (Briquet's syndrome) and sociopathy share a common etiology.

The widely recognized observation that somatization disorder is predominantly a disorder of women, whereas sociopathy is predominantly a disorder of men, raises the interesting possibility that, depending on the sex of the individual, the same etiologic and pathogenetic factors may lead to different, although sometimes overlapping, clinical pictures. As suggested above, future studies may show a familial aggregation involving borderline and multiple personality disorders as well as somatization disorder and antisocial personality. It may be established that many individuals with any or all of these four clinical conditions are suffering from a common disorder whose overt manifestations vary in accordance with gender and a variety of clinical and social circumstances.

Two studies (8, 9, 63) of adopted children whose biological parents showed antisocial behavior revealed greater-than-normal frequency in female offspring of Briquet's syndrome or somatization disorder or other multiple unexplained somatic complaints, thus supporting the hypothesis that these are related disorders. One of these studies was carried out in the United States; the other in Sweden.

DIFFERENTIAL DIAGNOSIS

Three psychiatric conditions must, at times, be considered in the differential diagnosis of these conditions: panic disorder, major depressive disorder, and schizophrenia.

As already noted, the characteristic symptoms of somatization disorder include many that are also seen in panic disorder and depression. If the patient is a young women with menstrual and sexual difficulties who presents with a full range of anxiety or depressive symptoms, she may nearly meet the diagnostic criteria. Age of onset, details of the symptom picture, course, and mental status will usually help clarify the diagnostic problem.

A number of patients with schizophrenia also meet the diagnostic criteria for Briquet's syndrome or somatization disorder. Also, an occasional patient with these latter conditions who does not show definite evidence of schizophrenia when first seen will, in time, develop the typical clinical picture of schizophrenia (69).

Unlike the situation in which the same patients may meet diagnostic criteria for sociopathy and hysteria, a situation in which family studies suggest that the disorders are associated, the overlap with schizophrenia is not accompanied by evidence of a familial association.

CLINICAL MANAGEMENT

The diagnosis of somatization disorder (based on Briquet's syndrome criteria) provides two advantages. (Whether the *DSM-IV* criteria will prove to be as satisfactory awaits more experience.) For patients with the full diagnostic picture, the physician can predict in over 90 percent of cases that the characteristic symptoms will continue through time and that other illnesses, which in retrospect could account for the original clinical picture, will not become evident. For patients who do not present with the full diagnostic picture, especially for those who have conversion symptoms and little else, the physician knows that in a substantial number of cases other disorders will become evident that do, in retrospect, account for the original clinical picture (46, 64). Many, perhaps most, of the patients whose symptoms resemble somatization disorder, but fail to meet the diagnostic criteria, will remain undiagnosed at follow-up. Enough of them, however, will turn out to have other serious medical, neurological, or psychiatric disorders to justify the kind of diagnostic open-mindedness that can lead to earlier recognition of the other illnesses.

Patients with these conditions are difficult to treat (2, 44). The typical clinical picture of recurrent, multiple, vague symptoms combined with doctor-shopping and frequent requests for time and attention can frustrate many physicians. Few of these patients referred for psychiatric treatment persist with such treatment (27). Thus the burden of caring for them continues to rest with other physicians. A controlled, randomized study indicates, however, that psychiatric consultation may be helpful in reducing the extent and cost of medical care (58).

The physician's major goal should be to avoid the complications described earlier. Success will depend on winning the patient's confidence without allowing her symptomatic behavior to exhaust the physician's sympathy. The patient and family can be told that the patient tends to experience symptoms that suggest other disorders, but that they are not medically serious. On this basis, the physician can approach each new complaint circumspectly and conservatively, especially with regard to elaborate or expensive diagnostic studies. As the physician grows familiar with the patient, the physician will become increasingly confident in his or her clinical judgments. Remembering that somatization disorder can "explain" many puzzling symptoms, the physician, always looking for objective evidence of other disorders, can avoid unnecessary hospitalization and surgery.

The physician should strive to substitute discussions of the patient's life problems, personality, and concerns for a quick-triggered response of ordering additional tests and X-rays or yet another drug. At the same time, the physician must recognize the limitations resulting from our lack of knowledge about the causes and mechanisms of the disorder.

REFERENCES

1. Arkonac, O., Guze, S. B. A family study of hysteria. N. Engl. J. Med. 268:239–242, 1963.
2. Bird, J. The behavioural treatment of hysteria. Brit. J. Psychiat. 134:129–137, 1979.
3. Blinder, M. G. The hysterical personality. Psychiatry 29:227–235, 1966.
4. Bliss, E. L. A symptom profile of patients with multiple personalities, including MMPI results. J. Nerv. Ment. Dis. 172:197–202, 1984.
5. Boor, M. The multiple personality epidemic. Additional cases and inferences regarding diagnosis, etiology, dynamics, and treatment. J. Nerv. Ment. Dis. 170:302–304, 1982.
6. Breuer, J., and Freud, S. Studies in Hysteria (Brill, A. A., trans.). New York: Nerv. Ment. Dis. Monogr., 1936.

7. Briquet, P. *Traité clinique et thérapeutique à l'hystére.* Paris: J-B. Ballière & Fils, 1859.

8. Cadoret, R. J. Psychopathology in adopted-away offspring of biologic parents with antisocial behavior. Arch. Gen. Psychiat. *35*:176–184, 1978.

9. Cadoret, R. J., Cunningham, L., Loftus, R., and Edwards, J. Studies of adoptees from psychiatrically disturbed biological parents. Ill. Medical symptoms and illness in childhood and adolescence. Am. J. Psychiat. *133*:1316–1318, 1976.

10. Carothers, J. C. Hysteria, psychopathy and the magic word. Mankind Q. *16*:93–103, 1975.

11. Chodoff, P. The diagnosis of hysteria: an overview. Am. J. Psychiat. *131*:1073–1078, 1974.

12. Chodoff, P., and Lyons, H. Hysteria: the hysterical personality and hysterical conversion. Am. J. Psychiat. *114*:734–740, 1958.

13. Cloninger, C. R., and Guze, S. B. Psychiatric illness and female criminality: the role of sociopathy and hysteria in the antisocial woman. Am. J. Psychiat. *127*:303–311, 1970.

14. Cloninger, C. R., and Guze, S. B. Female criminals: their personal, familial, and social backgrounds. Arch. Gen. Psychiat. *23*:554–558, 1970.

15. Cloninger, C. R., Martin, R. L., Guze, S. B., and Clayton, P. J. A prospective follow-up and family study of somatization in men and women. Am. J. Psychiat. *143*:873–878, 1986.

16. Cohen, M. E., Robins, E., Purtell, J. J., Altmann, M. W., and Reid, D. E. Excessive surgery in hysteria. JAMA *151*:977–986, 1953.

17. Coryell, W. A blind family history study of Briquet's syndrome. Further validation of the diagnosis. Arch. Gen. Psychiat. *37*:1266–1269, 1980.

18. Coryell, W., and Norten, S. G. Briquet's syndrome (Somatization Disorder) and primary depression: comparison of background and outcome. Compr. Psychiat. *22*:249–256, 1981.

19. Coryell, W. Diagnosis-specific mortality. Primary unipolar depression and Briquet's syndrome (somatization disorder). Arch. Gen. Psychiat. *38*:939–942, 1981.

20. De Figueiredo, J. M., Baiardi, J. J., and Long, D. M. Briquet syndrome in a man with chronic intractable pain. Johns Hopkins Med. J. *147*:102–106, 1980.

21. DeSouza, C., and Othmer, E. Somatization disorder and Briquet's syndrome. Arch. Gen. Psychiat. *41*:334–336, 1984.

22. Eysenck, H. *The Dynamics of Anxiety and Hysteria.* New York: Praeger, 1957.

23. Farley, J., Woodruff, Jr., R. A., and Guze, S. B. The prevalence of hysteria and conversion symptoms. Brit. J. Psychiat. *114*:1121–1125, 1968.

24. Gatfield, P. D., and Guze, S. B. Prognosis and differential diagnosis of conversion reactions. Dis. Nerv. Syst. *23*:623–631, 1962.

25. Greaves, G. B. Multiple personality. 165 years after Mary Reynolds. J. Nerv. Ment. Dis. *168*:577–596, 1980.

26. Guze, S. B., Cloninger, C. R., Martin, R. L., and Clayton, P. J. A follow-up and family study of Briquet's syndrome. Brit. J. Psychiat. *149*:17–23, 1986.

27. Guze, S. B., and Perley, M. J. Observations on the natural history of hysteria. Am. J. Psychiat. *119*:960–965, 1963.

28. Guze, S. B., Wolfgram, E. D., McKinney, J. K., and Cantwell, D. P. Psychiatric illness in the families of convicted criminals: a study of 519 first-degree relatives. Dis. Nerv. Syst. *28*:651–659, 1967.

29. Guze, S. B. The diagnosis of hysteria: what are we trying to do? Am. J. Psychiat. *124*:491–498, 1967.

30. Guze, S. B. The role of follow-up studies: their contribution to diagnostic classification as applied to hysteria. Semin. Psychiat. *2*:392–402, 1970.

31. Guze, S. B., Woodruff, Jr., R. A., and Clayton, P. J. Hysteria and antisocial behavior: further evidence of an assoication. Am. J. Psychiat. *127*:957–960, 1971.

32. Guze, S. B., Woodruff, R. A., and Clayton, P. J. A study of conversion symptoms in psychiatric outpatients. Am. J. Psychiat. *128*:643–646, 1971.

33. Hafeiz, H. B. Hysterical conversion: a prognostic study. Brit. J. Psychiat. *136*:548–551, 1980.

34. Hudziak, J. J., Boffeli, T. J., Kreisman, J. J., Battaglia, M. M., and Guze, S. B. A clinical study of borderline personality disorder: the significance of Briquet's syndrome (hysteria), somatization disorder, antisocial personality disorder and substance abuse disorders. Submitted for publication.

35. Kimble, R., Williams, J. G., and Agras, S. A comparison of two methods of diagnosing hysteria. Am. J. Psychiat. *132*:1197–1199, 1975.

36. Kroll, P., Chamberlain, K. R., and Halpern, J. The diagnosis of Briquet's syndrome in a male population. The Veterans Administration revisited. J. Nerv. Ment. Dis. *167*:171–174, 1979.

37. Lewis, D. O., and Shanok, S. S. Medical histories of delinquent and non-delinquent children: an epidemiologic study. Am. J. Psychiat. *134*:1020–1025, 1977.

38. Lilienfeld, S. O., Van Valkenburg, C., Larntz, K., and Akiskal, H. S. The relationship of histrionic personality disorder to antisocial personality and somatization disorders. Am. J. Psychiat. *143*:718–722, 1986.

39. Mai, F. M., and Merskey, H. Briquet's *Treatise on Hysteria*. A synopsis and commentary. Arch. Gen. Psychiat. *37*:1401–1405, 1980.

40. Mai, F. M., and Merskey, H. Historical review. Briquet's concept of hysteria: an historical perspective. Can. J. Psychiat. *26*:57–63, 1981.

41. Marsden, C. D. Hysteria—a neurologist's view. Psychol. Med. *16*:277–288, 1986.

42. Mohr, P. D., and Bond, M. J. A chronic epidemic of hysterical blackouts in a comprehensive school. Brit. Med. J. *284*:961–962, 1982.

43. Morrison, J. R. Early birth order in Briquet's syndrome. Am. J. Psychiat. *140*:1596–1597, 1983.

44. Murphy, G. E. The clinical management of hysteria. JAMA *247*:2559–2564, 1982.

45. North, C. S., Ryall, J. M., Ricci, D. A., and Wetzel, R. D. *Multiple Personalities, Multiple Disorders*. New York: Oxford University Press, 1993.

46. Perley, M. J., and Guze, S. B. Hysteria—the stability and usefulness of clinical criteria. N. Engl. J. Med. *266*:421–426, 1962.
47. Purtell, J. J., Robins, E., and Cohen, M. E. Observations on clinical aspects of hysteria. JAMA *146*:902–909, 1951.
48. Ries, R. K. Single case study. DSM-III differential diagnosis of Munchausen's syndrome. J. Nerv. Ment. Dis. *168*:629–632, 1980.
49. Robins, E., Purtell, J. J., and Cohen, M. E. "Hysteria" in men. N. Engl. J. Med. *246*:677–685, 1952.
50. Robins, E., Murphy, G., Wilkinson, R., Gassner, S., and Kayes, J. Some clinical considerations in the prevention of suicide based on a study of 134 successful suicides. Am. J. Public Health *49*:888–899, 1959.
51. Robins, L. *Deviant Children Grown Up.* Baltimore: Williams & Wilkins, 1966.
52. Rounsaville, B. J., Harding, P. S., and Weissman, M. M. Single case study. Briquet's syndrome in a man. J. Nerv. Ment. Dis. *167*:364–367, 1979.
53. Savill, T. D. *Lectures on Hysteria and Allied Vasomotor Conditions.* London: H. J. Glaisher, 1909.
54. Schmidt, E. H., O'Neal, P., and Robins, E. Evaluation of suicide attempts as guide to therapy. Clinical and follow-up study of 109 patients. JAMA *155*:549–557, 1954.
55. Simon, G. E., and Von Korff, M. Somatization and psychiatric disorder in the NIMH Epidemiologic Catchment Area Study. Am. J. Psychiat. *148*:1494–1500, 1991.
56. Slater, E. Diagnosis of "hysteria." Brit. Med. J. *1*:1395–1399, 1965.
57. Small, G. W., and Nicholi, Jr., A. M. Mass hysteria among schoolchildren. Early loss as a predisposing factor. Arch. Gen. Psychiat. *39*:721–724, 1982.
58. Smith, Jr., G. R., Monson, R. A., and Ray, D. C. Psychiatric consultation in somatization disorder. N. Engl. J. Med. *314*:1407–1413, 1986.
59. Spalt, L. Hysteria and antisocial personality. A single disorder? J. Nerv. Ment. Dis. *168*:456–464, 1980.
60. Stefansson, J. G., Messina, J. A., and Meyerowitz, S. Hysterical neurosis, conversion type: clinical and epidemiological considerations. Acta Psychiat. Scand. *53*:119–138, 1976.
61. Swartz, M., Blazer, D., Woodbury, M., George, L., and Landerman, R. Somatization disorder in a U.S. southern community: use of a new procedure for analysis of medical classification. Psychol. Med. *16*:595–609, 1986.
62. Vieth, I. *Hysteria. The History of a Disease.* Chicago: Univ. of Chicago Press, 1965.
63. von Knorring, A.-L. *Adoption Studies on Psychiatric Illness.* Umea University Medical Dissertations, Series no. 101. Sweden: Umea, 1983.
64. Watson, C. G., and Buranen, C. The frequency and identification of false positive conversion reactions. J. Nerv. Ment. Dis. *167*:243–247, 1979.
65. Weissman, M. M., Myers, J. K., and Harding, P. S. Psychiatric disorders in a U.S. urban community: 1975–76. Am. J. Psychiat. *135*:459–462, 1978.
66. Wetzel, R. D., Guze, S. B., Cloninger, C. R., Martin, R. L., and Clayton, P. J. Briquet's syndrome (hysteria) is both a somatoform and a "psychoform"

illness: a Minnesota Multiphasic Personality Inventory Study. Psychosom. Med. *56*:564–569, 1994.

67. Woerner, P. I., and Guze, S. B. A family and marital study of hysteria. Brit. J. Psychiat. *114*:161–168, 1968.

68. Woodruff, Jr., R. A. Hysteria: an evaluation of objective diagnostic criteria by the study of women with chronic medical illnesses. Brit. J. Psychiat. *114*:1115–1119, 1967.

69. Woodruff, Jr., R. A., Clayton, P. J., and Guze, S. B. Hysteria: studies of diagnosis, outcome, and prevalence. JAMA *215*:425–428, 1971.

70. Yutzy, S. H., Cloninger, C. R., Guze, S. B., Pribor, E. F., Martin, R. I., Kathol, R. G., Smith, G. R., and Strain, J. J. DSM-IV Field Trial: testing a New Proposal for Somatization Disorder. Am. J. Psychiat. *152*:97–101, 1995.

71. Ziegler, F. J., Imboden, J. B., and Meyer, E. Contemporary conversion reactions: clinical study. Am. J. Psychiat. *116*:901–910, 1960.

5

OBSESSIVE-COMPULSIVE
DISORDER

DEFINITION

Obsessions are persistent distressing thoughts or impulses experienced as unwanted and senseless but irresistible. *Compulsions* are acts resulting from obsessions. Obsessive-compulsive disorder (OCD) is a chronic illness dominated by obsessions and compulsions occurring in the absence of another psychiatric disorder. Obsessional neurosis was a synonym in vogue before *DSM-III* was published in 1980.

HISTORICAL BACKGROUND

The term "obsessional neurosis" apparently originated with Karl Westphal (1833–1890), a German neurologist who wrote about obsessional conditions and phobias. Kraepelin described obsessional neurosis (*Zwangsneurose*) in his textbooks in the early part of the twentieth century, and the same term was adopted by Freud, whose classical description of the clinical picture, published in 1917, follows (18):

> The obsessional neurosis takes this form: the patient's mind is occupied with thoughts that do not really interest him, he feels impulses

which seem alien to him, and he is impelled to perform actions which not only afford him no pleasure but from which he is powerless to desist. The thoughts (obsessions) may be meaningless in themselves or only of no interest to the patient; they are often only absolutely silly.

Recognition of obsessional traits, however, far antedated psychiatrists' description of the syndrome. In the early seventeenth century Richard Flecknoe, in discussing "enigmaticall characters," described one such character as an "irresolute Person" (27):

He hovers in his choice, like an empty Ballance with no waight of Judgement to incline him to either scale . . . everything he thinks on, is matter of deliberation . . . and he does nothing readily, but what he thinks not on . . . when he begins to deliberate, never makes an end. . . . Has some dull demon cryes, do not, do not still, when hee's on point of doing anything. . . . He plays at shall I, shall I? so long, till opportunity be past . . . and then repents at leisure.

In the seventeenth century obsessions were often referred to as "scruples," defined by Jermey A. Taylor (65) as

a great trouble of mind preceding from a little motive, and a great indisposition, by which the conscience though sufficiently determined by proper arguments, dares not proceed to action, or if it do, it cannot rest . . . some persons dare not eat for fear of gluttony, they fear that they shall sleep too much, and that keeps them waking, and troubles their heads more and then their scruples increase. When they are married they are afraid to do their duty, for fear it be secretly an indulgence to the flesh, and to be suspected of carnality, and yet they dare not omit it, for fear they should be unjust, and yet their fear that the very fearing it to be unclean should be a sin, and suspect that if they do not fear so it is too great a sign they adhere to Nature more than to the Spirit. . . . *Scruple is a little stone in the foot, if you set it upon the ground it hurts you; if you hold it up you cannot go forward; it is a trouble where the trouble is over, a doubt when doubts are resolved* . . . very often it hath no reason at all for its inducement.

The content of obsessions, today as in years past, is often religious. In his monograph *Of Religious Melancholy* (50), published in 1692, John Moore described "naughty and sometimes blasphemous thoughts which start in the mind while they are exercised in the worship of God despite all their endeavors to stiffle and suppress them." In fact, he wrote, "the more they struggle with them, the more they increase." Bishop Moore had difficulty understanding this state as the sufferers were "mostly good People," whereas "bad men . . . rarely know anything of these kinds of Thoughts." Like others, he argued that this was good reason "to judge them to be Distempers of the body rather than Faults of the Mind." He was particularly concerned about the phobic avoidances that could result from such obsessions and wrote, "I exhort you not to quit your Employment . . . for no business at all is as bad for you as too much: and there is always more Melancholy to be found in a Cloyster than in the Marketplace."

The obsessional fear of suffering from syphilis was also well recognized as a manifestation of mental illness by the clergy and later by psychiatrists. In the past, "superstition" has often been used to mean what we would consider an obsession. Samuel Johnson apparently had this in mind when he wrote that "the superstitious are often melancholic, and the melancholic almost always superstitious." As will be noted later, obsessions are common in depressive states and vice versa.

EPIDEMIOLOGY

Obsessive-compulsive disorder was once considered rare but a mid-1980 study suggested that the disorder may affect 2% of the general population, making it one of the more common forms of serious psychopathology (6, 40, 55, 57). Only a small proportion visit psychiatrists. Less than 5% of psychiatric inpatients and outpatients receive the diagnosis; according to some studies, obsessive-compulsive disorder occurs more frequently in women than in men (54).

When compared with all other psychiatric patients, obsessionals reportedly differed in the following ways: (a) they belong to higher social classes, (b) they make higher scores on intelligence tests, (c) they have a higher educational level (28, 45, 54, 59).

A recent comparison of prevalence rates of obsessive-compulsive disorder in seven countries found the rates to be remarkably consistent, falling in the 1 to 2% range (54).

CLINICAL PICTURE

When obsessionals finally seek medical attention (often years after their illness began), it may be because of depression, acute anxiety, exacerbation of obsessions, or social incapacity resulting from any of these conditions (10, 44, 53) (Table 5.1).

Table 5.1   Diagnostic criteria for Obsessive-Compulsive Disorder
(*DSM-IV*)

A. Either obsessions or compulsions:

Obsessions as defined by:

(1) Recurrent and persistent thoughts, impulses, or images that are experienced, at some time during the disturbance, as intrusive and inappropriate and that cause marked anxiety or distress

(2) The thoughts, impulses, or images are not simply excessive worries about real-life problems

(3) The person attempts to ignore or suppress such thoughts, impulses, or images, or to neutralize them with some other thought or action

(4) The person recognizes that the obsessional thoughts, impulses, or images are a product of his or her own mind (not imposed from without as in thought insertion)

Compulsions as defined by

(1) Repetitive behaviors (e.g., hand washing, ordering, checking) or mental acts (e.g., praying, counting, repeating words silently) that the person feels driven to perform in response to an obsession, or according to rules that must be applied rigidly

(2) The behaviors or mental acts are aimed at preventing or reducing distress or preventing some dreaded event or situation; however, these behaviors or mental acts either are not connected in a realistic way with what they are designed to neutralize or prevent or are clearly excessive

Table 5.1 *(Continued)*

B. At some point during the course of the disorder, the person has recognized that the obsessions or compulsions are excessive or unreasonable. NOTE: This does not apply to children

C. The obsessions or compulsions cause marked distress, are time consuming (take more than 1 hour a day), or significantly interfere with the person's normal routine, occupational (or academic) functioning, or usual social activities or relationships

D. If another psychiatric disorder is present, the content of the obsessions or compulsions is not restricted to it (e.g., preoccupation with food in the presence of an Eating Disorder; hair pulling in the presence of Trichotillomania; concern with appearance in the presence of Body Dysmorphic Disorder; preoccupation with drugs in the presence of a Substance Use Disorder; preoccupation with having a serious illness in the presence of Hypochondriasis; preoccupation with sexual urges or fantasies in the presence of a Paraphilia; or guilty ruminations in the presence of major Depressive Disorder)

E. The disturbance is not due to the direct physiological effects of a substance (e.g., a drug of abuse, a medication) or a general medical condition

---

A life event often seems associated with the onset of symptoms: the death of a relative, a sexual conflict, overwork, or pregnancy (28, 45). Just as often, however, no precipitating factors can be identified.

A common presenting complaint is the obsessional fear of injuring oneself or another person, often a child or close relative. Fearful of losing control, the patients may develop avoidances or rituals that lead in turn to social incapacity. Perhaps they will refuse to leave the house or will avoid sharp objects or wash repeatedly.

On reflection they may identify the obsessional idea as illogical, but not always. Sometimes the ideas are not, strictly speaking, illogical (germs do produce disease) and sometimes, even when obviously absurd, the ideas are not viewed as such. What distinguishes an obsession from a delusion is not so much insight (recognizing the idea's absurdity) as the person's struggle against the obsessional experience itself. He strives to free himself from the obsession but cannot and feels increasingly uncomfortable until the idea temporarily runs its course or the obsessional act has been completed (44).

The frequency with which obsessional symptoms appear in obsessional patients has been studied systematically by three groups, and their results indicate that the illness may assume one or more of the following forms (1, 15, 63):

Obsessional ideas: Thoughts that repetitively intrude into consciousness (words, phrases, rhymes) and interfere with the normal train of thought and causing distress to the person. Often the thoughts are obscene, blasphemous, or nonsensical.

Obsessional images: Vividly imagined scenes, often of a violent, sexual, or disgusting nature (images of a child being killed, cars colliding, excrement, parents having sexual intercourse) that repeatedly come to mind.

Obsessional convictions: Notions that are often based on the magical formula of thought equals act: "Thinking ill of my son will cause him to die." Unlike delusions, obsessional beliefs are characterized by ambivalence: The person believes and simultaneously does not believe. As Jaspers expressed it, there is a "constant going on between a consciousness of validity and non-validity. Both push this way and that, but neither can gain the upper hand" (35).

Obsessional rumination: Prolonged, inconclusive thinking about a subject to the exclusion of other interests. The subject is often religion or metaphysics—why and wherefore questions that are as unanswerable as they are endlessly ponderable. Indecisiveness in ordinary matters is very common: "Which necktie should I wear?" Doubt may lead to extremes in caution, both irksome and irresistible. "Did I turn off the gas?" "Lock the door?" "Write the correct address?" The patient checks and rechecks, stopping only when exhausted or on checking a predetermined "magical" number of times. Several studies suggest that obsessional doubts—*manie du doute*—may well be the most prominent feature in obsessional neurosis (1, 15, 60). As with other obsessions, ruminations are resisted. The person tries to turn his or her attention elsewhere, but cannot; often the more he or she tries, the more intrusive and distressing the thoughts become.

Obsessional impulses: Typically relates to self-injury (leaping from a window); injury to others (smothering an infant); or embarrassing behavior (shouting obscenities in church).

Obsessional fears: Often of dirt, disease, contamination; of potential weapons (razors, scissors); of being in specific situations or performing particular acts.

Obsessional rituals (compulsions): Repetitive, stereotyped acts of counting, touching, arranging objects, moving, washing, tasting, looking in specific ways. Compulsions are inseparable from the obsessions from which they arise. A compulsion is an obsession expressed as action. About one-quarter of patients display no compulsions (1).

Counting rituals are especially common. The person feels compelled to count letters or words or the squares in a tile floor or to perform arithmetical operations. Certain numbers, or their multiples, may have special significance (the person "must" lay down her pencil three times or step on every fifth sidewalk crack). Other rituals concern the performance of excretory functions and such everyday acts as preparing to go to bed. Also common are rituals involving extremes of cleanliness (handwashing compulsions, relentless emptying of ashtrays) and complicated routines assuring orderliness and punctuality. Women apparently have a higher incidence of contamination phobia and of compulsive cleaning behavior than do men (15).

According to a study of obsessionals (10), four kinds of rituals occur most frequently: counting, checking, cleaning, and avoidance rituals. Each occurred in half of the patients. Avoidance rituals were similar to those seen in phobic disorders (see Differential Diagnosis). An example can be seen in a patient who avoided anything colored brown. Her inability to approach brown objects greatly limited her activities.

Other rituals that occur less often consist of slowing, striving for completeness, and extreme meticulousness. With slowing, such simple tasks as buttoning a shirt or tying a shoelace might take up to fifteen minutes. Striving for completeness may be seen in dressing also. Asked why he spends so much time with a single button, the patient might reply that he was trying to prove to himself that he had "buttoned the button properly."

A common form of pathological meticulousness is a concern that objects be arranged in a special way. Pencils, for example, may have to be arranged so that the points are directed away from the patient. Students may spend so much time in arranging pencils, pens, erasers, and so on that they cannot do their work.

Rituals, ridiculous as they may seem to the patients, are accompanied by a profound dread and apprehension that assures their performance because they alone give relief. "I'll explode if I don't do it," a patient may say. Occasionally patients believe that failure to perform a given ritual will result in harm to themselves or others; often the ritual is as inexplicable to patients as it is to observers.

Obsessional symptoms often are accompanied by a dysphoric mood. The patient may be irritable, tense, depressed. This may lead to an erroneous diagnosis of affective disorder because the mood element at the time of examination may overshadow the obsessional content.

Obsessional symptoms rarely occur singly (41). As with most psychiatric illnesses, obsessional disorder presents a cluster of symptoms that, individually, are variable and inconstant over time but as a group maintain characteristics unique to the illness. Thus a patient may now have one set of obsessional impulses, phobias, and rituals and later another set, but the symptoms remain predominantly obsessional.

R. J. obsessed so much about eating contaminated food that he was thirty pounds underweight. He worried so much that he might gun the accelerator and run people over at an intersection that he always put the car in park. He was so compulsive that he copied serial numbers off dollar bills and dressed and undressed so many times in the morning that it was noon before he was ready to go to work as a school custodian.

Occasionally, however, a single obsession dominates the clinical picture.

A thirty-five-year-old banker, P. T., had an obsession concerning the length of his trousers. He would buy a pair of trousers but fail to convince himself that they were the correct length. He would then go back to the tailor repeatedly to have them adjusted—returning as many as a dozen times and stopping only when his embarrassment became acute as the tailor became more frustrated. Then he would adjust the length himself. He would stand endlessly before mirrors, trying to decide whether the length was correct. Whenever he crossed his leg and the pant was hiked up, showing a stretch of hose, he worried that there was too much hose showing or too little. Again he would alter the pants.

The obsession was making him miserable. He could not concentrate on his work. He repeatedly asked fellow employees whether they thought his pants were too long or too short and was convinced that they thought he was crazy (which perhaps they did). He had legitimate fears of losing his position at the bank. He started staying home more and more, hating himself for succumbing to what he recognized was a foolish fear. But he could not stop having the fear. It came to occupy most of his waking hours as he altered between studying the pant leg to see if it should be a millimeter shorter or longer and castigating himself for being a weak and feckless fellow in worrying about such matters.

Although P. T. had mild-to-moderate symptoms of depression, the obsession dominated his clinical picture. It had begun in his early twenties and had persisted more or less intensely since then. He had no other obsessions. In previous times the symptom would have been called a monomania.

NATURAL HISTORY

Most obsessionals develop their illness before age twenty-five (9). The median age of onset in one study (54) was twenty-three. Many obsessionals have clear-cut obsessional symptoms by age fifteen and the illness may begin as early as age six. Fewer than 15 percent of obsessionals develop their illness after age thirty-five (17, 28, 41, 51).

Though the mean age of onset of symptoms is roughly twenty in both sexes, the first psychiatric contact is made on the average about seven years later. If hospitalized, most patients are in their thirties by the time they enter a hospital. Rarely are obsessionals admitted to a psychiatric hospital for the first time after age forty (21).

The mode of onset may be acute or insidious (41). The course of obsession disorder may be unremitting (with or without social incapacity), episodic, or characterized by incomplete remissions that permit normal social functioning.

In one outpatient study, the majority of patients had episodic courses with exacerbations that usually lasted less than a year (53). Most investigators who study patients requiring hospitalization, however, have found the course to be steady, with exacerbations often attributed to fatigue or medical illness and with a tendency for the severity of the illness to wane gradually over many years (28, 45).

Obsessionals with mild symptoms requiring only outpatient therapy appear to have a rather good prognosis; as many as 60 to 80 percent are asymptomatic or improved one to five years after diagnosis (35, 53). Hospitalized cases as a group do less well. One-third or fewer are improved symptomatically on reexamination several years after discharge; two-thirds or more, however, are functioning as well socially as before hospitalization (28, 41). Between 5 and 10 percent of clear-cut obsessionals do have a course marked by progressive social incapacity (58). Favorable prognosis is reported to be associated with three factors: (a) mild or atypical symptoms, including predominance of phobic-ruminative ideas and absence of compulsions (28, 41); (b) short duration of symptoms before treatment is begun (53); and (c) good premorbid personality without childhood symptoms or abnormal personality traits (41, 42). The specific content of obsessions is not believed to have prognostic significance (Table 5.2).

Table 5.2 Follow-up studies of Obssesive-Compulsive Disorder

| Sample Characteristics | | | | Length of Follow-up | Condition on Follow-up (%) | | |
Author	Place	Pt. Source*	N†	(To Nearest Year)	Asymptomatic	Improved	Unimproved
Balslev-Olesen and Geert-Jorgensen (6)	Denmark	I, O	52	0–8	6	58	57
Coryell (13)	U.S.	I	36	1–32	22	57	22
Grimshaw (22)	England	O	97	1–14	40	24	35
Hastings (24)	U.S.	I	23	6–12	13	40	47
Ingram (28)	England	I	46	1–11	9	50	61
Kringlen (41)	Norway	I	85	13–20	4	45	45
Langfeldt (42)	Norway	I	27	1–11	26	41	33
Lewis (44)	England	I, O	50	>5	32	34	34
Lo (45)	Hong Kong	I, O	87	1–14	20	36	44
Luff and Garrod (46)	England	O	49	3	39	27	34
Pollitt (53)	England	I, O	66	0–15	24	48	28
Rennie (56)	U.S.	I	47	20	36	38	26
Rüdin (59)	Germany	I, O	130	2–26	12	26	61

*I = inpatient; O = outpatient

†Excluded are lobotomized cases and patients dead on follow-up. The sex ratio differs from study to study but approaches unity when all studies are combined

Source: Goodwin et al. (10)

COMPLICATIONS

Depression—often indistinguishable symptomatically from depression seen in major depression—is probably the most common complication of obsessional disorder.

Failure to marry also may be a complication of obsessional disorder, judging by three studies (28, 45, 59) that show a higher rate of celibacy among obsessionals than in the general population.

Despite the frequency with which suicide may figure in obsessional thinking (22, 28), obsessionals rarely commit suicide. In most studies less than 1 percent of the patients committed suicide.

Obsessional patients sometimes fear they will injure someone by an impulsive act. They fear they will lose control and embarrass themselves in some manner. They worry about becoming addicted to drugs prescribed by their physician. These fears are generally unwarranted (13). There is little evidence that obsessional disorder predisposes to homicide, criminal behavior, alcoholism, or drug addiction (28, 41).

Finally, obsessionals may fear they will "lose" their minds, become totally disabled, need chronic hospitalization. None of these events is a common complication of obsessional disorder. If schizophrenia is clearly ruled out at the beginning, obsessionals probably become schizophrenic no more often than nonobsessionals. They infrequently become totally disabled, and they usually do not require long-term hospitalization (22, 28, 53).

FAMILY HISTORY

Two studies comparing parents of obsessionals with parents of other psychiatric patients found the former group to be significantly more perfectionistic (7, 45), obstinate, pedantic, and parsimonious (41). Studies without controls have yielded similar findings (6, 44). Unfortunately, such attributes as perfectionism and obstinacy are vague and resist quantification. Even in controlled studies, it is unclear whether observer bias has been suffi- ciently eliminated to render the results meaningful. A more re- cent study found no increased prevalence of personality disorders—including compulsive personalities—in first-degree relatives of patients with OCD (8, 9).

Psychiatric illness in the families of obsessionals has been stud- ied by several investigators. Many obsessionals have close rela- tives with psychiatric illness (6, 8, 26, 58). In one study, about 30 percent of the siblings of obsessionals had been treated for psychi- atric symptoms (about one-quarter as inpatients) (44) and in another study, about 10 percent of the first-degree relatives of obsessionals had received psychiatric treatment (58).

Obsessional illness may occur with greater frequency in the families of obsessionals than in the families of other patients (or in the general population), but so do other psychiatric illnesses, and the extent of increased risk is uncertain (9, 31). One study comparing the families of obsessionals with those of other psychi- atric and medical patients found not only a higher incidence of obsessional disorder in the families of obsessionals (8 percent of parents, 7 percent of siblings) but also a higher incidence of other psychopathology: For example, about 8 percent had manic de- pressive disease (6). In another study (19), *no* instances of obses- sive compulsive disorder were found in 174 relatives of 10 se- verely obsessive-compulsive patients, although 12 percent of first-degree relatives had been hospitalized for psychiatric illness. A review of eleven studies (8) of relatives of persons with OCD suggested that family members have increased rates of anxiety disorders *in general* but not of OCD in particular. Some evidence suggests a link to Tourette's syndrome (37, 43, 52). About half of people with Tourette's syndrome also have obsessive-compulsive symptoms.

Moreover, in one study, relatives of patients with Tourette's syndrome had an increased rate of OCD whether the Tourette's probands had OCD symptoms or not. No increase in other anxiety disorders was found among the family members of Tourette's patients (52). This was unexpected. The association between

OCD and Tourette's syndrome is firmly established but family studies of the disorders yield conflicting results.

Studies of twins with obsessional illness indicate that monozygotic twins are more concordant for obsessional illness than dizygotic twins (29). About 80 to 90 percent of monozygotic twins are concordant for obsessional illness versus a concordance rate in dizygotic twins of no more than 50 percent and probably much lower. This does not prove the existence of genetic factors in obsessional illness; all of the twin pairs were raised together and identical twins may emulate each other more than fraternal twins. However, in instances where twins have little contact, environmental explanations seem implausible, as illustrated by the following case histories adapted from a published report (49).

The "W" Twins

Jean, a housewife, developed her symptoms at twenty-four when she acquired a fear of contamination by dirt with severe washing and cleansing rituals. At the time of her referral to this hospital three years later she was washing her hands between sixty and eighty times per day, spending twelve hours a day cleaning and disinfecting her house, and using up to twenty quarts of liquid disinfectant a week. Her daughter, aged two-and-a-half years, was not toilet trained and was restricted to one room of the house in order to avoid spread of contamination, and her husband had been obliged to give up sports for fear that his soiled sports clothes would introduce dirt to their home. On admission to the hospital the skin of her hands was roughened, red, cracked, and bleeding.

Jill, the co-twin, a social worker, developed her symptoms at twenty-two when she and Jean were leading separate lives and had little contact with each other. Her traits of neatness and cleanliness became more pronounced and she developed rituals concerned with washing up the crockery and cutlery which had to be started immediately when a meal was finished, any delay resulting in severe anxiety; the washing of the dishes and utensils had to proceed in a specific order and failure to comply with the routine, or an attempt by others to relieve her of her task, provoked great discomfort. She attempted to resist carrying out her rituals, which she considered silly and unnecessary, but the time spent on them increased and interfered with her social life.

Their father, a retired clerk, was fastidiously neat and orderly in his habits but neither he nor other family members had received psychiatric treatment. Their early development and childhood were unremarkable, and at school both did well academically. They attended separate universities. Both were normally outgoing and sociable and both had personality traits of orderliness, determination, and conscientiousness. Neither had suffered any previous illness and they only learned of their similar obsessional problems after Jean began treatment.

The "K" Twins

Linda, a secretary, began having obsessional thoughts at twenty-five when she felt envious of a roommate who had formed a close relationship with a man. Aware of her envy and associated guilt, she began to think of imaginary pleasant scenes of herself with her friend, but within a few weeks these thoughts became recurrent, intrusive, and difficult to resist and were no longer associated with relief of unpleasanat feelings. Obsessional thoughts troubled her to a varying degree for several years, with exacerbations during times of stress or unhappiness. Often she would have to repeat a conversation in her mind and, if interrupted before it was completed, she felt bound to repeat the whole conversation again. Sometimes she was compelled to touch an object to signify completion of an obsessional thought and this sometimes had a magical aspect; for example, if the object was a clock, the numbers indicating the time became her "lucky numbers" for the rest of the day.

Ann, the co-twin, an actress, also developed obsessional thoughts in her mid-twenties. She was not in regular contact with Linda at this time and only years later learned of her similar difficulties. Ann also used "good thoughts" to counter anxiety which was usually caused by parental disapproval of her career. The thoughts soon developed an obsessional quality and were associated with compulsive behavior. For example, if a "bad thought" occurred to her while speaking on the telephone, after the call was ended she felt compelled to repeat the conversation and create "good thoughts." If she passed a shop window and could not recall its contents she would have to go back and check them and she often spent hours arranging clothing in her wardrobe according to the color or type of garment. Although she considered her obsessions to be irrational, any attempts to resist them gave rise to the fears of impending disaster.

The father was an accountant described as being "compulsively neat." Their mother had older twin sisters who both had a life-long phobia of birds.

DIFFERENTIAL DIAGNOSIS

Obsessions occur in children, in healthy adults, and in patients with a variety of psychiatric and medical illnesses.

The rituals and superstitions of children—avoidance of sidewalk cracks, insistence on a given routine, carrying of amulets and charms—may resemble the compulsive acts of obsessional disorder, but with a difference: Children usually do not complain about these acts, which seem natural to them and produce little distress. Nor do obsessional children view the behavior as unreasonable.

Only a small proportion of children manifesting obsessional behavior can be classified by usual standards as having obsessional disorder. It is not known whether children who are exceptionally ritualistic and superstitious have a greater risk of developing obsessional disorder than their less-obsessional peers.

Many adult obsessionals give a history of obsessional symptoms in childhood (21, 45, 59), but the commonness of such symptoms and the influence of retrospective distortion make such data hard to interpret. Obsessionals commonly cite phobias and rituals as childhood symptoms (28, 41, 45). They rarely give a history of stealing, truancy, or tantrums in childhood (41, 45).

Obsessional personality (called obsessive-compulsive personality disorder in *DSM-IV*) is more a description than a diagnosis. No investigator has followed a group of clearly defined obsessional personalities over time to determine their fate; hence the label has no predictive value and is not in this sense a diagnosis. The individual with an obsessional personality is punctual, orderly, scrupulous, meticulous, and dependable. He is also rigid, stubborn, pedantic, and something of a bore. He has trouble making up his mind, but once made up, is single-minded and obstinate (49).

Many individuals with obsessional disorder have obsessional personalities antedating the illness (41, 53, 59), although one study (9) found no relationship between obsessional disorder and obsessional personality. The proportion of obsessional personalities who develop obsessional disorder, depression, or other psychiatric illness is not known.

Phobias are commonly associated with obsessional disorder, and obsessionals often have anxiety symptoms. Obsessional phobias have a compulsive quality and are almost always accompanied by rituals as well as other obsessional phenomena (41). The phobias of phobic disorders, on the other hand, are characterized primarily by simple avoidance of the anxiety-provoking object or situation.

Obsessions and depression occur together so commonly that discriminating symptom from illness may be difficult. The difficulty is compounded by the fact that obsessionals may develop a depression as florid as that seen in major depression or bipolar illness. During the depression the obsessional symptoms may remain unchanged, worsen, or disappear. Similarly, after the depression the obsessions may be worse, better, or unchanged (the last being the most common outcome) (19).

Episodes of depression, in a substantial number of cases, are accompanied by obsessions (19). These are usually ruminative in nature, characterized by guilt and self-deprecation, and mild by comparison with the depressed mood. In more atypical depressions, however, obsessions may dominate the picture. According to one study, one-third of depressives have obsessional personality traits premorbidly and during remissions (44). Obsessional traits apparently precede depression as often as they precede obsessional disorder (44).

Obsessional disorder in some instances may be as cyclical as bipolar disorder, with alternating remissions and exacerbations having no apparent relation to life events (28, 45, 53). The history may suggest affective disorder, the symptoms obsessional disorder. Some clinicians treat patients with cyclical obsessions as if they had depressions, that is, with antidepressant drugs or electrotherapy.

In distinguishing between obsessional disorder and major depression, the following points may be helpful: Compared with depressives and bipolars who have obsessional symptoms, obsessionals who develop a depression do so at an earlier age, have more depressive episodes in their history, exhibit obsessional symptoms episodically during each depression, have a lower rate of attempted suicide, and lack a history of mania (19).

Family history is of diagnostic value when it includes clear-cut depressions, mania, suicide, or alcoholism, which are found more regularly in the families of depressives than in the families of patients with any other illness (69).

Mistaking obsessional disorder for schizophrenia is not unusual, especially in the early stages of the illness. Error may arise from difficulty in distinguishing obsessions from delusions and from equating bizarreness or disablement with schizophrenia. Early onset and insidious development are common in both illnesses.

Schizophrenia is characterized by delusions, hallucinations, and *formal* thought disorder (form referring to the flow and connections of thought). Obsessional disorder is primarily a disorder of thought *content.* The speech of obsessionals is understandable; their ideas are weird. The fact that obsessionals recognize they are weird is one of the chief distinctions between obsessional neurosis and schizophrenia.

According to one study, obsessions occur in schizophrenia in about 3 percent of cases, usually early in the course and almost always in the paranoid type (62). When obsessions and schizophrenia symptoms occur together, schizophrenia is usually the most appropriate diagnosis.

Obsessions have been observed in the following organic condition: encephalitis lethargia—especially during oculogyric crises; early stages of arteriosclerotic dementia; post-encephalitic states; hearing loss with tinnitus; and hypothyroidism (21).

Each of these conditions may be accompanied by the sense that one's mind is working independently, that it is not an integrated part of oneself (44), and by repetitive behavior resembling compulsions. However, the "forced thinking" and "organic orderliness" (20) occasionally observed in brain-damaged patients are said to be less well organized than those that occur in obsessional disorder, and they also lack the sense of internal compulsion that distinguishes the latter condition.

The hallmarks of organic brain disease—confusion, disorientation, memory loss—are not seen in obsessional disorder. Their presence makes the diagnosis comparatively simple. Past history; neurological examination; blood, urine, and spinal fluid studies; plus special imaging techniques help establish the specific cause.

CLINICAL MANAGEMENT

The data on obsessional disorder justify a certain measure of optimism about its natural course. Spontaneous improvement often occurs, and the patient can be informed of this. She can be reassured that her impulses to commit injury or socially embarrassing acts almost certainly will not be carried out and that she will not—as she often fears—lose her mind. If she needs to be hospitalized, she can be assured that the hospitalization is unlikely to be a long one.

Obsessionals are rarely helped by psychotherapy alone. "Insight" therapy may even by contraindicated. "A searching, interpretive, in-depth approach," wrote one therapist, "in many instances facilitates an introspective obsessive stance" (48). Pessimism about psychotherapy for obsessional disorder is reflected by the scarcity of publications on the subject. Of several hundred articles listed in *Index Medicus* that pertain to therapies for obsessional disorder, only 16 percent are studies of psychotherapy. By far the largest number are studies of behavioral treatments.

Behavior therapy derives from learning theory. According to learning theory, obsessional thoughts are conditioned responses to anxiety-provoking stimuli. Compulsions are established when the individual discovers that the compulsive act reduces the anxiety attendant on obsessional thought. The reduction in anxiety reinforces the compulsive act.

The techniques of behavior therapy are manifold, but their ap-

plication to obsessional disorder usually involves a single princi-
ple: The patient must be exposed to the fear-inducing stimulus.
After repeated exposure, the fear disappears because, at bottom, it
is unfounded. As fear subsides, so do the obsessions and compulsions. The various techniques for achieving this goal bear such
names as desensitization, flooding, implosion, paradoxical intention, operant shaping, and cognitive rehearsal (5, 11, 12, 16, 17,
38).

More than a dozen studies indicate that behavior therapy produces relief from compulsive rituals in many patients; the relief is
maintained for at least two to three years following treatment (47,
48). There is less evidence that obsessions are relieved by behavior therapy. The type of behavior therapy producing the best results is called "in vivo exposure." "In vivo" means the patients
repeatedly confront the actual source of the anxiety that evokes
the ritual. For example, compulsive handwashers might be asked
to touch the sole of a dirty shoe and otherwise force themselves to
handle dirty objects. The compulsive tidier and checker of windows might be asked to untidy his or her possessions and deliber-
ately refrain from checking rituals. In many patients, the anxiety-
evoking stimulus eventually will be tolerated without evoking
rituals.

Exposure therapy takes up to thirty sessions in the therapist's
office plus self-exposure homework, sometimes with relatives co-
operating as exposure cotherapists. Some patients are too apprehensive to submit to such an ordeal. Others are too depressed. But
as Marks points out (48), the evidence supporting the efficacy of
exposure therapy for compulsive rituals is impressive.

Many drugs also have been used in the treatment of obsessional
disorder. They include phenothiazines, monoamine oxidase inhibitors (MAOIs), lysergic acid diethylamide (LSD), L-trypto-
phan, and tricyclic antidepressants (32). With the exception of
chlorimipramine, a tricyclic antidepressant, the only evidence for
efficacy of the above agents has come from single case reports or
open trials. Double-blind, placebo-controlled studies (2, 4, 30,

48, 66) of chlorimipramine have indicated antiobsessional effects from this drug. There has been only one negative report (56).

Until recently, chlorimipramine was clearly the drug that showed the most promise as a specific antiobsessional agent. There has been much speculation about its mode of action. Chlorimipramine inhibits serotonin reuptake and thus potentiates serotonergic activity, the latter believed to have a mood-altering effect (14, 23, 32, 34, 64). Tryptophan, the amino acid precursor of serotonin, is reported to relieve obsessional symptoms (3), supporting the idea that serotonin in some way is related to obsessional thinking. (Tryptophon has been withdrawn from the market.)

With the introduction of selective serotonin-reuptake inhibitors (SSRIs), the role of serotonin and OCD has received more attention. One SSRI, fluoxetin (Prozac), has won FDA approval for the treatment of OCD; other SSRIs will probably receive similar approval. It is not clear why these drugs are effective. Studies of blood serotonin concentration in OCD patients have produced mixed results, one (23) showing that OCD patients had *higher* pretreatment blood levels of serotonin than controls. This contradicts the idea that the mechanism of action of SSRIs is to *increase* serotonin levels. Imaging studies suggest that SSRIs may normalize cerebral metabolism, said to be subnormal in OCD (64).

Monoamine oxidase inhibitors (MAOIs) *are* available in the United States, and single case reports with phenelzine sulfate (33) and tranylcypromine sulfate (36) describe marked improvement in obsessional patients. Clorgyline, in a double-blind comparison with chlorimipramine, proved ineffective (30). In other anxiety disorders such as phobic states, MAOIs have been found to be effective (68), so these drugs still show promise.

Benzodiazepines relieve anxiety accompanying obsessions, and antidepressants relieve depression seen with the disorder. Except for chlorimipramine, and SSRIA, neither group seems to reduce the obsessional thinking.

In summary, the literature indicates that in vivo exposure is the most effective treatment for compulsive rituals and that some antidepressants are promising drugs for obsessional ideation. Behavior therapy has one strong advantage over drugs: The improvement persists after the treatment ends. Studies agree that chlorimipramine is effective only while the drug is being taken.

A word about electroshock therapy and lobotomy. The former is viewed by much of the general public and some physicians as a more drastic treatment than, say, antidepressant drugs, but this is arguable. Lobotomy has fallen into disrepute, more justifiably. In any case, there has been only one study of EST for obsessive-compulsive disorder.

The study suggests that EST is less effective for depression associated with obsessional disorder than for primary depression (59). In this series, half the obsessionals receiving electroconvulsive therapy (ECT) improved and half did not.

Five follow-up studies (22, 25, 41, 53, 67) indicate that lobotomy produces symptomatic improvement in obsessional disorder superior to that which occurs spontaneously. The more "typical" the obsessional illness, one investigator found, the more likely this was true (41). For a small minority of patients, therefore, lobotomy may warrant consideration. Before undertaking such irreversible treatment, evaluation by two or more psychiatrists is highly desirable. There is general agreement that, if used at all, lobotomy should be reserved for those severely ill obsessional patients with classical symptoms (especially rituals) who fail to respond to other treatments and are totally disabled by their illness.

REFERENCES

1. Akhtar, S., Wig, N., Varma, V., Pershad, D., and Verma, S. A phenomenological analysis of symptoms in obsessive-compulsive neurosis. Brit. J. Psychiat. *127*:342–348, 1975.

2. Ananth, J., Pecknold, J. C., Van Den Steen, M., and Engelsmann, F. Double-blind comparative study of clorimipramine and amitriptyline in obsessive neurosis. Prog. Neuropsychopharmacol. *5*:257–262, 1981.

3. Ananth, J. Clorimipramine in obsessive-compulsive disorder: a review. Psychosomatics. *24*:723–727, 1983.

4. Ananth, J. Clorimipramine: an antiobsessive drug. Can. J. Psychiat. *3*:253–258, 1986.

5. Baer, L. Behavior therapy for obsessive compulsive disorder in the office-based practice. J. Clin. Psychiat. *54(Suppl. 6)*:10–15. 1993.

6. Balslev-Olesen, T., and Geert-Jorgensen, E. The prognosis of obsessive-compulsive neurosis. Acta Psychiat. Scand. *34*:232–241, 1959.

7. Brown, F. W. Heredity in the psychoneuroses. Proc. R. Soc. Med. *35*:785–790, 1942.

8. Black, D. W., Noyes, R., Goldstein, R. B., and Blum, N. A family study of obsessive-compulsive disorder. Arch. Gen. Psychiat. *49*:362–368, 1992.

9. Black, D. W., Noyes, R., Pfohl, B., Goldstein, R. B., and Blum, N. Personality disorder in obsessive-compulsive volunteers, well comparison subjects, and their first-degree relatives. Am. J. Psychiat. *150*:8, 1993.

10. Burke, K. C., Burke, J. D., Regier, D. A., and Rae, D. S. Age at onset of selected mental disorders in five community populations. Arch. Gen. Psychiat. *47*:511–518, 1990.

11. Carney, R. M. Behavior therapy and the anxiety disorders: some conceptual and methodological issues. Psychiat. Dev. *3*:65–81, 1985.

12. Cobb, J. Behaviour therapy in phobic and obsessional disorders. Psychiat. Dev. *1*:351–365, 1983.

13. Coryell, W. Obsessive-compulsive disorder and primary unipolar depression: comparisons of background, family history, course, and mortality. J. Nerv. Ment. Dis. *169*:220–224, 1981.

14. DeVeaugh-Geiss, J., Katz, R., Landau, P., Goodman, W., and Rasmussen, S. Clinical predictors of treatment response in obsessive compulsive disorder: exploratory analyses from multicenter trials of clomipramine. Psychopharmacol. Bull. *26(1)*:54–59, 1990.

15. Dowson, J. The phenomenology of severe obsessive-compulsive neurosis. Brit. J. Psychiat. *131*:75–78, 1977.

16. Fals-Stewart, W., Marks, A. P., and Schafer, J. A comparison of behavioral group therapy and individual behavior therapy in treating obsessive-compulsive disorder. J. Nerv. Ment. Dis. *181(3)*:189–193, 1993.

17. Foa, E. B., Steketee, G. S., Ozarow, B. J. Behavior therapy with obsessive-compulsives: from theory to treatment. In *Obsessive-Compulsive Disorders: Psychological and Pharmacological Treatments*, Mavissakalian, M (ed.), 49–129. New York: Plenum, 1985.

18. Freud, S. Notes upon a case of obsessional neurosis. In *Standard Edition of the Complete Psychological Works of Sigmund Freud*, vol. 10, 153. London: Hogarth Press, 1955.

19. Gittleson, N. L. The phenomenology of obsessions in depressive psychosis. Brit. J. Psychiat. *112*:261–264, 1966.

20. Goldstein, K. *After Effects of Brain Injuries in War. Their Evaluation and Treatment.* New York: Grune & Stratton, 1942.

21. Goodwin, D. W., Guze, S. B., and Robins, E. Follow-up studies in obsessional neurosis. Arch. Gen. Psychiat. *20*:182–187, 1969.

22. Grimshaw, L. The outcome of obsessional disorder: a follow-up study of 100 cases. Brit. J. Psychiat. *111*:1051–1056, 1965.

23. Hanna, G. L., Yuwiler, A., and Cantwell, D. P. Whole blood serotonin in juvenile obsessive-compulsive disorder. Biol. Psychiat. *29*:738–744, 1991.

24. Hastings, D. W. Follow-up results in psychiatric illness. Am. J. Psychiat. *114*:1057–1065, 1958.

25. Hay, P., Sachdev, P., Cumming, S., Smith, J. S., Lee, T., Kitchener, P., and Matheson, J. Treatment of obsessive-compulsive disorder by psychosurgery. Acta. Psychiat. Scand. *87(3)*:197–207, 1993.

26. Hoover, C. F., and Insel, T. R. Families of origin in obsessive-compulsive disorder. J. Nerv. Ment. Dis. *172*:207–215, 1984.

27. Hunter, R., and Macalpine, I. *Three Hundred Years of Psychiatry*, pp. 1535–1860. London: Oxford Univ. Press, 1963.

28. Ingram, I. M. Obsessional illness in mental hospital patients. J. Ment. Sci. *107*:382–402, 1961.

29. Inouye, E. Similar and dissimilar manifestations of obsessive-compulsive neurosis in monozygotic twins. Am. J. Psychiat. *131*:1171–1175, 1965.

30. Insel, T. R., Murphy, D. L., Cohen, R. M., et al. Obsessive-compulsive disorder: a double-blind trial of chlorimipramine and clorgyline. Arch. Gen. Psychiat. *40*:605–612, 1983.

31. Insel, T. R. Obsessive-compulsive disorder. Psychiat. Clin. North Am. *8*:105–117, 1985.

32. Insel, T. R., and Winslow, J. T. Neurobiology of obsessive compulsive disorder. Psychiatr. Clin. North Am. *15(4)*:813–824, 1992.

33. Jain, V. K., Swinson, R. P., and Thomas, J. E. Phenelzine in obsession neurosis. Brit. J. Psychiat. *117*:237–238, 1970.

34. James, W. A., and Lippmann, S. B. Clomipramine for obsessive-compulsive disorder: prescribing guidelines. South Med. J. *84*:1243–1245, 1991.

35. Jaspers, K. *General Psychopathology*. Chicago: Univ. of Chicago Press, 1963.

36. Jenike, M. A. Rapid response of severe obsessive-compulsive disorder to tranylcypromine. Am. J. Psychiat. *138*:1249–1250, 1981.

37. Jenike, M. Obsessive compulsive disorder: a question of a neurologic lesion. Compr. Psychiat. *25*:298–304, 1984.

38. Jenike, M. A., and Rauch, S. C. Managing the patient with treatment-resistant obsessive compulsive disorder: current strategies. J. Clin. Psychiat. *55(Suppl. 3)*:11–17, 1994.

39. Kahn, R. S., Westenberg, H. G. M., and Jolles, J. Zimelidine treatment of obsessive-compulsive disorder. Acta Psychiat. Scand. *69*:259–261, 1984.

40. Karno, M., Golding, J. M., Sorenson, S. B., and Burnam, M. A. The epidemiology of obsessive-compulsive disorder in five US communities. Arch. Gen. Psychiat. *45*:1094–1099, 1988.

41. Kringlen, E. Obsessional neurotics: a long-term follow-up. Brit. J. Psychiat. *111*:709–722, 1965.

42. Langfeldt, G. Studier av Tvangsfernomenenes forelomist, genese, klinik og prognose. Norsk Laegeforen *13*:822–850, 1938.

43. Leckman, J. F., and Cohen, D. J. Recent advances in Gilles de la Tourette syndrome: implications of clinical practice and future research. Psychiat. Dev. *1*:301–316, 1983.

44. Lewis, A. J. Problems of obsessional illness. Proc. R. Soc. Med. *29*:325–336, 1936.

45. Lo, W. H. A follow-up study of obsessional neurotics in Hong Kong Chinese. Brit. J. Psychiat. *113*:823–832, 1967.

46. Luff, M. C., and Garrod, M. The after results of psychotherapy in 500 adult cases. Brit. Med. J. *11*:54–59, 1935.

47. Marks, I., Hodgson, R., and Rachman, S. Treatment of chronic obsessive-compulsive neurosis by in-vivo exposure. Brit. J. Psychiat. *127*:349–364, 1975.

48. Marks, I. M. Review of behavioral psychotherapy, I: obsessive-compulsive disorders. Am. J. Psychiat. *138*:584–592, 1981.

49. McGuffin, P., and Mawson, D. Obsessive-compulsive neurosis: two identical twin pairs. Brit. J. Psychiat. *137*:285–287, 1980.

50. Moore, J. *Of Religious Melancholy*. London: Published by Her Majesty's Special Command, 1692.

51. Orloff, L. M., Battle, M. A., Baer, L., Ivanjack, L., Pettit, A. R., Buttolph, M. L., and Jenike, M. A. Long-term follow-up of 85 patients with obsessive-compulsive disorder. Am. J. Psychiat. *151*:441–442, 1994.

52. Pauls, D. L., Leckman, J. F., and Cohen, D. J. Evidence against a genetic relationship between Tourette's syndrome and anxiety, depression, panic and phobic disorders. Brit. J. Psychiat. *164*:215–221, 1994.

53. Pollitt, J. Natural history of obsessional states: a study of 150 cases. Brit. Med. J. *1*:194–198, 1957.

54. Rasmussen, S. A., and Eisen, J. L. Epidemiology of obsessive compulsive disorder. J. Clin. Psychiat. *51*:10–13, 1990.

55. Rasmussen, S. A., and Tsuang, M. T. The epidemiology of obsessive compulsive disorder. J. Clin. Psychiat. *45*:450–457, 1984.

56. Rennie, T. A. C. *Prognosis in the Psychoneurosis: Benign and Malignant Developments, Current Problems in Psychiatric Diagnosis*, 66–79. New York: Grune & Stratton, 1953.

57. Robins, L. N., Helzer, J. E., Weissman, M. M., Orvaschel, H., Gruenberg, E., Burke, J. D., and Regier, D. A. Lifetime prevalence of specific psychiatric disorders in three sites. Arch. Gen. Psychiat. *41*:949–967, 1984.

58. Rosenberg, C. M. Familial aspects of obsessional neurosis. Brit. J. Psychiat. *113*:405–413, 1967.

59. Rüdin, G. Ein Beitrag zur Frage der Zwangskrankheit, insbesondere ihrer heriditaren Beziehungen. Arch. Psychiat. Nervenkr. *191*:14–54, 1953.

60. Schilder, P. Depersonalization. In *Introduction to Psychoanalytic Psychiatry*. Nerv. Ment. Dis. Monogr., Series 50, 1928.

61. Skoog, G. Onset of anancastic conditions. Acta Psychiat. Scand. *41(Suppl. 184)*:131, 1965.

62. Stengel, E. A study of some clinical aspects of the relationship between obsessional neurosis and psychotic reaction types. J. Ment. Sci. *91*:129, 1945.

63. Stern, R., and Cobb, J. Phenomenology of obsessive-compulsive neurosis. Brit. J. Psychiat. *132*:233–239, 1978.

64. Swedo, S. E., Pietrini, P., Leonard, H. L., Schapiro, M. B., Rettew, D. C., Goldberger, E. L., Rapoport, S. I., Rapoport, J. L., and Grady, C. L. Cerebral glucose metabolism in childhood-onset obsessive-compulsive disorder. Arch. Gen. Psychiat. *49*:690–694, 1992.

65. Taylor, J. *Ductor Dubitantium, or the Rule of Conscience.* London: Royston, 1660.

66. Thoren, P., Asberg, M., Cronholm, B., et al. Clorimipramine treatment of obsessive compulsive disorder: a controlled clinical trial. Arch. Gen. Psychiat. *37*:1281–1289, 1980.

67. Tippin, J., and Henn, F. Modified leukotomy in the treatment of intractable obsessional neurosis. Am. J. Psychiat. *139*:1601–1603, 1982.

68. Tyrer, P., Candy, J., and Kelly, D. Phenelzine in phobic anxiety: a controlled trial. Psychol. Med. *3*:120–124, 1973.

69. Winokur, G., Clayton, P. J., and Reich, T. *Manic Depressive Illness.* St. Louis: C. V. Mosby, 1969.

6

PHOBIC
DISORDERS

DEFINITION

A phobia is an intense, recurrent, unreasonable fear of a specific object, activity, or situation that results in a compelling desire to avoid the dreaded object, activity, or situation. A phobic disorder is a chronic condition dominated by one or more phobias. *DSM-III-R* subdivides phobias into specific phobias (e.g., fear of animals), social phobias (e.g., fear of public speaking), and agoraphobia. The last is often characterized by multiple phobias involving a fear of being in places where help might not be available in the event of a panic attack.

HISTORICAL BACKGROUND

Phobos was a Greek god who frightened one's enemies. His likeness was painted on masks and shields for this purpose. "Phobos," or "phobia," came to mean fear or panic (37).

"Phobia" first appeared in medical terminology in Rome two thousand years ago, when hydrophobia was used to describe a symptom of rabies. Though the term was not used in a psychiatric sense until the nineteenth century, phobic fears and behavior

153

were described in medical literature long before that. Hippocrates described at least two phobic persons. One was "beset by terror" whenever he heard a flute, whereas the other could not go beside "even the shallowest ditch," yet could walk in the ditch itself (25).

Robert Burton in *The Anatomy of Melancholy* distinguishes "morbid fears" from "normal" fears (10). Demosthenes's stage fright was normal, whereas Caesar's fear of sitting in the dark was morbid. Burton believed that morbid fears had little connection with willpower.

The term "phobia" appeared increasingly in descriptions of morbid fears during the nineteenth century, beginning with syphilophobia, defined in a medical dictionary published in 1848 as "a morbid dread of syphilis giving rise to fancied symptoms of the disease." Numberous theories were advanced to explain phobias, including poor upbringing (33).

In 1871 Westphal described three men who feared public places and labeled the condition agoraphobia, "agora" coming from the Greek word for place of assembly or marketplace (80). Excellent review articles on the historical development of the concept of phobia have been written by Errera (15) and Marks (33). They give Westphal credit for describing phobia in terms of a syndrome rather than an isolated symptom. Westphal even prescribed a treatment for the condition, suggesting that companionship, alcohol, or the use of a cane would be helpful.

Later authorities compiled long lists of phobias, naming each in Greek or Latin terms after the object or situation feared. Thus, as Nemiah points out, "the patient who was spared the pangs of taphaphobia (fear of being buried alive) or ailurophobia (fear of cats) might yet fall prey to belonophobia (fear of needles), siderodromophobia (fear of railways), or triskaidekaphobia (fear of thirteen at table), and pantaphobia was the diagnostic fate of that unfortunate soul who feared them all" (55).

Since the late nineteenth century there has been a continuing controversy over the relationship of phobias to other psychiatric disorders. Janet and Kraepelin, for example, sometimes spoke of phobias and obsessions as though they were synonymous. Others, such as Henry Maudsley and Melanie Klein, considered phobias to be a manifestation of affective illness (37, 72).

As noted, *DSM-III-R* classifies agoraphobia as a subtype of panic disorder. Regardless of the controversy, clinicians agree that phobias may occur in a variety of psychiatric conditions, but particular types of phobias are the primary manifestation of specific phobic disorders.

The prevalence of phobic disorders varies according to the sample being surveyed, the interview being employed, and the choice of diagnostic criteria. In the mid-1990s data began appearing from the latest survey using a structured psychiatric interview and a national probability sample in the United States (28). *DSM-III-R* criteria were used and the sample was drawn from the national population of noninstitutionalized civilians between the ages of 15 and 54. The interview, called the Composite International D Interview, was administered face to face by nonclinicians. A total of 8,098 respondents participated in the survey. The survey research center at the University of Michigan administered the interviews and analyzed the data.

The study yielded high rates for the three major types of phobia. Eleven percent of men gave a history of social phobia and 15% of women, for a total prevalence rate of social phobia of 13%. Rates of simple (specific) phobia were somewhat lower, which may come as a surprise since many authorities have viewed simple phobias as ubiquitous, especially in childhood and particularly in women. (Simple phobia would include fear of snakes and heights.) Seven percent of the men reported having simple phobias at some point in their life and 15% of the women, for a total prevalence rate of 11%. Agoraphobia (without panic disorder) also was reported to have a higher prevalence rate than had been found in other studies, with 3.5% of the men reporting agoraphobia and 7% of the females, for a total rate of 5.3% in both sexes.

These figures were for lifetime prevalence, meaning the respondents had been asked whether they had had a particular disorder at any time in their lives (remembering the respondents were between 15 and 54 at the time they were interviewed). They also were asked whether they had experienced the disorders in the 12-month period before the interview. In all categories there was a much lower prevalence of the phobic disorders in the year preceding the interview. In general, the figures for the 12-month period were about half of what they had been for lifetime. This has implications for the course of phobic disorders that contradict clinical observation and most studies. Phobias are believed to be chronic conditions. The finding that half of the subjects had experienced phobias in the past but not in the past 12 months suggests they are either episodic or temporary. Most phobic individuals never receive treatment for their phobias and therefore drugs or psychotherapy cannot be given credit for most of the decrease in prevalence when 12 months is compared to lifetime.

When broken down by demographic variables, this latest study (28) also contradicted earlier reports. One earlier report, for example, held that blacks were nearly twice as likely to have simple phobias and agoraphobia as whites. This difference did not show up in the survey.

One possible explanation for the higher prevalence was that in the survey respondents were shown three lists of twenty feared objects and situations, while interviewers in previous studies often presented no list. The validity of this study will probably never be tested because different criteria will be used and a different interview administered in future national surveys. This is a common problem in epidemiological studies and it means that the findings must be viewed tentatively.

Earlier studies had shown an association of alcoholism with social phobias and agoraphobia, and this association seems to hold up in the latest study. It appears that alcoholics have a high rate of phobia, one-third suffering from disabling phobias and another third from milder phobias. Several studies have confirmed an association of alcoholism with social phobias and agoraphobia (32, 58).

In clinical samples, two other reasons may explain the discrepancy in prevalence data concerning phobias: (a) some physicians may include what others consider normal fears in their statistics and (b) people tend to be secretive about phobias. Many people are embarrassed about their phobias and keep them secret. It is not unusual in psychiatric practice to see patients for long periods and then have them describe, almost in passing, a phobia that has plagued them for years.

CLINICAL PICTURE

Phobias can be distinguished from "normal" fears by their intensity, duration, irrationality, and the disablement resulting from avoidance of the feared situation.

DSM-V divides phobic disorders into three types: specific, social, and agoraphobia (Tables 6.1, 6.2, 6.3).

Table 6.1 Diagnostic criteria for Specific Phobia (*DSM-IV*)

A. Marked and persistent fear that is excessive or unreasonable, cued by the presence or anticipation of a specific object or situation (e.g., flying, heights, animals, receiving an injection, seeing blood)

B. Exposure to the phobic stimulus almost invariably provokes an immediate anxiety response, which may take the form of a situationally bound or situationally predisposed Panic Attack. NOTE: In children, the anxiety may be expressed by crying, tantrums, freezing, or clinging

C. The person recognizes that the fear is excessive or unreasonable. NOTE: In children, this feature may be absent

D. The phobic situation(s) is avoided or else is endured with intense anxiety or distress

E. The avoidance, anxious anticipation, or distress in the feared situation(s) interferes significantly with the person's normal routine, occupational (or academic) functioning, or social activities or relationships, or there is marked distress about having the phobia

F. In individuals under age 18 years, the duration is at least 6 months

G. The anxiety, Panic Attacks, or phobic avoidance associated with the specific object or situation is not better accounted for by another mental disorder, such as Obsessive-Compulsive Disorder (e.g., fear of dirt in someone with an obsession about contamination), Post-

(Continued)

Table 6.1 Diagnostic criteria for Specific Phobia (*DSM-IV*) (*Continued*)

traumatic Stress Disorder (e.g., avoidance of stimuli associated with a severe stressor), Separation Anxiety Disorder (e.g., avoidance of school), Social Phobia (e.g., avoidance of social situations because of fear of embarrassment), Panic Disorder With Agoraphobia, or Agoraphobia Without History of Panic Disorder

Specify type:

ANIMAL TYPE: if the fear is cued by animals or insects. This subtype generally has a childhood onset

NATURAL ENVIRONMENT TYPE: if the fear is cued by objects in the natural environment, such as storms, heights, or water. This subtype generally has a childhood onset

BLOOD-INJECTION-INJURY TYPE: if the fear is cued by seeing blood or an injury or by receiving an injection or other invasive medical procedure. This subtype is highly familial and is often characterized by a strong vasovagal response

SITUATIONAL TYPE: if the fear is cued by a specific situation such as public transportation, tunnels, bridges, elevators, flying, driving, or enclosed places. This subtype has a bimodal age-at-onset distribution, with one peak in childhood and another peak in the mid-20s. This subtype appears to be similar to Panic Disorder With Agoraphobia in its characteristic sex ratios, familial aggregation pattern, and age at onset

OTHER TYPE: if the fear is cued by other stimuli. These stimuli might include the fear or avoidance of situations that might lead to choking, vomiting, or contracting an illness; "space" phobia (i.e., the individual is afraid of falling down if away from walls or other means of physical support); and children's fears of loud sounds or costumed characters

---

Table 6.2 Diagnostic criteria for Social Phobia (*DSM-IV*)

A. A marked and persistent fear of one or more social or performance situations in which the person is exposed to unfamiliar people or to possible scrutiny by others. The individual fears that he or she will act in a way (or show anxiety symptoms) that will be humiliating or embarrassing. NOTE: In children, there must be evidence of the capacity for age-appropriate social relationships with familiar people and the anxiety must occur in peer settings, not just in interactions with adults

Table 6.2 *(Continued)*

B. Exposure to the feared social situation almost invariably provokes anxiety, which may take the form of a situationally bound or situationally predisposed Panic Attack. NOTE: In children, the anxiety may be expressed by crying, tantrums, freezing, or shrinking from social situations with unfamiliar people

C. The person recognizes that the fear is excessive or unreasonable. NOTE: In children, this feature may be absent

D. The feared social or performance situations are avoided or else are endured with intense anxiety or distress

E. The avoidance, anxious anticipation, or distress in the feared social or performance situation(s) interferes significantly with the person's normal routine, occupational (academic) functioning, or social activities or relationships, or there is marked distress about having the phobia

F. In individuals under age 18 years, the duration is at least 6 months

G. The fear or avoidance is not due to the direct physiological effects of a substance (e.g., a drug of abuse, a medication) or a general medical condition and is not better accounted for by another mental disorder (e.g., Panic Disorder With or Without Agoraphobia, Separation Anxiety Disorder, Body Dysmorphic Disorder, a Pervasive Developmental Disorder, or Schizoid Personality Disorder)

H. If a general medical condition or another mental disorder is present, the fear in criterion A is unrelated to it, e.g., the fear is not of Stuttering, trembling in Parkinson's disease, or exhibiting abnormal eating behavoir in Anorexia Nervosa or Bulimia Nervosa

Specify if:
GENERALIZED: if the fears include most social situations (e.g., intiating or maintaining conversations, participating in small groups, dating, speaking to authority figures, attending parties). NOTE: Also consider the additional diagnosis of Avoidant Personality Disorder

A *specific phobia* (formerly called *simple phobia*) is an isolated fear of a single object or situation, leading to avoidance of the object or situation. The fear is irrational and excessive but not always disabling because the object or situation can sometimes be easily avoided (e.g., snakes, if you are a city dweller). Impairment

Table 6.3   Diagnostic criteria for Agoraphobia (*DSM-IV*)

A. Anxiety about being in places or situations from which escape might be difficult (or embarrassing) or in which help may not be available in the event of having an unexpected or situationally predisposed Panic Attack or panic-like symptoms. Agoraphobic fears typically involve characteristic clusters of situations that include being outside the home alone; being in a crowd or standing in a line; being on a bridge; and traveling in a bus, train, or automobile

B. The situations are avoided (e.g., travel is restricted) or else are endured with marked distress or with anxiety about having a Panic Attack or panic-like symptoms, or require the presence of a companion

C. The anxiety or phobic avoidance is not better accounted for by another mental disorder, such as Social Phobia (e.g., avoidance limited to social situation because of fear of embarrassment), Specific Phobia (e.g., avoidance limited to a single situation like elevators), Obsessive-Compulsive Disorder (e.g., avoidance of dirt in someone with an obsession about contamination), Post-traumatic Stress Disorder (e.g., avoidance of stimuli associated with a severe stressor), or Separation Anxiety Disorder (e.g., avoidance of leaving home or relatives)

---

may be considerable if the phobic object is common and cannot be avoided, such as a fear of elevators in someone who must use elevators at work.

A person with a specific phobia typically is no more (or less) anxious than anyone else until exposed to the phobic object or situation. Then he or she becomes overwhelmingly uncomfortable and fearful, sometimes having symptoms associated with a panic attack (palpitations, sweating, dizziness, difficulty breathing). The phobic person also fears the *possibility* of confronting the phobic stimulus. Called "anticipatory anxiety," this leads to avoidance of situations in which the stimulus might be present.

Some common specific phobias are fear of animals, heights, closed spaces, wind, storms, lightning, loud noises, driving a car, flying in airplanes, riding in subways, hypodermic needles, and blood. Less common ones include fear of running water and of going to the hairdresser. There is even the case of the tennis player who wore gloves because he was afraid of fuzz, and tennis balls are fuzzy. Phobias can develop toward almost any object or situation.

Animal phobias are perhaps the most common specific phobias or at least the most commonly studied. They occur often in childhood and are usually transient. Among adults, women are subject to animal phobias more often than men. The phobia usually involves only one kind of animal but may lead to frequent distress with mild social disablement if the animals are domestic, such as dogs or cats (21).

Fear of heights is another common phobia. The fear may be totally unrealistic. The person may be close enough to the ground, so that a fall would not cause injury. Some phobics will not walk down a flight of stairs if they see the open stairwell. Some will not look out a window from the second floor or above, particularly if the window goes from floor to ceiling. Others will not cross a bridge on foot, though they may go by car.

A fear of heights is really a fear of falling—and a fear of falling is really a fear of loss of support (33). More exactly, it is fear of loss of *visual* support. Hence, the person looking out a window experiences no fear if the window is waist-high. A car offers the same protection.

Behind the fear of losing visual support there seems to be a fear of being *drawn* over the edge of the height. The high-up window, the car's doors, provide a sense of protection that no amount of reasoning with oneself can give. The fear of losing support need not even involve heights.

While running for a bus, a woman suddenly felt dizzy and had to hold on to a lamppost for support. This recurred and gradually the patient became terrified to walk anywhere without holding on to a wall or furniture to support her—she was "furniture bound." (33)

Social phobias are another form of isolated phobia that generally lead to only mild forms of impairment. These include fear of eating in public, public speaking, urinating in the presence of others, or other behaviors that may be embarrassing but do not generally lead to total avoidance of the situations. Occasionally, severe handicap may result.

The young wife of a business executive refused to entertain associates of her husband with a dinner party or attend dinner parties in restaurants or someone else's home. Her husband made excuses for her but felt his career was being damaged by their lack of social life. At first her explanation for refusing to join in dinner parties was that it was a waste of time or too much trouble. Later she confessed, tearfully and with much embarrassment, that she was afraid of being *unable* to eat if strangers were watching. Questioned by her concerned husband, she said she was afraid that once food was in her mouth she would be unable to swallow it and then find herself in the embarrassing situation of not knowing where to dispose of the food. She was also afraid that she would gag on the food and possibly vomit.

She could eat in front of her husband with no difficulty until she told him about the phobia and then became concerned that *he* was watching her eat and expecting her to gag or vomit. From then on she ate alone in the kitchen. The marriage survived, but barely (21).

Other social phobias include a fear of practicing musical instruments because the neighbors will hear mistakes; a fear of swimming or undressing in front of others because of shame at one's appearance; and a fear of criticism from superiors.

Unlike specific and social phobias, *agoraphobia* has a complex clinical picture involving various combinations of symptoms, including phobias for the following:

1. *Public transportation:* trains, buses, subways, airplanes. When crowded, these vehicles may be intolerable to agoraphobics. Waiting in line is almost as bad, whether for a bus or a movie.

2. *Other confining Places:* tunnels, bridges, elevators, the hairdresser or barber's chair, and the dentist's chair. These fears belong to the category of claustrophobia, but most people with claustrophobia have only a single phobia and are not agoraphobics. Paradoxically, agoraphobics may also be fearful of open spaces such as empty parking lots.

3. *Being home alone.* Some agoraphobics require constant companionship, to the despair of friends, neighbors, and family.

4. *Being away from home* or another "safe" place where help cannot be readily obtained if needed. The agoraphobic is sometimes comforted just knowing there is a police officer or a doctor somewhere nearby.

In recent years, largely because of observations made by Klein and associates (30, 31), clinicians have come to realize that most agoraphobics give a history of panic attacks preceding the onset of phobias. This has led to the conceptualization of agoraphobia as a complication of panic disorder. According to Klein, agoraphobics experience one or more *spontaneous panic attacks* that lead to *anticipatory anxiety* that in turn leads to *phobic avoidance.* The latter explains why the "housebound housewife" becomes housebound: far better to experience a panic attack in the relative safety of one's home than in places or situations from which escape might be difficult (or embarrassing) or in which help might not be available. A bridge phobia may not involve a fear of bridges per se. Instead, it may reflect a fear of experiencing panic on a bridge. Phobias about buses, trains, or airplanes may arise from concern that a panic attack might occur in a vehicle from which escape is impossible or embarrassing.

Klein's concept

panic attack $\longrightarrow$ anticipatory anxiety $\longrightarrow$ phobic avoidance

is a concept now shared by many clinicians that led to a departure from conventional nomenclature in *DSM-III-R.* Instead of being listed under phobic disorders, as occurred in previous manuals, *DSM-III-R* adopted Klein's view of the disorder and described agoraphobia as a subtype of panic disorder. Depending on which symptoms predominate—the panic attacks or phobias—agoraphobia may fall in one of three categories: Panic Disorder with Agoraphobia, Panic Disorder without Agoraphobia, and Agoraphobia without History of Panic Disorder. (The term "panic disorder" first received official recognition in *DSM-III,* replacing the term "anxiety neurosis" and a host of synonyms for this term [see chapter 3].) *DSM-IV* continues the practice of separating agoraphobia/panic disorder into three categories.

Klein concedes that agoraphobics do not always give a history of panic disorder. However, he maintains that even those who do not give this history still experience "limited symptom attacks," which he views as milder forms of panic (27). Klein gave an example of what he meant by "limited symptom attacks," citing "patients with sudden dizzy feelings who feel as though their heads are floating off their shoulders and that they might fall down." Such patients may not experience a fully developed panic attack, involving cardiorespiratory symptoms. Some symptoms seen in "limited symptom attacks" may lead to confusion of anxiety states with Meniere's disease.

In fact, when agoraphobia was first described in the nineteenth century by neurologists, they referred to it by a German word meaning "dizziness in public places," probably caused by a disorder of the eye muscles. (One patient compared the sensation to standing on a boat in a rough sea, or being drunk.) From personal experience the essayist, E. B. White described the symptoms humorously (12):

> I will be walking along the street, say, and will take three normal steps in a forward direction: then, as I am about to set my foot down for the fourth step, the pavement moves an inch or two to the right and drops off three-quarters of an inch, and I am not quick enough for it. This results in my jostling somebody on my left, or hitting the corner of the Fred F. French building a glancing blow. It was fun for a few days, but I have recovered from the first fine ecstasy of dizziness, and am getting bored with it. Once I sidled into a police horse, and he gave me back as good as I gave him.

White saw a doctor who "partly by stealth, partly by cunning," gained entrance into his middle ear, hoping to discover there the secret of the dizziness.

Agoraphobics have other psychiatric symptoms than panic attacks and phobias. They tend to be anxious people. They are subject to depression and often experience an eerie feeling called "depersonalization." The feeling is hard to define and appears to be an unpleasant, scary sense of being unreal, strange, and disembodied, cut off from one's surroundings.

Agoraphobia is the most disabling of the phobic disorders. When severe, it can be as disabling as the most crippling forms of schizophrenia. Although agoraphobics almost never require chronic hospitalization, they are sometimes unable to leave home for months or years at a time. The more extreme cases may confine themselves to a single room or spend most of their time in bed. Even milder cases involve restrictions in social functioning. Victims are unable to visit friends and neighbors or go on family outings. They recruit other people to do their shopping and take their children to school. They postpone seeing the dentist and may cut their own hair. Fortunately, new treatments—behavioral and pharmacological—have provided relief for many (see Clinical Management).

NATURAL HISTORY

In three studies (2, 14, 38) phobic individuals have been followed for long periods to see what happens to them and their phobias. Here are the conclusions:

Simple phobias that begin in childhood and early adolescence tend to improve and eventually disappear. Five years after onset, about half of the young victims are symptom-free and almost all are improved.

Phobias that begin after adolescence continue for longer periods, with about half of patients improved after five years but only about 5 percent symptom-free. In the older group, the phobia gradually becomes more severe in about one-third of patients. About 20 percent are impaired in their work or social functioning because of the phobia.

Gender has little influence on the outcome of simple phobia: Women do as well (or poorly) as men, and age of onset is the most important prognostic indicator.

Simple phobias as a group have a more favorable prognosis than the other phobic disorders. They almost always involve a single isolated phobia, whereas social phobias more often involve two or more phobias and agoraphobia invariably involves multiple phobias.

Most social phobias first occur in adolescence or the early twenties. They rarely begin before puberty or after age thirty. Unlike simple phobias and agoraphobia, which affect women more often than men, social phobias affect both sexes equally (34, 74). They are the most common type of phobia in men. Most social phobias develop over several months, stabilizing after a period of years with a gradual diminution of severity in middle life. Most begin without any apparent precipitating event.

Agoraphobia usually develops in the middle or late twenties, almost never occurring before eighteen or after thirty-five. Of the three types of phobia, agoraphobia has the latest age of onset; simple phobia occurs most often in childhood and social phobia most often in adolescence (28, 48).

Simple phobias seem more strongly related to the occurrence of a single traumatic event than do social phobias. The onset of agoraphobia is particularly obscure. Agoraphobics rarely associate the onset of their phobias with a single frightening event, but vividly recall their *first* panic attack. Freud reported this first. In agoraphobia, he wrote, "We often find a recollection of a state of panic; and what the patient actually fears is a repetition of such an attack under those special conditions in which he believes he cannot escape it" (19).

Agoraphobics rarely have an explanation for the first anxiety attack. "It came out of the blue," they tend to say. They associate future anxiety attacks with other unpleasant possibilities—a fainting spell, a sudden illness, something embarrassing—but their real reason for staying in the house and avoiding open spaces and public places is to avoid another attack. What makes the prospect of an anxiety attack especially frightening is the unexplained nature of the first attack: If it happened for no obvious reason once, it could happen again for no obvious reason.

The first anxiety attack often occurs against a background of worry and unhappiness: job dissatisfaction, a domestic crisis, a serious medical illness, a death in the family. The relationship of nonspecific stress and the onset of agoraphobia has led some to call agoraphobia the "calamity syndrome." Nevertheless, agoraphobics do not associate the first anxiety attack with a *specific* stress that would justify panic. Isaac Marks quotes a patient as saying (33):

> I was standing at the bus stop wondering what to cook for dinner when suddenly I felt panicky and sweaty, my knees felt like jelly, and I had to hold on to the lamppost and I was afraid I would die. I got on the bus and was terribly nervous, but just managed to totter home. Since than I haven't liked to go out on the street and have never been on a bus again.

Marks comments:

> In such cases the primary event is anxiety which arose within the patient for no accountable reason. The phobia developed secondarily as the anxiety is attached to the immediate environment prevailing when the internal anxiety happens to surge. First comes the panic without relationship to the surroundings, the surroundings are then attached or "conditioned" to the anxiety and agoraphobia has begun.

One-half to three-quarters of mild or moderately disabled agoraphobics recover or substantially improve five to ten years after the illness begins. The severely disabled housebound patient may remain that way indefinitely. Some cases are short-lived but nobody knows how many. If the symptoms of agoraphobia persist for a year, they are almost certain to last much longer (33).

COMPLICATIONS

Social, occupational, and marital disability are the main complications of phobias (58). In isolated phobias the disability tends to be mild and is limited to responses to the phobic object or situation. Agoraphobics suffer greater impairment, sometimes to the point of being totally housebound.

In several series of patients, frigidity and other sexual maladjustments have been reported in association with agoraphobia. The frigidity often antedates the phobias (62, 78).

Agoraphobics occasionally have an affective syndrome indistinguishable from primary affective disorder except for the prior history of chronic phobias. Suicide does not appear to be a complication of phobic disorder. At least seven studies (8, 32, 42, 48, 57, 71, 74) indicate that agoraphobics and people with social phobias are particularly susceptible to alcohol dependence, but the National Comorbidity Survey (28) found high rates of anxiety disorders, including phobia, in the general population (20% of men and 30% of women had *some* anxiety disorder) and the prevalance rates among alcoholics is often found to be no higher, so it is no longer possible to conclude that alcoholics are more prone to these disorders than nonalcoholics.

In recent years, much attention has been focused on the relationship between mitral valve prolapse and anxiety disorders. It has been reported that as many as 50 percent of patients with panic disorder have mitral valve prolapse, which is considerably higher than the 4- to 17-percent prevalence reported in general population studies (12, 22, 26, 44). Kantor and associates found that 44 percent of twenty-five agoraphobic women had mitral valve prolapse compared with 17 percent of twenth-three age-matched controls (26).

FAMILY AND GENETIC STUDIES

Six studies (23, 27) have addressed the question of whether phobias aggregate in families. Five of the studies provided some evidence of familial aggregation. Only in agoraphobia, however, has there been consistent evidence of a specific phobia running true to type. Most studies show increased rates of agoraphobia in families of agoraphobics but not of social or simple phobias. One study found significantly higher rates for simple but not social phobia in relatives of affected versus control probands.

Three twin studies (27) but no adoption studies have addressed the nature–nurture issue. The largest twin study, in which more than 2,000 twins were interviewed, showed varying degrees of heritability for the different phobias (27). At one end of the spectrum was agoraphobia, which had the latest age of onset, the highest rates of comorbidity (as with affective disorder), the highest heritability, and the least evidence of environmental influences. At the other end of the continuum were simple phobias, which had the earliest age of onset, the lowest rates of comorbidity, the lowest heritability, and the strongest evidence of environmental influence. On nearly all of these measures, social phobia was intermediate between agoraphobia and simple phobias. The twins in this study were all women, and there is no way to know at this time whether the results apply equally to men (27).

One study revealed that 35 percent of the fathers of agoraphobics were alcoholic compared to 10 percent of fathers of controls (21). Affective disorders were more common in the first-degree relatives of the nonanxious controls (10 percent) than in the families of agoraphobics (7 percent), disputing the view that agoraphobia is a variant of affective disorder. In another study of sixty agoraphobics, 12 percent of the relatives had the illness, a rate significantly higher than in the general population (51).

Several studies indicate that phobics come from stable families in which the mothers may be overprotective (62, 78).

DIFFERENTIAL DIAGNOSIS

Phobias occur in psychiatric conditions other than phobic disorders, notably obsessional disorder and panic disorder. Because all three conditions begin early in life and have a chronic though sometimes fluctuating course, distinguishing them may be difficult. This is particularly true of agoraphobia when multiple phobias occur together with panic attacks, obsessional thinking, and other nonphobic psychiatric symptoms.

Panic disorder patients often have phobias, but the most conspicuous feature of panic disorder is anxiety attacks unrelated to external situations in which the subjective experience of fear is accompanied by cardiorespiratory symptoms. Obsessive-compulsive disorder is manifested by a panoply of obsessional symptoms, including checking and counting rituals, repetitive ideas relating to the possibility of harming oneself or others, and other recurrent thoughts.

Like patients with other anxiety disorders, phobics may become depressed and develop the full range of affective symptoms, physiological and subjective. When the phobias preceding the affective episode are isolated and nonincapacitating, it may be legitimate to view the affective disorder as "primary." With regard to agoraphobia, depressions commonly occur during the course of the illness and probably should be considered "secondary" (without giving this nosologic distinction etiological connotations). Some British authors consider agoraphobia an atypical form of affective disorder. Many of the symptoms of primary affective disorder may have phobic qualities such as fearfulness of social situations and disease.

When phobic-like symptoms occur in schizophrenia, they are usually bizarre and unaccompanied by insight.

Excessive worriers are sometimes diagnosed as having Generalized Anxiety Disorder. Despite the term, this often takes the form of anxiety about specific events such as work or school disturbance. The person is restless, easily tired, irritable, and has trouble concentrating as well as some sleep difficulty. People with this condition are seldom disabled and their fears (which are usually chronic) are distinguishable from phobia by their shifting focus and absence of avoidance behavior. About 5 percent of the population are afflicted by the disorder at some time in their lives (81).

CLINICAL MANAGEMENT

Regardless of the theoretical orientation of the therapist, it is generally agreed that at some point the phobic patient must confront the feared situation. Freud observed that "one can hardly ever master a phobia if one waits till the patient lets the analysis influence him to give it up. One succeeds only when one can induce them through the influence of the analysis to go about alone and to struggle with their anxiety while they make the attempt" (19).

Most treatments have been designed to reduce the phobic anxiety to the extent that the patient can tolerate exposure to the phobic situation. These treatments include drugs, psychotherapy, and behavior modification techniques.

A number of double-blind, placebo-controlled studies have demonstrated the efficacy of imipramine hydrochloride (61, 68, 83–85) and phenelzine sulfate (52, 76) in the treatment of phobic disorders, particularly agoraphobia associated with panic attacks. Uncontrolled clinical observations suggest that other antidepressants may also be effective.

In 1983 two additional large studies of imipramine and phenelzine were published, one by Klein and his colleagues in New York (31, 85) and the other by Marks and his British colleagues (40). They arrived at somewhat different conclusions. The New York group found that imipramine is effective in the treatment of panic attacks in agoraphobic patients; not all agoraphobics, however, have panic attacks. Furthermore, dynamically oriented supportive psychotherapy was reported to be as effective as behavior therapy, as long as both led to confrontation with the phobic situation. In contrast, the British group reported that imipramine was not superior to placebo in preventing panic attacks in the agoraphobic patient and that in vivo exposure (exposure to real-life phobic stimuli) was a specific and potent treatment for agoraphobia. The doses of imipramine and the schedule of administration were different in the two studies, and this may explain the discrepancy.

Imipramine and other tricyclic antidepressants as well as phenelzine and other monoamine oxidase inhibitors (MAOIs) may only be effective in preventing panic attacks when the patient is taking the medication (30, 40); there is some disagreement on this point. In one study (46), agoraphobic patients treated with imipramine remained symptom-free for at least six months after the drug was discontinued. Marks et al. (40) found that patients treated with in vivo exposure were much improved six weeks after the drug and behavioral treatment, but there was no benefit for the group treated only with phenelzine after the drug had been discontinued. Klein sometimes finds improvement persisting after imipramine is stopped. He also has switched from imipramine to desipramine because the latter has fewer anticholinergic side effects and greater patient compliance (31).

Klein (30) distinguishes between the panic component of agoraphobia and the anticipatory anxiety patients experience between panic attacks. Using higher doses of imipramine than did the British group, Klein reported a high rate of success in preventing panic attacks but no success in relieving anticipatory anxiety. Benzodiazepines have been suggested as an effective treatment for the latter.

Buspirone, the nonbenzodiazepine anxiolytic introduced in late 1986, however, may be the drug of choice for anticipatory anxiety. Unlike the benzodiazepines, which produce mild physical dependence, buspirone (75) apparently produces none and is as effective as the benzodiazepines in relieving anxiety.

In a review (34) Liebowitz and his coauthors called attention to several studies in which patients with social phobias have received relief with beta-adrenergic receptor blockers. Antidepressants of the MAOI class have also been recommended for social phobia; so have clonidine (66), benzodiazepines (64), and buspirone (42). Liebowitz calls social phobia the "neglected anxiety disorder." Treatments for the problem began to emerge in the mid-1980s.

Before the emphasis on pharmacotherapy, the most popular approach to the treatment of simple and social phobias involved behavioral techniques based on learning theory. Of these, "systematic desensitization," introduced by Wolpe, has been most widely used and studied (82). Nearly twenty studies, most of them controlled, indicate that systematic desensitization produces at least temporary relief of isolated phobias but is less effective in agoraphobia (4, 56, 59).

The method consists of training patients to relax and then gradually exposing them to more and more intensive versions of the phobic stimulus. This requires that patients imagine the feared events, starting with events that produce minimal anxiety and then progressing through a "hierarchy" to imagine events of maximal fearfulness. At this point, they are expected to confront the phobic situation in reality and by relaxation be able to tolerate it. The approach is based on the concept of "reciprocal inhibition" that holds that two mutually incompatible emotions such as fear and pleasure cannot be simultaneously experienced. Therefore, relaxation, being "pleasurable," theoretically cancels the sensation of fear if the latter is not overwhelming.

A variation of this approach consists of "flooding" the individual with the phobic stimulus at maximal intensity without progressing through a hierarchy. Flooding is apparently most effective with in vivo exposure. If the person is afraid of heights, the therapist may take him to the roof of a tall building and have him lean over the guardrail. The patient will be terrified. Terror, however, is not an emotion that can be sustained indefinitely, and, with continued exposure, he will find his anxiety diminishing.

Real-life flooding is often hard to arrange, so therapists fall back on imaginary flooding. After learning what frightens the patient the most, the therapist asks the patient to visualize his most frightening scene and helps by describing the scene. The therapist watches for signs of anxiety in the patient and repeats the scenes that produce the most anxiety. As with real-life flooding, the therapist keeps it up until the anxiety level falls. A recent comparison of imipramine and flooding in sixty-two agoraphobic patients indicated that imipramine had superior effects (45).

Some therapists embellish flooding by describing exaggerated catastrophic scenes to the patient. The patient who is afraid to drive is asked to imagine that she is driving a school bus that plunges over a cliff with everyone killed. The patient who is frightened of speaking out at a small meeting is told to imagine that she is the keynote speaker at a convention in Madison Square Garden. This is called *implosion therapy.*

What works best? There are studies showing that flooding is better than systematic desensitization; studies showing that systematic desensitization is better than flooding; and studies showing that both have the same effect or no effect (21, 49). What almost all studies show is that real-life exposure is superior to imaginary exposure.

REFERENCES

1. Agras, S., Sylvester, D., and Oliveau, D. The epdiemiology of common fears and phobia. Compr. Psychiat. *10*:151–156, 1969.
2. Agras, S., Chapin, H. N., and Oliveau, D. C. The natural history of phobia, course and prognosis. Arch. Gen. Psychiat. *26*:315–317, 1972.
3. Ayd, Jr., F. J. Antidepressant, 1959. Psychosomatics *1*:31, 1960.
4. Barlow, D. H. Comorbidity in social phobia: implications for cognitive-behavioral treatment. Bull. Menninger Clin. *58:2*(*Suppl. A*):A43–A57, 1994.
5. Bates, H. D. Predictive power of the reinforcement survey schedule; near null results. Newsl. Res. Psychol. *12*:113–116, 1970.
6. Berg, I. School phobia in the children of agoraphobic women. Brit. J. Psychiat. *128*:86–89, 1976.
7. Berg, I., Butler, A., and Pritchard, J. Psychiatric illness in the mothers of school phobic adolescents. Brit. J. Psychiat. *125*:466–467, 1974.
8. Bowen, R. C., Cipywynk, D., D'Arcy, D., and Keegan, D. Alcoholism, anxiety disorders, and agoraphobia. Alcoholism Clin. Exp. Res. *8*:48–50, 1984.
9. Buglass, D., Clarke, J., Henderson, A. S., Kreitman, N., and Presley, A. S. A study of agoraphobic housewives. Psychol. Med. *7*:73–86, 1977.
10. Burton, R. *The Anatomy of Melancholy* (1621), vol. 1, 11th ed. London, 1813.
11. Dally, P. J., and Rohde, P. Comparison of antidepressant drugs in depressive illnesses. Lancet *1*:18, 1961.
12. Darsee, J. R., Mikolich, J. R., Nicoloff, N. B., et al. Prevalence of mitral valve prolapse in presumably healthy young men. Circulation *59*:619–622, 1979.
13. Elledge, S. *E. B. White, a Biography*. New York: Oxford Univ. Press, 1984.
14. Emmelkamp, P. M. G., and Kuipers, A. C. M. Agoraphobia: a follow-up study four years after treatment. Brit. J. Psychiat. *134*:342–355, 1979.
15. Errera, P. Some historical aspects of the concept of phobia. Psychiat. Q. *36*:325–336, 1962.
16. Errera, P., and Coleman, J. V. A long-term follow-up study of neurotic patients in a psychiatric clinic. J. Nerv. Ment. Dis. *136*:267, 1963.
17. Frankel, F., and Orne, M. Hypnotizability and phobic behavior. Arch. Gen. Psychiat. *33*:1259–1261, 1976.
18. Frazier, S. H., and Carr, A. C. Phobic reactions. In *Comprehensive*

Textbook of Psychiatry. Freedman, A. M., and Kaplan, H. E. (eds.). Baltimore: Williams & Wilkins, 1967.

19. Freud, S. *Collected Papers,* vol. 2. New York: Basic Books, 1950.
20. Goldman, D. Clinical experience with newer antidepressant drugs and some related electroencephalographic observations. Ann. N.Y. Acad. Sci. *80*:687, 1959.
21. Goodwin, D. W. *Phobia: The Facts.* London: Oxford Univ. Press, 1983.
22. Gorman, J. M., Fyer, A. F., Gliklich, J., et al. Mitral valve prolapse and panic disorder: effect of imipramine. In *Anxiety Revisited.* Klein, D. F., and Rabkin, J. G. New York: Raven Press, 1981.
23. Gruppo Italiano Disturbi d'Ansia. Familial analysis of panic disorder and agoraphobia. J. Affective Dis. *17*:1–8, 1989.
24. Harris, E. L., Noyes, R., Crowe, R. R., and Chaudhry, D. R. A family study of agoraphobia: report of a pilot study. Arch. Gen. Psychiat. *40*:1065–1070, 1983.
25. Hippocrates on Epidemics, V, Section LXXXII.
26. Kantor, J. S., Zitrin, C. M., and Zeldis, S. M. Mitral valve prolapse syndrome in agoraphobic patients. Am. J. Psychiat. *127*:467–469, 1980.
27. Kendler, K. S., Neale, M. C., Kessler, R. C., Heath, A. C., and Eaves, L. J. The genetic epidemiology of phobias in women. Arch. Gen. Psychiat. *49*:273–281, 1992.
28. Kessler, R. C., McGonagle, K. A., Zhao, S., Nelson, C. B., Hughes, M., Eshleman, S., Wittchen, H., and Kendler, K. S. Lifetime and 12-month prevalence of DSM-III-R psychiatric disorders in the United States. Arch. Gen. Psychiat. *51*:8–19, 1994.
29. Klein, D. F. The delineation of two drug-responsive anxiety syndromes. Psychopharmacologia *5*:397, 1964.
30. Klein, D. F., Zitrin, C. M., Woerner, M. G., and Ross, D. C. Treatment of phobias. II. Behavior therapy and supportive psychotherapy: are there any specific ingredients? Arch. Gen. Psychiat. *40*:139–145, 1983.
31. Klein, D. F. Interview. Currents *4*:5–10, 1985.
32. Kushner, M. G., Sher, K. J., and Beitman, B. D. The relation between alcohol problems and the anxiety disorders. Am. J. Psychiat. *147*:685–695, 1990.
33. Lang, P. J. Fear reduction and fear behaviour. "Problems in treating a construct." In *3d Conference on Research in Psychotherapy.* Chicago, June 1966.
34. Liebowitz, M. R., Gorman, T. M., Fyer, A. T., and Klein, D. F. Social phobia: review of a neglected anxiety disorder. Arch. Gen. Psychiat. *42*:729–736, 1985.
35. Marks, I. M., Birley, J. L. T., and Gelder, M. G. Modified leucotomy in severe agoraphobia: a controlled serial inquiry. Brit. J. Psychiat. *112*:757–769, 1966.
36. Marks, I. M. Agoraphobic syndrome (phobic anxiety state). Arch. Gen. Psychiat. *23*:538–553, 1970.
37. Marks, I. M. The classification of phobic disorders. Brit. J. Psychiat. *116*:377–386, 1970.

38. Marks, I. M. Phobic disorders four years after treatment: a prospective follow-up. Brit. J. Psychiat. *118*:683–688, 1971.

39. Marks, I. M., Boulougouris, J., and Marset, P. Flooding versus desensitization in the treatment of phobic patients: a crossover study. Brit. J. Psychiat. *119*:353–375, 1971.

40. Marks, I. M., Gray, S., Cohen, D., Hill, R., Mawson, D., Ramm, E., and Stern, R. S. Imipramine and brief therapist-aided exposure in agoraphobics having self-exposure homework. Arch. Gen. Psychiat. *40*:153–162, 1983.

41. Marks, I. Are there anticompulsive or antiphobic drugs? Review of the evidence. Brit. J. Psychiat. *143*:338–347, 1983.

42. Marshall, J. R. The diagnosis and treatment of social phobia and alcohol abuse. Bull. Menninger Clin. *58:2(Suppl. A)*:A58–A66, 1994.

43. Mavissakalian, M., Michelson, L., and Dealy, R. S. Pharmacological treatment of agoraphobia: imipramine versus imipramine with programmed practice. Brit. J. Psychiat. *143*:348–355, 1983.

44. Mavissakalian, M., Salerni, R., Thompson, M. E., and Michelson, L. Mitral valve prolapse and agoraphobia. Am. J. Psychiat. *140*:1612–1614, 1983.

45. Mavissakalian, M., and Michelson, L. Agoraphobia: relative and combined effectiveness of therapist-assisted in vivo exposure and imipramine. J. Clin. Psychiat. *47*:117–122, 1986.

46. Mavissakalian, M., and Perel, J. M. Protective effects of imipramine maintenance treatment in panic disorder with agoraphobia. Am. J. Psychiat. *149*:1053–1057, 1992.

47. Mathews, A., Johnston, D., Lancashire, M., Munby, M., Shaw, P., and Gelder, M. Imaginal flooding and exposure to real phobic situations: treatment outcome with agoraphobic patients. Brit. J. Psychiat. *129*:362–371, 1976.

48. Mathews, A. M., Gelder, M. G., and Johnston, D. W. *Agoraphobia: Nature and Treatment.* New York: Guilford Press, 1981.

49. Mavissakalian, M., and Barlow, D. H. (eds.). *Phobia: Psychological and Pharmacological Treatment.* New York: Guilford Press, 1981.

50. McConaghy, N. Results of systematic desensitization with phobias reexamined. Brit. J. Psychiat. *117*:89–92, 1970.

51. Moran, C., and Andrews, G. The familial occurrence of agoraphobia. Brit. J. Psychiat. *146*:262–267, 1985.

52. Montjoy, C., Roth, M., Garside, R., and Leitch, I. A clinical trial of phenelzine in anxiety depressive and phobic neuroses. Brit. J. Psychiat. *131*:486–492, 1977.

53. Mullaney, J. A., and Trippett, C. J. Alcohol dependence and phobias: clinical description and relevance. Brit. J. Psychiat. *135*:565–573, 1979.

54. Nemiah, J. D. Phobic disorder. In *Comprehensive Textbook of Psychiatry*, 3rd ed. Freedman, A. M., and Kaplan, H. E. (eds.). Baltimore: Williams & Wilkins, 1980.

55. Paul, G. L. Outcome of systematic desensitization: 1. Background and procedures, and uncontrolled reports of individual treatments. In *Behavior*

Therapy: Appraisal and Status. Franks, C. M. (ed.). New York: McGraw-Hill, 1969.

56. Paul, G. L. Outcome of systematic desensitization: 2. Controlled investigations of individual treatment, technique variations, and current status. In *Behavior Therapy: Appraisal and Status.* Franks, C. M. (ed.). New York: McGraw-Hill, 1969.

57. Quitkin, F. M., and Rabkin, J. G. Hidden psychiatric diagnosis in the alcoholic. In *Alcoholism and Clinical Psychiatry.* Solomon, J. (ed.), 130–131. New York: Plenum, 1982.

58. Regier, D. A., Farmer, M. E., Rae, D. S., Locke, M. Z., Keith, S. J., Judd, L. L., and Goodwin, F. K. Comorbidity of mental disorders with alcohol and other drug abuse: results from the Epidemiologic Catchment Area (ECA) study. JAMA *264*:2511–2518, 1990.

59. Rimm, D. C., and Masters, J. C. *Behavior Therapy: Techniques and Empirical Findings,* 2nd ed. New York: Academic Press, 1979.

60. Roberts, A. H. Housebound housewives: a follow-up study of a phobic anxiety state. Brit. J. Psychiat. *110*:191–197, 1964.

61. Rosenbaum, J. F., and Pollock, R. A. The psychopharmacology of social phobia and comorbid disorders. Bull. Menninger Clin. *58:2(Suppl. A)*:A67–A83, 1994.

62. Ross, H. E., Glaser, F. B., and Germanson, T. The prevalence of psychiatric disorders in patients with alcohol and other drug problems. Arch. Gen. Psychiat. *45*:1023–1031, 1988.

63. Roth, M. The phobic-anxiety-depersonalisation syndrome. Proc. R. Soc. Med. *52*:587, 1959.

64. Sbarbaro, J. A., Mehlman, D. J., Wu, L., et al. A prospective study of mitral valvular prolapse in young men. Chest *75*:555–559, 1979.

65. Schatzberg, A. F. Overview of anxiety disorders: prevalence, biology, course, and treatment. J. Clin. Psychiat. *52(Suppl. 7)*:5–9, 1991.

66. Shafar, S. Aspects of phobic illness—a study of 90 personal cases. Brit. J. Med. Psychol. *49*:221–236, 1976.

67. Shapiro, M. B., Marks, I. M., and Fox, B. A therapeutic experiment on phobic and affective symptoms in an individual psychiatric patient. Brit. J. Soc. Clin. Psychol. *2*:81–93, 1963.

68. Shaw, H. A simple and effective treatment for flight phobia. Brit. J. Psychiat. *130*:229–232, 1977.

69. Sheehan, D. V., Ballenger, J., and Jacobsen, G. Treatment of endogenous anxiety with phobic, hysterical, and hypochondriacal symptoms. Arch. Gen. Psychiat. *37*:51–59, 1980.

70. Sheehan, D. V., Sheehan, K. E., and Minichiello, W. E. Age of onset of phobic disorders: a reevaluation. Compr. Psychiat. *22*:544–553, 1981.

71. Sim, M., and Houghton, H. Phobic anxiety and its treatment. J. Nerv. Ment. Dis. *143*:484–491, 1966.

72. Smail, P., Stockwell, T., Canter, S., and Hodgson, R. Alcohol dependence and phobic anxiety states: I. A prevalence study. Brit. J. Psychiat. *144*:53–57, 1984.

73. Snaith, R. P. A clinical investigation of phobias. Brit. J. Psychiat. *114*:673–698, 1968.

74. Solyom, L., Ledwidge, B., and Solyom, C. Delineating social phobia. Brit. J. Psychiat. *149*:464–470, 1986.

75. Stockwell, T., Smail, P., Hodgson, R., and Canter, S. Alcohol dependence and phobic anxiety states: II. A retrospective study. Brit. J. Psychiat. *144*:58–63, 1984.

76. Sussman, N. Treatment of anxiety with buspirone. Psychiatr. Ann. *17*:114–120, 1987.

77. Tyrer, P., Candy, J., and Kelly, D. Phenelzine in phobic anxiety: a controlled trial. Psychol. Med. *3*:120–124, 1973.

78. Tyrer, P., and Steinberg, D. Symptomatic treatment of agoraphobia and social phobias: a follow-up study. Brit. J. Psychiat. *127*:163–168, 1975.

79. Webster, A. S. The development of phobias in married women. Psychol. Monogr. *67*:367, 1953.

80. West, E. D., and Dally, P. J. Effects of iproniazid in depressive syndromes. Brit. Med. J. *1*:1491, 1959.

81. Westphal, C. Die Agoraphobie: eine neuropathische Erscheinuung. Arch. Psychiat. Nervenk. *3*:138–171, 219–221, 1871–72.

82. Wittchen, H., Zhao, S., Kessler, R. C., and Eaton, W. W. DSM-III-R generalized anxiety disorder in the national comorbidity survey. Arch. Gen. Psychiat. *51*:355–364, 1994.

83. Wolpe, J. *Psychotherapy by Reciprocal Inhibition.* Stanford: Stanford Univ. Press, 1958.

84. Zitrin, C. M., Klein, D., and Woerner, M. G. Behavior therapy, supportive psychotherapy, imipramine and phobias. Arch. Gen. Psychiat. *35*:307–316, 1978.

85. Zitrin, C. M., Klein, D. F., and Woerner, M. G. Treatment of agoraphobia with group exposure in vivo and imipramine. Arch. Gen. Psychiat. *37*:63–72, 1980.

86. Zitrin, C. M., Klein, D. F., Woener, M. G., and Ross, D. C. Treatment of phobias. I. Comparison of imipramine hydrochloride and placebo. Arch. Gen. Psychiat. *40*:125–138, 1983.

7

ALCOHOLISM

DEFINITION

Alcoholism has been defined by Keller and his associates (66) as the "repetitive intake of alcoholic beverages to a degree that harms the drinker in health or socially or economically, with indication of inability consistently to control the occasion or amount of drinking." A synonym for alcoholism recommended by the World Health Association (23, 47) and *DSM-IV* (Table 7.1) is *alcohol dependence.*

DSM-IV distinguishes alcohol dependence from alcohol abuse (Table 7.2). The abuse category is for problems resulting from drinking. In addition to these problems, the dependence category includes alcohol-seeking behavior, tolerance to alcohol, and alcohol withdrawal (Table 7.1). Since alcohol dependence can be diagnosed in the absence of tolerance or withdrawal, there is minimal difference between dependence and abuse as defined by *DSM-IV.* Abuse can be viewed as a milder form of dependence, but the validity of distinguishing between dependence and abuse can be questioned. It is hard to imagine individuals having serious problems from drinking without having some degree of tolerance and at least severe hangovers, which can be viewed as mild forms of withdrawal (since hangovers are relieved by alcohol, as is withdrawal). The term "alcoholism" is still widely used and there is no reason to believe that it will be used less in the future. For

179

Table 7.1   Diagnostic criteria for Substance Dependence (*DSM-IV*)*

A maladaptive pattern of substance use, leading to clinically significant impairment of distress, as manifested by three (or more) of the following, occurring at any time in the same 12-month period:

(1) Tolerance, as defined by either of the following:

   (*a*) A need for markedly increased amounts of the substance to achieve intoxication or desired effect

   (*b*) Markedly diminished effect with continued use of the same amount of the substance

(2) Withdrawal, as manifested by either of the following:

   (*a*) The characteristic withdrawal syndrome for the substance (refer to criteria A and B of the criteria sets for Withdrawal from the specific substances)

   (*b*) The same (or a closely related) substance is taken to relieve or avoid withdrawal symptoms

(3) The substance is often taken in larger amounts or over a longer period than was intended

(4) There is a persistent desire or unsuccessful efforts to cut down or control substance use

(5) A great deal of time is spent in activities necessary to obtain the substance (e.g., visiting multiple doctors or driving long distances), use the substance (e.g., chain-smoking), or recover from its effects

(6) Important social, occupational, or recreational activities are given up or reduced because of substance use

(7) The substance use is continued despite knowledge of having a persistent or recurrent physical or psychological problems that is likely to have been caused or exacerbated by the substance (e.g., current cocaine use despite recognition of cocaine-induced depression, or continued drinking despite recognition that an ulcer was made worse by alcohol consumption)

*Criteria for alcohol dependence and abuse are the same as for any substance of abuse (e.g., opiates, cocaine; see chapter 8)

Table 7.2 Diagnostic criteria for Substance Abuse (*DSM-IV*)

A. A maladaptive pattern of alcohol use leading to clinically significant impairment or distress, as manifested by one (or more) of the following, occurring with a 12-month period:

   (1) Recurrent substance use resulting in a failure to fulfill major role obligations at work, school, or home (e.g., repeated absences or poor work performance related to substance use; substance-related absences, suspensions, or expulsions from school; neglect of children or household)

   (2) Recurrent substance use in situations in which it is physically hazardous (e.g., driving an automobile or operating a machine when impaired by substance use)

   (3) Recurrent substance-related legal problems (e.g., arrests for substance-related disorderly conduct)

   (4) Continued substance use despite having persistent or recurrent social or interpersonal problems caused or exacerbated by the effects of the substance (e.g., arguments with spouse about consequences of intoxication, physical fights)

this reason, the term "alcoholism" is retained in this chapter, referring to both alcohol dependence and alcohol abuse, when the abuse, as defined in Table 7.2, is severe.

HISTORICAL BACKGROUND

Six millennia ago at the Sumerian trading post of Godin Tepe in what is now western Iran people were drinking beer and wine. In 1992, chemists analyzed a residue in pottery jars found in the ruins of Godin Tepe and identified it as wine or beer. A scientist said, "I think a lot of serious drinking was going on there." The Sumerians were among the first people to develop a complex, literate society of prospering city-states based on irrigation, agriculture, and widespread trade (43).

Beer-making began almost as soon as (or even before) Mesopotamians domesticated barley to make bread in the early transition to agriculture around 8000 B.C. A longstanding debate in archaeology centers on the question of which came first after the domestication of barley: beer or bread?

There is other evidence that alcohol goes back at least to Paleolithic times. This derives from etymology as well as from studies of Stone Age cultures that survived into the twentieth century.

Available to Paleolithic man, presumably, were fermented fruit juice (wine), fermented grain (beer), and fermented honey (mead). Etymological evidence suggests that mead may have been the earliest beverage of choice. The word "mead" derives—by way of *mede* (Middle English) and *meodu* (Anglo-Saxon)—from ancient words of Indo-European stock, such as *methy* (Greek) and *madhu* (Sanskrit). In Sanskrit and Greek, the term means both "honey" and "intoxicating drink." The association of honey rather than grain or fruit with intoxication may indicate its greater antiquity as a source of alcohol (100).

All but three of the numerous Stone Age cultures that survived into modern times have been familiar with alcohol. "The three exceptions," Berton Roueché writes, "are the environmentally underprivileged polar peoples, the intellectually stunted Australian aborigines, and the comparably lackluster primitives of Tierra del Fuego" (100). Early European explorers of Africa and the New World invariably discovered that alcohol was important in the local cultures. The Indians of eastern North America, for instance, were using alcohol in the form of fermented birch and sugar maple sap (100).

Alcohol was used medicinally and in religious ceremonies for thousands of years, but it also has a long history of recreational use. Noah, according to the Old Testament, "drank of the wine and was drunken." Mesopotamian civilization provided one of the earliest clinical descriptions of intoxication and one of the first hangover cures. In *The History of Medicine* (106), Sigerist translates a Mesopotamian physician's advice: "If a man has taken strong wine, his head is affected and he forgets his words and his speech becomes confused, his mind wanders and his eyes have a set expression; *to cure him,* take licorice, beans, oleander . . . to be compounded with oil and wine before the approach of the goddess Gula [or sunset], and in the morning before sunrise and before anyone has kissed him, let him take it, and he will recover."

Roueché notes that "one of the few surviving relics of the Seventeenth Egyptian Dynasty, which roughly coincided with the reign of Hammurabi, is a hieroglyphic outburst of a female courtier. 'Give me eighteen bowls of wine!' she exclaims for posterity. 'Behold, I love drunkenness!'" (100). So did other Egyptians of that era. "Drunkenness was apparently not rare," Sigerist remarks, "and seems to have occurred in all layers of society from the farmers to the gods (or ruling class). Banquets frequently ended with the guests, men and women, being sick, and this did not in any way seem shocking" (106).

Descriptions of drunkenness fill the writings of antiquity, but so do pleas for moderation. Dynastic Egypt apparently invented the first temperance tract (100). Moderation was recommended by no less an authority than Genghis Khan: "A soldier must not get drunk oftener than once a week. It would, of course, be better if he did not get drunk at all, but one should not expect the impossible." The Old Testament condemns drunkenness, but not alcohol. "Give strong drink unto him that is ready to perish," the Book of Proverbs proclaims, "and wine unto those that be of heavy hearts. Let him drink, and forget his poverty, and remember his misery no more."

The "strong drink" of the Bible was probably undiluted wine. Where Proverbs states, "She hath mingled her wine," it refers to a mixture of wine and water.

Alexander the Great was one of the long line of heavy-drinking generals. According to Plutarch, Alexander was under the influence of alcohol at the time of the burning of the royal palace at Persepolis in 330 B.C., seven years before his death. With torch in hand, a drunken Alexander led revellers in a procession in honor of Dionysus and threw the first firebrand, an act he bitterly regretted when sober. The final year of Alexander's life was punctuated by drunken binges and his death may have been hastened by alcohol withdrawal.

Plutarch describes a debauch in 325 B.C. involving Alexander and his Macedonian army: "Not a single helmet, shield or spear was to be seen, but along the whole line of march the soldiers kept dipping their cups, drinking-horns or earthenware goblets into huge casks and mixing bowls and toasting one another, some drinking as they marched, others sprawled by the wayside" (100).

Not only foot soldiers depended on booze. For centuries no British sailor went to sea without his quota of rum.

The process of distillation was discovered about A.D. 800 in Arabia. ("Alcohol" comes from the arabic *alkuhl*, meaning essence.) For centuries distilled alcohol was used in medicine, but by the seventeenth century it had also become a drug of abuse on a large scale. By the late seventeenth century the annual worldwide production of distilled liquors, chiefly gin, was enormous.

Ancient and classical writers used words that are universally translated as "drunkenness." The people who had it were drunkards. In the fourteenth century Chaucer used *dronkelewe* to mean addiction to alcohol as a mental illness (13). By the nineteenth century "inebriety" was the favored descriptor; those who manifested it were not merely inebriated—they were inebriates. A Swedish public health authority, Magnus Huss, in 1849 coined the term "alcoholism." The word caught on: Danish has *alkoholisme;* Dutch, *alcoholisme;* English, *alcoholism;* Finnish, *alkoholismi;* German, *alkoholismus;* Italian, *alcolismo;* Norwegian, *alcoholisme;* Polish, *alkoholizm;* Portuguese, *alcoolismo;* Russian, *alkogolism;* Serbo-Croatian, *alkoholizam;* Slovene, *alkoholizem;* Spanish, *alcoholismo;* Swedish, *alkoholism* (65).

The "disease concept" of alcoholism originated in the writings of Benjamin Rush and the British physician Thomas Trotter (101), and during the last half of the nineteenth century the notion that alcoholism was a disease became popular with physicians. In the 1830s, Dr. Samuel Woodward, the first superintendent of Worcester State Hospital, Massachusetts, and Dr. Eli

Todd of Hartford, Connecticut, suggested establishing special institutions for inebriates. The first was opened in Boston in 1841. In 1904 the Medical Temperance Society changed its name to the American Medical Association for the Study of Inebriety and Narcotics. The *Journal of Inebriety*, established in 1876, was founded on the "fact that inebriety is a neurosis and psychosis." During Prohibition, however, the concept of alcoholism as a disease lost its vogue (58).

With repeal of the Eighteenth Amendment, the disease concept was revived. Pioneering studies performed at the Yale School of Alcohol Studies and the writings of E. M. Jellinek were largely responsible for the popularization of this concept in the twentieth century. In the mid-1960s the U.S. government began supporting alcoholism research on a rather large scale; by the 1980s the federal government and most state governments were sponsoring treatment programs for alcoholics, and a large number of proprietary hospitals for alcoholism spanned the continent, many of them less profitable because of the advent of managed care.

Epidemiology

Alcohol has been the "intoxicant of choice" in Judeo-Christian culture. "To drink is a Christian diversion / Unknown to the Turk and the Persian," wrote Congreve 300 years ago. It was not *totally* unknown to the Turk and the Persian, but it is true that they favored other intoxicants, notably the products of the poppy and hemp plant.

One of the myths of our times is that the "stresses" of modern living have produced a society unusually reliant on alcohol. This is not true. Per capita consumption in the United States was highest, at an estimated six or seven gallons a year per person (computed in absolute alcohol—200 proof), in the early 1800s when whiskey and cider were the favorite beverages (100). One reason was that whiskey is more portable than grain, and cider more portable than apples. Portability was important before trains came along.

Today, in the United States, the reported consumption of alcohol (pure alcohol) is a little less than three gallons per year per person over age 14 (87). This figure is based on tax data. Untaxed sales, such as those on military installations, are not included, so per capita consumption may be underestimated. Also, because consumption estimates are based on the resident population, when residents of one state cross into another state to purchase lower-priced alcoholic beverages, the result is a higher per capita consumption figure for the state in which sales occur. Washington, D.C., and states with high rates of tourism and business travel have higher reported consumption rates because sales to transients are calculated as consumption by the resident population.

International comparisons are difficult at best. However, it appears that "wine countries" such as France and Italy consume more alcohol than do countries where distilled spirits are favored. Israel has the lowest per capita consumption. Ireland, contrary to its popular image, has a lower consumption rate than the United Kingdom. The United States ranks in the middle with regard to alcohol consumption and Russia (if you can believe the figures) is in the lower third (87).

Most adults in the United States are light drinkers. About 35 percent abstain, 55 percent drink less than three drinks per week, and only 11 percent consume an average of one ounce or more of alcohol per day (87).

Drinking patterns vary by age and sex. For both men and women, the prevalence of drinking is highest and abstention is lowest in the twenty-one- to thirty-four-year age range. Four to five times more males are "heavy" drinkers compared to females at all ages. For ages sixty-five years and older, abstainers exceed drinkers in both sexes and only 7 percent of men and 2 percent of women are considered heavy drinkers (87). "Heavy" drinking is defined by the U.S. government as consuming 14 or more drinks per week.

The level of consumption varies markedly in different segments of the population. In the United States consumption is greatest in the Northeast, lowest in the South. Young males drink more than any other group in the United States (43).

The proportion of adolescents who report drinking increases steadily with age, reaching 80 to 90 percent among the oldest schoolchildren. By that time as many girls report having "ever" drunk as boys.

Most alcohol is consumed by a small percentage of people: 70 percent of the drinking population consume only 20 percent of the total alcohol consumed; 30 percent of drinkers consume 80 percent of the alcohol; and 10 percent consume 50 percent (87).

Consumption must be distinguished from alcoholism. Is the latter increasing?

It could be decreasing (11, 12). In 1795 the distinguished American physician Benjamin Rush estimated that 4,000 Americans died each year from "over-indulgence in ardent spirits." Since the population of the country was about four million, this gives a rate of 100 per 100,000. The officially recorded rate of death from alcoholism in the United States today is two per 100,000. Granting that Dr. Rush's estimate is suspect, alcoholism in the United States still may be less prevalent today than it was 200 years ago.

There are several problems in estimating the prevalence of alcoholism (61). One is that few researchers agree on the precise definition of alcoholism (85). Also, when a household survey is done, the alcoholics, more than most people, are not home.

A third reason to be skeptical about prevalence estimates is that ax-grinding is a potent factor in the production of statistics. Government officials spend much of their time trying to wring money out of reluctant legislators and some are caught in the dilemma of, on the one hand, wanting the prevalence of alcoholism to be low to show they are doing a good job and, on the other hand, wanting it to be high to inspire lawmakers to spend more money on the problem. In the late 1960s, for example, the U.S. government announced that there were five million American alcoholics. Now it is said that there are fourteen million. This increase coincides with increased efforts by the national government to study and treat alcoholism (61).

Alcohol problems are correlated with a history of school difficulty (80). High school dropouts and individuals with a record of frequent truancy and delinquency appear to have a particularly high risk of alcoholism.

Individuals in certain occupations are more vulnerable to alcoholism than those doing other types of work. Waiters, bartenders, longshoremen, musicians, authors, and reporters have relatively high cirrhosis rates; accountants, mail carriers, and carpenters have relatively low rates (78).

CLINICAL PICTURE

Alcoholism is a behavioral disorder. The specific behavior that causes problems is the consumption of large quantities of alcohol on repeated occasions. The motivation underlying this behavior is often obscure (3). When asked why they drink excessively, alcoholics occasionally attribute their drinking to a particular mood such as depression or anxiety or to situational problems. They sometimes describe an overpowering "need" to drink, variously described as a craving or compulsion. Just as often, however, the alcoholic is unable to give a plausible explanation of his excessive drinking (75).

Like other drug dependencies, alcoholism is accompanied by a preoccupation with obtaining the drug in quantities sufficient to produce intoxication over long periods. It is especially true early in the course of alcoholism that the patient may deny this preoccupation or attempt to rationalize his need by assertions that he drinks no more than his friends. As part of this denial or rationalization, alcoholics tend to spend their time with other heavy drinkers.

An alcoholic named David writes (43):

My need was easy to hide from myself and others (maybe I'm kidding myself about the others). I only associated with people who drank. I married a woman who drank. There were always reasons to drink. I was low, tense, tired, mad, happy. I probably drank as often because I was happy as for any other reason. And occasions for drinking—when drinking was appropriate, expected—were endless, Football games, fishing trips, parties, holidays, birthdays, Christmas, or merely Saturday night. Drinking became interwoven with everything pleasurable—food, sex, social life. When I stopped drinking, these things, for a time, lost all interest for me, they were so tied to drinking.

As alcoholism progesses and problems from drinking become more serious, alcoholics may drink alone, sneak drinks, hide the bottle, and take other measures to conceal the seriousness of their condition. This is almost always accompanied by feelings of guilt and remorse, which in turn may produce more drinking, temporarily relieving the feelings. Remorse may be particularly intense in the morning, when the patient has not had a drink for a number of hours, and this may provoke morning drinking (59):

> For years [David writes], I drank and had very little hangover, but now the hangovers were gruesome. I felt physically bad—headachy, nauseous, weak, but the mental part was the hardest. I loathed myself. I was waking early and thinking what a mess I was, how I had hurt so many others and myself. The words "guilty" and "depression" sound superficial in trying to describe how I felt. The loathing was almost physical—a dead weight that could be lifted in only one way, and that was by having a drink, so I drank, morning after morning. After two or three, my hands were steady, I could hold some breakfast down, and the guilt was gone, or almost.

Prolonged drinking, even if initiated to relieve guilt and anxiety, commonly produces anxiety and depression (19). The full range of symptoms associated with depression and anxiety disorders—including terminal insomnia, low mood, irritability, and anxiety attacks with chest pain, palpitations, and dyspnea—often appear. Alcohol temporarily relieves these symptoms, resulting in a vicious cycle of drinking-depression-drinking, which may ultimately result in a classical withdrawal syndrome. Often the patient makes a valiant effort to stop drinking and may succeed for a period of several days or weeks, only to fall off the wagon again:

> At some point I was without wife, home or job. I had nothing to do but drink. The drinking was now steady, days on end. I lost appetite and

missed meals (besides money was short). I awoke at night, sweating and shaking, and had a drink. I awoke in the morning vomiting and had a drink. It couldn't last. My ex-wife found me in my apartment shaking and seeing things, and got me in the hospital. I dried out, left, and went back to drinking. I was hospitalized again, and this time stayed dry for six months. I was nervous and couldn't sleep, but got some of my confidence back, and found a part-time job. Then my ex-boss offered my job back and I celebrated by having a drink. The next night I had two drinks. In a month I was drinking as much as ever and again unemployed.

Repeated experiences like this easily lead to feelings of despair and hopelessness. By the time patients consult a physician, they have often reached rock bottom. Their situation seems hopeless and, after years of heavy drinking, their problems have become so numerous that they feel nothing can be done about them. At this point, they may be ready to acknowledge their alcoholism, but feel powerless to stop drinking. But many do stop—permanently—as will be discussed later.

Alcohol is one of the few psychoactive drugs that produce, on occasion, classical amnesia. Nonalcoholics, when drinking, also experience this amnesia (blackouts), but much less often, as a rule, than do alcoholics (35). These episodes of amnesia are particularly distressful to alcoholics because they may fear that they have unknowingly harmed someone or behaved imprudently while intoxicated (43):

A thirty-nine-year-old salesman awoke in a strange hotel room. He had a mild hangover but otherwise felt normal. His clothes were hanging in the closet: he was clean-shaven. He dressed and went down to the lobby. He learned from the clerk that he was in Las Vagas and that he had checked in two days previously. It had been obvious that he had been drinking, the clerk said, but he hadn't seemed very drunk. The date was Saturday the fourteenth. His last recollection was of sitting in a St. Louis bar on Monday the ninth. He had been drinking all day and was drunk, but could remember everything perfectly until about three P.M., when "like a curtain dropping," his memory went blank. It remained blank for approximately five days. Three years later, those five days were still a blank. He was so frightened by the experience that he abstained from alcohol for two years.

Studies of blackouts (35, 108) indicate that the amnesia is anterograde. During a blackout, individuals have relatively intact remote and immediate memory but they experience a specific short-term memory deficit in which they are unable to recall events that happened five or ten minutes before. Because their other intellectual faculties are well preserved, they can perform complicated acts and appear normal to the casual observer. Present evidence suggests that alcoholic blackouts represent impaired consolidation of new information rather than repression motivated by a desire to forget events that happened while drinking (35).

Sometimes, however, a curious thing happens: The drinker recalls things that happened during a previous drinking period that, when sober, he had forgotten. For example, alcoholics often report hiding money or alcohol when drinking, forgetting it when sober, and having their memory return when drinking again (35):

> A forty-seven-year-old housewife often wrote letters when she was drinking. Sometimes she would jot down notes for a letter and start writing it but not finish it. The next day, sober, she would be unable to decipher the notes. Then she would start drinking again, and after a few drinks the meaning of the notes would become clear and she would resume writing the letter. "It was like picking up the pencil where I had left off."

Anecdotal reports suggest that benzodiazepine medication combined with alcohol increases the likelihood of a blackout occurring with smaller amounts of alcohol than is usually required (84). Benzodiazepines taken orally produce a mild impairment of short-term memory (69) but are not associated with blackouts of the type produced by alcohol (unless given intravenously).

By the time alcoholics consult a physician, they have often developed medical and social complications from drinking (see Complications).

IDENTIFYING THE ALCOHOLIC

Before alcoholism can be treated, it first must be recognized. Physicians are in a particularly good position to identify a drinking problem early: They can do a physical examination and order laboratory tests. Here are some hints of a drinking problem:

1. Arcus senilis—a ringlike opacity of the cornea—occurs commonly with age, causes no visual disturbance, and is considered an innocent condition. The ring forms from fatty material in the blood. Alcohol increases fat in the blood and more alcoholics are reported to have the ring than others their age (25).
2. A red nose (acne rosacea) suggests the owner has a weakness for alcoholic beverages. Often, however, people with red noses are teetotalers or even rabid prohibitionists, and they resent the insinuation.
3. Red palms (palmer erythema) are also suggestive but not diagnostic of alcoholism.
4. Cigarette burns between the index and middle fingers or on the chest and contusions and bruises should raise suspicions of alcoholic stupor.
5. Painless enlargement of the liver may suggest a larger alcohol intake than the liver can cope with. Severe, constant upper abdominal pain and tenderness radiating to the back indicates pancreatic inflammation, and alcohol sometimes is the cause.
6. Reduced sensation and weakness in the feet and legs may occur from excessive drinking.
7. Laboratory tests provide other clues. More than half of alcoholics have increased amounts of gamma-glutamyl transpeptidase (GGT) in their blood, which is unusual in nonalcoholics (11). After GGT, elevations in the following tests are most often associated with heavy drinking: mean corpuscular volume, uric acid, triglycerides, aspartate aminotransferase, and urea (123).

Another approach is to use a wide range of commonly available blood chemistry tests and subject them to quadratic discriminant analysis (102). Each value may be in the normal range, but in toto they produce a distinctive "fingerprint" that is highly specific for detecting recent heavy drinking. Whether it is a useful test for alcoholism per se is not known.

In their search for signs of alcohol abuse, physicians sometimes slip into a moralistic attitude that alienates the patient. For personal reasons, physicians may believe any drinking is wrong, but they still should be aware of new findings that suggest moderate drinking may actually contribute to longevity (2, 4, 67). Turner and associates (111) in their review of the "beneficial" effects of alcohol surveyed a number of well-designed studies that indicated the risk of coronary heart disease is lower in persons who use alcohol moderately than in abstainers. Increased levels of high-density lipoproteins (HDL)—a negative risk factor for myocardial infarction—are associated with moderate and even (in some studies) heavy alcohol use (30). Moderate drinking is defined by Turner et al. as an intake that exceeds neither 0.8 g/kg of ethanol per day (up to a limit of 80 g) nor an average of 0.7 g/kg for three successive days.

None of this should be interpreted as encouragement of immoderate use of alcohol. For alcoholics, no level of intake is considered beneficial. Moreover, uncertainties exist concerning both the effects of moderate drinking on the unborn child and the relationship of moderate drinking to automobile accidents.

NATURAL HISTORY

The natural history of alcoholism seems to be somewhat different in men and women (92). In men the onset is usually in the late teens or twenties, the course is insidious, and the alcoholic may not be fully aware of his dependency on alcohol until his thirties. The first hospitalization usually occurs in the late thirties or forties (22).

In men symptoms of alcoholism rarely occur for the first time after age forty-five (43). If they do occur, the physician should be alerted to the possibility of primary affective disorder or brain disease.

Alcoholism has a higher "spontaneous" remission rate than is often recognized. The incidence of first admissions to psychiatric hospitals for alcoholism drops markedly in the sixth and seventh decades, as do first arrests for alcohol-related offenses. Although the mortality rate among alcoholics is perhaps two to three times that of nonalcoholics, this is probably insufficient to account for the apparent decrease in problem drinking in middle and late middle life (22).

Women alcoholics have been studied less extensively than men alcoholics, but the evidence suggests that the course of the disorder is more variable in women. The onset often occurs later and spontaneous remission apparently is less frequent (92). Women alcoholics are also more likely to have a history of depression (103).

On the basis of questionnaire data obtained from alcoholics, Jellinek promulgated the view that manifestations of alcoholism follow a natural chronological order, with blackouts being one of the early "prodromal" symptoms of the illness (59). Later studies (35) have challenged this view, and it is now believed that problems from drinking may occur in various sequences and that blackouts have no special significance as a sign of incipient alcoholism. Frequently, after years of heavy problem-free drinking, a person may experience a large number of problems in a brief period. Table 7.3 shows the mean age of onset of alcohol problems in an unselected series of hospitalized men alcoholics.

Patterns of drinking also are variable, and it is a mistake to associate one particular pattern exclusively with alcoholism. Jellinek (58) divided alcoholics into various "species," depending on their pattern of drinking. One species, the so-called "gamma alcoholic," is common in America and conforms to the stereotype of the Alcoholics Anonymous member. Gamma alcoholics have problems with "control": Once they begin drinking, they are unable to stop until poor health or depleted financial resources prevent them from continuing. Once the bender is terminated, however, the person is able to abstain from alcohol for varying lengths of time. Jellinek contrasted the gamma alcoholic with a species of alcoholic common in France. He has "control" but is "unable to abstain"; he *must* drink a given quantity of alcohol every day, although he has no compulsion to exceed this amount. He may

Table 7.3 Onset of Alcoholic manifestations among all subjects ($N = 100$)

Manifestation	Present (%)	Mean Age at Onset	Percentage of Subjects Reporting Manifestation (By Age at First Occurrence)*										
			<20	20–24	25–29	30–34	35–39	40–44	45–49	50–54	55–59	60–64	65–70
1. Frequent drunks	98	27	18	17	21	18	13	7	3		1	1	
2. Weekend drunks	82	28	11	18	21	32	6	8	2		1	1	
3. Morning drinking	84	31	2	17	15	25	17	9	11	1	1		
4. Benders	76	31	7	14	18	21	13	9	12	5	1		1
5. Neglecting meals	86	32	2	11	14	29	15	10	10	6	1		1
6. "Shakes"	88	33	1	11	15	24	17	9	16	3	2		
7. Job loss from drinking	69	34	3	7	19	19	26	7	9	6	3	1	
8. Separation or divorce from drinking	44	34		16	7	23	14	20	14	7			
9. Blackouts	64	35	2	6	16	28	25	8	9	3	3		
10. Joined AA	39	36		8	8	28	20	15	8	10	3		
11. Hospitalization for drinking	100	37	1	3	14	18	20	13	14	9	6	1	1
12. Delirium tremens	45	38		2	11	11	40	16	7	11	2		

*Figures rounded off to nearest whole number for ease of perusal. Sums may therefore not equal 10 percent

Goodwin et al. (36)

not recognize that he has an alcohol problem until, for reasons beyond his control, he has to stop drinking, whereupon he experiences withdrawal symptoms.

Although these pure types of alcoholism do exist, many individuals who do not conform to the stereotypes still have serious drinking problems. Among American alcoholics, one drink does *not* invariably lead to a binge; a person may drink moderately for a long time before his or her drinking begins to interfere with health or social functioning (112).

COMPLICATIONS

Because alcoholism is defined by the problems it creates, symptoms and complications inevitably overlap. For present purposes, we will consider social and medical complications separately.

Alcoholics have a high rate of marital separation and divorce (43). They often have job troubles, including frequent absenteeism and job loss. They also have a high frequency of accidents—in the home, on the job, and while driving automobiles. About 40 percent of highway fatalities in the United States involve a driver who has been drinking (107). Nearly half of convicted felons are alcoholic (43) and about half of police activities in large cities are associated with alcohol-related offenses. About 10 percent of pilots killed in private plane crashes had been drinking, according to the Federal Aviation Commission (*New York Times*, April 9, 1995).

Medical complications fall into three categories: (a) acute effects of heavy drinking, (b) chronic effects of heavy drinking, and (c) withdrawal effects.

Consumption of very large amounts of alcohol can lead directly to death by depressing the respiratory center in the medulla. Acute hemorrhagic pancreatitis occasionally occurs from a single heavy drinking episode.

Nearly every organ system can be affected, directly or indirectly, by chronic, heavy use of alcohol. Gastritis and diarrhea are common reversible effects. Gastric ulcer may also occur, although the evidence that alcohol direclty produces ulceration is equivocal (122).

The most serious effect of alcohol on the gastrointestinal tract is liver damage. After many years of study, however, it is still not clear whether alcohol alone has a direct toxic effect on the liver (43). At present, it appears that cirrhosis results from the combined effect of alcohol and diet plus other factors, possibly including heredity. Human and animal studies indicate that a single large dose of alcohol combined with a diet rich in fat produces a fatty liver (72, 116). Conversely, alcohol together with fasting can result in a fatty liver. The connection between fatty liver and cirrhosis, however, is unclear. The fatty changes in the liver after acute alcohol intoxication are reversible. Most patients with Laennec's cirrhosis in western countries are excessive drinkers. Most severe alcoholics, however, do not develop cirrhosis (probably less than 10 percent).

Studies show that force-feeding baboons with large amounts of alcohol over long periods results in cirrhosis (73). However, not all baboons develop cirrhosis, and these studies leave unresolved the question of the direct role of alcohol in producing cirrhosis. One complication in interpreting the finding is that a large intake of alcohol also produces a malabsorption syndrome. Therefore, although the baboons had adequate diets, it is likely that important food constituents, including vitamins, were not fully absorbed during the drinking periods.

Alcoholism is associated with pathology of the nervous system, principally owing to vitamin deficiencies and not to a direct toxic effect of alcohol. Peripheral neuropathy, the most common neurological complication, apparently results from multiple vitamin B deficiencies (114). It is usually reversible with adequate nutrition. Retrobulbar neuropathy may lead to amblyopia (sometimes called "tobacco-alcohol amblyopia"), which is also usually reversible with vitamin therapy.

Other neurological complications include anterior lobe cerebellar degenerative disease (99) and the Wernicke-Korsakoff syndrome (115). The latter results from thiamine deficiency (43). The acute Wernicke stage consists of ocular disturbances (nystagmus or sixth-nerve palsy), ataxia, and confusion. It usually clears in a few days but may progress to a chronic brain syndrome (Korsakoff's psychosis). Short-term memory loss (anterograde amnesia) is the most characteristic feature of Korsakoff's psychosis. "Confabulation" (narration of fanciful tales) may also occur. The Wernicke-Korsakoff syndrome is associated with necrotic lesions of the mammillary bodies, thalamus, and other brain-stem areas. Thiamine corrects early Wernicke signs rapidly and *may* prevent development of an irreversible Korsakoff dementia. Once the dementia is established, thiamine does not usually help.

A 48-year-old divorced housepainter has been admitted to the hospital with a history of 30 years of heavy drinking. He has had two previous admissions for detoxification but the family states that he has not had a drink in several weeks and shows no sign of alcohol withdrawal. He looks malnourished, however, and on examination is found to be ataxic and [to] have a bilateral sixth cranial nerve palsy. He appears confused and mistakes one of his physicians for a dead uncle.

Within a week the patient walks normally and there is no sign of a sixth nerve palsy. He seems less confused and can now find his way to the bathroom without direction. He remembers the names and birthdays of his siblings but has difficulty naming the past five presidents.

More strikingly, he has great difficulty in retaining information for longer than a few minutes. He can repeat back a list of numbers immediately after he has heard them, but a few minutes later does not recall being asked to perform the task. Shown three objects (keys, comb, ring), he cannot recall them three minutes later. He does not seem worried about this. Asked if he can recall the name of his doctor, he replies, "Certainly," and proceeds to call the doctor "Dr. Masters" (not his name) whom he claims he first met in the Korean War. He tells a long untrue story about how he and "Dr. Masters" served as fellow soldiers in the Korean War.

The patient is calm, alert, friendly. One could be with him for a short period and not realize he has a severe memory impairment, in view of his intact immediate memory and spotty but sometimes impressive remote memory. His amnesia, in short, is largley anterograde. Although treated with high doses of thiamine, the short-term memory deficit persists and appears to be irreversible. (44)

Whether excessive use of alcohol produces cortical atrophy has been debated for many years (18). MRI and computerized tomography (CT) scans of alcoholics have been contradictory, some showing cerebral atrophy (24, 57, 94), some showing none (53), and one showing *reversible* atrophy (8) and restoration of glucose metabolism in PET scans (121). In a 1987 study, computer technology was used to count brain cells in alcoholics who came to autopsy; alcoholics had fewer neurons in the frontal cortex than did nonalcoholics (50). If confirmed by further studies, this would support the long-held but poorly documented view that excessive use of alcohol produces cortical atrophy of the frontal lobes. The extensive psychometric literature on intellectual impairment in alcoholics is also contradictory (40). Most studies performed soon after drinking bouts show intellectual deficits, but the deficits vary from study to study. The most consistent results have involved use of the categories test of the Halstead Battery, indicating that alcoholics have difficulty in "conceptual shifting." Many of the deficits found in alcoholics undergoing detoxification are reversible (96). No studies have reported a decline in alcoholics' IQs.

Other medical complications of alcoholism include cardiomyopathy, thrombocytopenia and anemia, and myopathy. Two studies showed an increase in breast cancer in women who were light or moderate drinkers (51, 124). Having not previously been reported, the association awaits further study for confirmation. It has also been reported that alcoholics have an increased risk of stroke (33). This could be related to alcohol-induced hypertension, although the relationship between alcohol and sustained hypertension remains controversial (77). The effect of alcohol on stroke was lost when adjusted for smoking in another study (49).

A possible teratogenic effect of alcohol had been suspected for centuries, but it was not until the work of Lemoine in 1968 (71) and the independent observations of Jones and Smith in 1973 (62) that a distinct dysmorphic condition associated with maternal alcoholism during pregnancy was described in the medical literature. The abnormalities most typically associated with alcohol teratogenicity can be grouped into four categories: central nervous system dysfunction, birth deficiencies, a characteristic cluster of facial abnormalities, and variable major and minor malformations (16). Animal studies have now demonstrated specific teratogenic properties of ethyl alcohol in a variety of species, many of the abnormalities being similar to those described in man (14, 16).

According to an Associated Press story (April 6, 1995), the percentage of babies born with health problems because their mothers drank alcohol during pregnancy increased sixfold from 1979 through 1993. Commenting on the article, the Centers for Disease Control and Prevention said that researchers did not know whether the increase meant improved diagnosis by doctors or whether more pregnant women are drinking. In any case, since the Centers began tracking cases, the rate increased from one per 10,000 births in 1979 to 6.7 per 10,000 births in 1993. Over the fifteen years, 2,023 cases were reported among the 9.4 million births. Far more women drink during pregnancy than have fetal alcohol syndrome babies, and nobody knows how much alcohol harms a fetus. Still, many doctors are advocating no drinking at all during pregnancy.

The term "alcohol withdrawal syndrome" is preferable to "delirium tremens" (DTs). The latter refers to a specific manifestation of the syndrome. The most common withdrawal symptom is tremulousness, which usually occurs only a few hours after cessation of drinking and may even begin while the person is still drinking ("relative abstinence"). Transitory hallucinations also may occur. If so, they usually begin twelve to twenty-four hours after drinking stops (114).

After a week of heavy drinking and little food, a 30-year-old newspaper reporter tried to drink a morning cup of coffee and found that his hands were shaking so violently he could not get the cup to his mouth. He managed to pour some whisky into a glass and drank as much as he could. His hands became less shaky but now he was nauseated and began having "dry heaves." He tried repeatedly to drink but could not keep the alcohol down. He felt ill and intensely anxious and decided to call a doctor friend. The doctor recommended hospitalization.

On admission, the patient had a marked resting and exertional tremor of the hands, and his tongue and eyelids were tremulous. He also had feelings of "internal" tremulousness. Lying in the hospital bed, he found the noises outside his window unbearably loud and began seeing "visions" of animals and, on one occasion, a dead relative. He was terrified and called a nurse, who gave him a tranquilizer. He became quieter and his tremor was less pronounced. At all times he realized that the visual phenomena were "imaginary." He always knew where he was and was oriented otherwise. After a few days the tremor disappeared and he no longer hallucinated. He still had trouble sleeping but otherwise felt back to normal and vowed never to drink again. (44)

Grand mal convulsions (rum fits) occur occasionally, sometimes as long as two or three days after drinking stops. As a rule, alcoholics experiencing convulsions do not have epilepsy; they have normal electroencephalograms (EEGs) when not drinking and experience convulsions only during withdrawal (79).

Delirium tremens is infrequent and when it does occur is often associated with an intervening medical illness. For a diagnosis of delirium tremens, gross memory disturbance should be present in addition to other withdrawal symptoms such as agitation and vivid hallucinations. Classically, delirium tremens begins two or three days after drinking stops and subsides within one to five days (114). One must always suspect intercurrent medical illness when delirium occurs during withdrawal. The physician should be particularly alert to hepatic decompensation, pneumonia, subdural hematoma, pancreatitis, and fractures.

So-called "chronic alcoholic hallucinosis" refers to the peristence of hallucinations, usually auditory, for long periods after other abstinence symptoms subside and after the patient has stopped heavy drinking (116). This occurs rarely; after seventy-five years of debate concerning the etiology, it has not been resolved whether drinking actually produces the condition.

Suicide is an important complication of alcoholism. About one-quarter of suicides are alcoholic, predominantly white men over age thirty-five. Apparently alcoholics (unlike patients with primary affective disorder) are especially likely to commit suicide after loss of a wife, close relative, or other serious interpersonal disruption (36).

FAMILY STUDIES

Every family study of alcoholism regardless of country of origin has shown much higher rates of alcoholism among the relatives of alcoholics than in the general population. According to a number of studies, about 25 percent of fathers and brothers of alcoholics are themselves alcoholics (17).

Not everything that runs in families is inherited, however (113). Speaking French, for example, runs in families and is not inherited. How does one separate nature from nurture in familial illnesses?

Two methods are used in psychiatric research. One is to compare identical and fraternal twins. If identical twins are more often concordant for alcoholism than fraternal twins, this would point to a genetic influence. Another way is to study adopted persons who have alcoholism in the biological family but not in the family of upbringing. Both approaches have been applied to alcoholism. Here, briefly, are the results.

Twin Studies

A Swedish investigator (64) found that identical twins were significantly more concordant for alcoholism than fraternal twins—the more severe the alcoholism the greater the difference. Among younger persons in a Finnish study (90), there was a difference between identical and fraternal twins with regard to alcohol problems, but there was no difference in the total sample. A third study, in England (86), showed no difference between identical and fraternal twins. A recent study (9) involved analyzing a large number of Veterans Administration records. The results supported a genetic factor; identical twins were more often concordant for alcoholism than fraternal twins. In summary, two twin studies produced results consistent with a genetic influence, one did not, and a fourth was equivocal.

Adoption Studies

The first adoption study of alcoholism was published in 1944 (98). It showed no difference in drinking behavior between children of alcoholics and children of nonalcoholics, both sets in their early twenties. The sample size was small and no criteria were presented for the diagnosis of alcoholism. It was not clear whether the biological parents were alcoholic by today's definition.

A small flurry of adoption studies began in the early 1970s, ushered in by a study comparing adult half-siblings of alcoholics with adult full-siblings (104). The assumption behind the study was that if genetic factors were important, full-siblings would more often be alcoholic than half-siblings. This did not prove to be the case. However, the study did find that half-siblings, predictably, were from broken families, and this afforded the opportunity to compare the incidence of alcoholism in offspring with alcoholism in biological parents and in parents of upbringing. Having a biological father who was alcoholic was highly correlated with alcoholism in the sons, but there was no correlation with alcoholism in the surrogate fathers. The study, in short, failed to prove its central hypothesis but ended up as a kind of adoption study suggesting that biological factors were more important than environmental factors in producing alcohol problems.

In the decade after the half-sibling study, the resuls from three separate adoption studies in Denmark, Sweden, and the United States (Iowa) were published (6, 7, 40). The studies produced remarkably similar findings: (a) Sons of alcoholics were three or four times more likely to be alcoholic than were sons of nonalcoholics, whether raised by their alcoholic biological parents or by nonalcoholic adoptive parents; and (b) sons of alcoholics were no more susceptible to nonalcoholic adult psychiatric disturbances (e.g., depression, sociopathy) than were sons of nonalcoholics where both groups were raised by nonalcoholic adoptive parents. The Iowa study (6, 7) did find a higher rate of childhood conduct disorder in the male offspring of alcoholics, an association later supported by several studies that have documented a history of hyperactive syndrome or conduct disorder in the childhood of alcoholics (39, 109).

The Concept of Familial Alcoholism

Toward the end of the 1970s, investigators began taking note of something rather obvious but often overlooked in recent years: Many alcoholics do not have alcoholism in the family. In most studies, about half of hospitalized alcoholics give a family history of alcoholism and about half do not. In the past few years, a number of investigators have compared the two groups. Two consistent findings have emerged (48): (a) "familial alcoholics" (as they are called) show the first signs of dependence at a younger age than do nonfamilial alcoholics; (b) familial alcoholics have a more severe form of dependence with a more rapid, fulminating course.

Other differences are reported less consistently. Several studies (7, 48) indicate that familial alcoholics are less likely to have other psychiatric illnesses than nonfamilial alcoholics. In this sense, familial alcoholism is synonymous with "primary" alcoholism. An exception to the general rule that *familial* equals *primary* is the finding by two groups that familial alcoholics more often have antisocial personalities (52, 93). This is still controversial. There is more agreement that familial alcoholics often have a history of childhood hyperactivity and/or conduct disorder (109).

We now have sufficient grounds for tentatively viewing familial and nonfamilial alcoholism as separate conditions. One study even suggests that this variable may be a predictor of treatment outcome: Nonfamilial alcoholics more often appeared to return to "controlled" drinking after treatment than familial alcoholics (83). Obviously, more studies are needed before this should influence clinical management in any way. That family history should be included as a potentially important variable in future research on alcoholism, however, is clear.

DIFFERENTIAL DIAGNOSIS

Chronic excessive use of alcohol produces a wide range of psychiatric symptoms that, in various combinations, can mimic other psychiatric disorders. Therefore, while a person is drinking heavily and during the withdrawal period, it is difficult to determine whether he or she suffers from a psychiatric condition other than alcoholism.

Many alcoholics also use other drugs, and it may be difficult to determine which symptoms are produced by alcohol and which by barbiturates, amphetamines, and so on. If a patient has been drinking heavily and not eating, he may become hypoglycemic (28), and this condition may produce symptoms resembling those seen in withdrawal (81).

A psychiatric condition commonly associated with alcoholism is primary affective disorder (46). Female alcoholics apparently suffer more often from primary affective disorder than do male alcoholics. The diagnosis of primary affective disorder usually can be made by past history or by observing the patient during long periods of abstinence. According to one study, about one-third of patients with manic depressive illness drink more while depressed and another third drink less (10). Studies indicate that small amounts of alcohol administered to a depressed patient relieve depressive symptoms, but large amounts worsen depression (43).

Many sociopaths drink to excess, although how many would be considered "alcoholic" is uncertain (118, 121). A follow-up study of convicted felons, about half of whom had alcohol problems, indicates that sociopathic drinkers have a higher "spontaneous" remission rate than do nonsociopathic alcoholics (97). When sociopaths reduce their drinking, their criminal activities are correspondingly reduced.

Various personality disorders have been associated with alcoholism, particularly those in which "dependency" is a feature. The consensus at present is that alcoholism is not connected with a particular constellation of personality traits. Longitudinal studies help little in predicting what types of individuals are particularly susceptible to alcoholism (63, 80).

CLINICAL MANAGEMENT

The treatment of alcoholism and the management of alcohol withdrawal symptoms present separate problems.

In the absence of serious medical complications, the alcohol withdrawal syndrome is usually transient and self-limited; the patient recovers within several days regardless of treatment (114). Insomnia and irritability may persist for longer periods (32).

Treatment for withdrawal is symptomatic and prophylactic. Relief of agitation and tremulousness can be achieved with a variety of drugs, including barbiturates, paraldehyde, chloral hydrate, the phenothiazines, and the benzodiazepines. Currently, the benzodiazepines (e.g., chlordiazepoxide) are widely considered the drugs of choice for withdrawal. They have little, if any, synergistic action with alcohol and, compared with barbiturates and paraldehyde, relatively little abuse potential. They can be administered parenterally to intoxicated patients without apparent risk and continued orally during the withdrawal period. There is some evidence that mortality is increased when the phenothiazines are used, reportedly from hypotension or hepatic encephalopathy.

Administration of large doses of vitamins—particularly the B vitamins—is obligatory, given the role of these vitamins in preventing peripheral neuropathy and the Wernicke-Korsakoff syndrome. The B vitamins are water-soluble and there is no apparent danger in administering them in large doses.

Unless the patient is dehydrated because of vomiting or diarrhea, there is no reason to administer fluids parenterally. Contrary to common belief, alcoholics usually are not dehydrated; actually, they may be overhydrated from consumption of large volumes of fluid (89). During the early stages of withdrawal, hyperventilation may cause respiratory alkalosis and this, together with hypomagnesemia, has been reported to produce withdrawal seizures (81). If the individual has a history of withdrawal seizures, diphenylhydantoin (Dilantin) may be prescribed, although there is no evidence that it prevents withdrawal seizures.

If patients develop delirium, they should be considered dangerous to themselves and others, and protective measures should be taken. Ordinarily, tranquilizers will calm the patient sufficiently to control agitation, and restraints will not be necessary. Administration of intravenous barbiturates may be necessary for severe agitation. Most important, if delirium occurs, further exploration should be conducted to rule out serious medical illness missed in the original examination. When a patient is delirious, an attendant should always be present. It is sometimes helpful to have a friend or relative present.

The treatment of alcoholism should not begin until withdrawal symptoms subside. Treatment has two goals: (a) sobriety and (b) amelioration of psychiatric conditions associated with alcoholism. A small minority of alcoholics are eventually able to drink in moderation, but for several months after a heavy drinking bout total abstinence is desirable for two reasons. First, the physician must follow the patient, sober, for a considerable period to diagnose a coexistent psychiatric problem. Second, it is important for the patient to learn that he or she can cope with ordinary life problems without alcohol. Most relapses occur within six months of discharge from the hospital; they become less and less frequent after that (34).

For many patients, disulfiram (Antabuse) is helpful in maintaining abstinence. By inhibiting aldehyde dehydrogenase, the drug leads to an accumulation of acetaldehyde if alcohol is consumed. Acetaldehyde is highly toxic and produces nausea and hypotension. The latter condition in turn produces shock and may be fatal. In recent years, however, Antabuse has been prescribed in a lower dosage (250 mg) than was employed previously and no deaths from its use have been reported for a number of years. One study indicates the dose is irrelevant; the deterrent effect is psychological and not dose dependent (29).

Discontinuation of Antabuse after administration for several days or weeks still deters drinking for a three- to five-day period because the drug requires that long to be excreted. Thus, it may be useful to give patients Antabuse during office visits at three- to four-day intervals early in the treatment program.

Until recent years it was recommended that patients be given Antabuse for several days and be challenged with alcohol to demonstrate the unpleasant effects that follow. This procedure was not always satisfactory because some patients showed no adverse effects after considerable amounts of alcohol were consumed and other patients became very ill after drinking small amounts of alcohol. At present, the alcohol challenge test is considered optional. The principal disadvantage of Antabuse is not that patients drink while taking the drug but that they stop taking the drug after a brief period. This, again, is a good reason to give the drug on frequent office visits during the early crucial period of treatment.

In recent years, a wide variety of procedures, both psychological and somatic, have been tried in the treatment of alcoholism. None has proven definitely superior to others (93). There is no evidence that intensive psychotherapy helps most alcoholics. Nor are tranquilizers or antidepressants usually effective in maintaining abstinence or controlled drinking (21, 45). Aversive conditioning techniques have been tried, using such agents as apomorphine and emetine to produce vomiting (120), succinylcholine to produce apnea (15), and electrical stimulation to produce pain (56). The controlled trials required to show that these procedures are effective have not been conducted, but a high rate of success has been reported for the apomorphine treatment in well-motivated patients (43).

Although we do not know how many alcoholics benefit from participation in Alcoholics Anonymous, most clinicians agree that alcoholics should be encouraged to attend their meetings on a trial basis.

In three double-blind studies, lithium carbonate was found superior to placebo in reducing drinking in depressed alcoholics (27, 68, 82). There was a high dropout rate in all three studies. A fourth study failed to confirm the efficacy of lithium for alcoholism (43).

In early 1995 the Department of Health and Human Services approved a drug called naltrexone (Revia) for the treatment of alcoholism. In a letter circulated to physicians the department reported that naltrexone, an opiate antagonist, appears to reduce craving for alcohol in alcoholics. In two double-blind, placebo-controlled studies (neither published), naltrexone reduced the rate of patient relapse by about one-half (43). In addition, patients who received naltrexone reported fewer drinking days and less severe alcohol-related problems than patients treated with a placebo. Pending further studies, these results cannot be viewed as conclusive but are encouraging.

Many reports in recent years have indicated that alcoholic patients benefit as much from brief outpatient services as they do from inpatient care (43). For more than two decades in the United States treatment of alcoholism was concentrated at facilities modeled after the so-called "Minnesota Plan." Patients were admitted for a period of several weeks and spent from early morning to late evening participating in group therapy, AA meetings, individual therapy, and educational activities, as well as a good deal of walking and mild exercise. Sometimes patients spent time on the "hot seat" where their faults were dissected enthusiastically by the other patients. The treatment philosophy was based on principles of AA, including the need for total abstinence. The treatment was expensive, costing up to $25,000. While insurance companies picked up the bill, the system became increasingly popular and even small cities would have at least one alcoholism and drug inpatient facility. Then insurers became aware of the lack of evidence supporting the effectiveness of long-term hospitalization and began curtailing reimbursements. Until more evidence is obtained that inpatient treatment is superior to outpatient counseling, this trend will probably contine.

In conclusion, it should be emphasized that relapses are characteristic of alcoholism and that physicians treating alcoholics should avoid anger or excessive pessimism when such relapses occur. Alcoholics see nonpsychiatric physicians as often as they see psychiatrists (probably more often), and there is evidence that general practitioners and internists are sometimes more helpful (32). This may be particularly true when the therapeutic approach is warm but authoritarian, with little stress on "insight" or "understanding." Since the cause of alcoholism is unknown, "understanding," in fact, means acceptance of a particular theory. That may provide temporary comfort but probably rarely provides lasting benefit.

REFERENCES

1. Abel, E. L., and Sokol, R. J. Incidence of fetal alcohol syndrome and economic impact of FAS-related anomalies. Drug Alcohol Depend. *19*:51–70, 1987.
2. Anderson, K. M., Casteeli, W. P., and Levy, D. Cholesteroal and mortality: 30 years of follow-up from the Framingham study. JAMA *257*:2176–2180, 1987.
3. Anderson, P., Cremona, A., Paton, A., Turner, C., and Wallace, P. The risk of alcohol addiction. Addiction *88*:1493–1508, 1993.
4. Baum-Baucker, C. The health benefits of moderate alcohol consumption: a review of the literature. Drug Alcohol Depend. *15*:207–227, 1985.
5. Blum, E. M., and Blum, R. H. *Alcoholism.* San Francisco: Jossey-Bass, 1969.
6. Cadoret, R. J., and Gath, A. Inheritance of alcoholism in adoptees. Brit. J. Psychiat. *132*:252–258, 1978.
7. Cadoret, R. J., Cain, C. A., and Grove, W. M. Development of alcoholism in adoptees raised apart from alcoholic biologic relatives. Arch. Gen. Psychiat. *37*:561–563, 1979.
8. Carlen, P. L., Wortzman, G., Holgate, R. C., Wilkinson, D. A., and Ranking, J. G. Reversible cerebral atrophy in recently abstinent chronic alcoholics measured by computed tomography scans. Science *200*:1076–1078, 1978.
9. Carmelli, D., Heath, A., and Robinette, D. Genetic analysis of drinking behavior in World War II veteran twins. Genet. Epidemiol. *10*:3, 201–213, 1993.
10. Cassidy, W. L., Flanagan, N. B., Spellman, M., and Cohen, M. E. Clinical observations in manic-depressive disease: a quantitative study of 100 manic depressive patients in 50 medically sick controls. JAMA *164*:1535–1546, 1953.
11. Centers for Disease Control and Prevention. Deaths and hospitalizations from chronic liver disease and cirrhosis—United States, 1980–1989. JAMA *269*:5, 1993.

12. Centers for Disease Control and Prevention. Reduction in alcohol-related traffic fatalities—United States, 1990–1992. JAMA *271*:2, 100, 1994.

13. Chaucer, G. *The Canterbury Tales: The Pardoner's Tale*. In *The Student's Chaucer*, Skeats, W. W. (ed.). New York: Oxford Univ. Press, 1900.

14. Chernoff, G. F. The fetal alcohol syndrome in mice: an animal model. Teratology *15*:223–230, 1977.

15. Clancy, J., Vanderhoof, E., and Campbell, P. Evaluation of an aversive technique as a treatment for alcoholism. Q. J. Stud. Alcohol *28*:476–485, 1967.

16. Clarren, S. K., and Smith, D. W. The fetal alcohol syndrome. N. Engl. J. Med. *298*:1063–1067, 1978.

17. Cotton, N. S. The familial incidence of alcoholism: a review. J. Stud. Alcohol. *40*:89–116, 1979.

18. Courville, C. *The Effects of Alcohol on the Nervous System of Man*. Los Angeles: San Lucas (privately printed), 1955.

19. Davis, D. Mood changes in alcoholic subjects with programmed and free-choice experimental drinking. In *Recent Advances in Studies of Alcoholism*. Washington, D.C.: U.S. GPO, 1971.

20. Daoust, M., Compagnon, P., Legrand, E., and Mocaer, E. Tianeptine, a specific serotonin uptake enhancer, decreases ethanol intake in rats. Alcohol. *27*:1, 15–17, 1992.

21. Ditman, K. S. Review and evaluation of current drug therapies in alcoholism. Int. J. Psych. *3*:248–258, 1967.

22. Drew, L. R. H. Alcoholism as a self-limiting disease. Q. J. Stud. Alcohol *29*:956–967, 1968.

23. Edwards, G., Gross, M. M., Keller, M., Moser, J., and Room, R. (eds.) *Alcohol-Related Disabilities*, WHO Offset Publ., no. 32. Geneva: WHO, 1977.

24. Epstein, P. S., Pisani, V. D., and Fawcett, J. A. Alcoholism and cerebral atrophy. Alcohol. Clin. Exp. Res. *1*:61–65, 1977.

25. Ewing, J. A., and Rouse, B. A. Corneal arcus as a sign of possible alcoholism. Alcohol. Clin. Exp. Res. *4*:104, 1980.

26. Ewing, J., Shilling, P., Smith, T., Irwin, M., Schuckit, M., and Kelsoe, J. Lack of association between an RFLP near the D_2 dopamine receptor gene and severe alcoholism. Biol. Psychiat. *31*:285–290, 1992.

27. Fawcett, J., Clark, D. C., Aagesen, C. A., Pisani, V. D., Tilkin, J. F., Sellers, D., McGuire, M., and Gibbons, R. D. A double-blind placebo-controlled trial of lithium carbonate therapy for alcoholism. Arch. Gen. Psychiat. *44*:248–256, 1987.

28. Freinkel, N., and Arky, R. A. Effects of alcohol on carbohydrate metabolism in man. Pscyhosom. Med. *28*:551–563, 1966.

29. Fuller, R. K., and Williford, W. O. Life-table analysis of abstinence in a study evaluating the efficacy of disulfiram. Alcohol. Clin. Exp. Res. *4*:298, 1980.

30. Gaziano, J., Buring, J., Breslow, J., Goldhaber, S., Rosner, B., Van Denburgh, M., Willett, W., and Hennekens, C. Moderate alcohol intake, increased levels of high-density lipoprotein and its subfractions, and de-

creased risk of myocardial infarction. N. Engl. J. Med., *329*:25, 1829–1834, 1993.

31. Gelernter, J., Goldman, D., and Risch, N. The A1 allele at the D_2 dopamine receptor gene and alcoholism. JAMA *269*:13, 1673–1677, 1993.

32. Gerard, D. L., and Saenger, G. *Out-Patient Treatment of Alcoholism*. Toronto: Univ. of Toronto Press, 1966.

33. Gill, J. S., Zezulka, A. V., Shipley, M. J., Gill, S. K., and Bevers, D. J. Stroke and alcohol consumption. N. Engl. J. Med. *315*:1041–1046, 1986.

34. Glatt, M. M. An alcoholic unit in a mental hospital. Lancet *2*:397–398, 1959.

35. Goodwin, D. W. Blackouts and alcohol-induced memory dysfunction. In *Recent Advances in Studies of Alcoholism*. Washington, D.C.: U.S. DHEW, 1971.

36. Goodwin, D. W. Alcohol in suicides and homicides. Q. J. Stud. Alcohol *34*:144–156, 1973.

37. Goodwin, D. W., Schulsinger, F., Hermansen, L., Guze, S. B., and Winokur, G. Alcohol problems in adoptees raised apart from alcoholic biological parents. Arch. Gen. Psychiat. *28*:238–242, 1973.

38. Goodwin, D. W., Schulsinger, F., Möller, N., Hermansen, L., Winokur, G., and Guze, S. B. Drinking problems in adopted and nonadopted sons of alcoholics. Arch. Gen. Psychiat. *31*:164–169, 1974.

39. Goodwin, D. W., Schulsinger, F., Hermansen, L., Guze, S. B., and Winokur, G. Alcoholism and the hyperactive child syndrome. J. Nerv. Ment. Dis. *160*:349–353, 1975.

40. Goodwin, D. W., and Hill, S. Y. Chronic effects of alcohol and other psychoactive drugs on intellect, learning and memory. In *Chronic Effects of Alcohol and Other Psychoactive Drugs on Cerebral Function*. Toronto: Addict. Res. Foundation Press, 1975.

41. Goodwin, D. W., Schulsinger, F., Möller, N., Mednick, S., and Guze, S. B. Psychopathology in adopted and nonadopted daughters of alcoholics. Arch. Gen. Psychiat. *34*:1005–1009, 1977.

42. Goodwin, D. W. Alcoholism and heredity: a review and hypothesis. Arch. Gen. Psychiat. *36*:57–61, 1979.

43. Goodwin, D. W. *Alcoholism: The Facts*. New York: Oxford Univ. Press, 1995.

44. Goodwin, D. W. In *DSM-III Case Book*, Spitzer, R. L., Skodol, A. E., Gibbon, M., and Williams, J. B. W. (eds.). Washington, D. C.: American Psychiatric Association, 1981.

45. Goodwin, D. W. Drug therapy of alcoholism. In *Psychopharmacology*, vol. I. Grahame-Smith, D. G., Hippius, H., and Winokur, G. (eds.) Amsterdam: Excerpta Medica, 1982.

46. Goodwin, D. W. Alcoholism and affective disorders. In *Alcoholism and Clinical Psychiatry*, N.Y. Academy of Medicine (ed.). New York: Plenum Press, 1982.

47. Goodwin, D. W. On defining alcoholism and taking stands. J. Clin. Psychiat. *43*:394–395, 1982.

48. Goodwin, D. W. Familial alcoholism. Subst. Alcohol Actions Misuse *4*:129–136, 1983.

49. Gorelick, P. B., Rodin, M. B., Langenberg, P., Hier, D. B., Costigan, J., Gomez, I., and Spontak, S. Is acute alcohol ingestion a risk factor for ischemic stroke? Results of a controlled study in middle-aged and elderly stroke patients at three urban medical centers. Stroke *18*:359–364, 1987.

50. Harper, C., Kril, J., and Daly, J. Are we drinking our neurones away? Brit. Med. J. *294*:534–536, 1987.

51. Harvey, E. B., Schairer, C., Brinton, L. A., Hoover, R. N., and Fraumeni, J. F. Alcohol consumption and breast cancer. J. Natl. Cancer Inst. *78*:657–661, 1987.

52. Hesselbrock, V. M., Stabenau, J. R., Hesselbrock, M. N., Meyer, R. E., and Babor, T. F. The nature of alcoholism in patients with different family histories for alcoholism. Neuropsychopharmacol. Biol. Psychiat. *6*:607–614, 1982.

53. Hill, S. Y., Reyes, R. B., Mikhael, M., and Ayre, F. A comparison of alcoholics and heroin abusers: computerized transaxial tomography and neuropsychological functioning. In *Currents in Alcoholism*, Sexias, F. (ed.). New York: Grune & Stratton, 1977.

54. Hill, S., and Steinhauer, S. Event-related potentials in women at risk for alcoholism. Alcohol *10*:5, 349–354, 1993.

55. Hrubec, Z., and Omenn, G. S. Evidence of genetic predisposition to alcoholic cirrhosis and psychosis: twin concordances for alcoholism and its biological end points by zygosity among male veterans. Alcohol. Clin. Exp. Res. *5*:207–215, 1981.

56. Hsu, J. J. Electroconditioning therapy of alcoholics. Q. J. Stud. Alcohol *26*:449–459, 1965.

57. Jacobson, R. The contributions of sex and drinking history to the CT brain scan changes in alcoholics. Psychol. Med. *16*:547–559, 1986.

58. Jellinek, E. M. *The Disease Concept of Alcoholism.* New Haven, Conn.: College & University Press, 1960.

59. Jellinek, E. M. Phases of alcohol addiction. Q. J. Stud. Alcohol *13*:673–684, 1952.

60. Kendler, K., Heath, A., Neale, M., Kessler, R., and Eaves, L. A population-based twin study of alcoholism in women. JAMA *268*:14, 1877–1882, 1992.

61. Kessler, R., McGonagle, K., Zhao, S., Nelson, C., Hughes, M., Eshleman, S., Wittchen, H., and Kendler, K. Lifetime and 12-month prevalence of DSM-III-R psychiatric disorders in the United States: results from the national comorbidity survey. Arch. Gen. Psychiat. *51*:1, 8–19, 1994.

62. Jones, K. L., Smith, D. W., Ulleland, C. M., et al. Pattern of malformation in offspring of chronic alcoholic mothers. Lancet *1*:1267–1271, 1973.

63. Jones, M. C. Personality correlates and antecedents of drinking patterns in adult males. J. Consult. Clin. Psychol. *32*:2–12, 1968.

64. Kaij, L. *Studies on the Etiology and Sequels of Abuse of Alcohol.* Lund, Sweden: Univ. of Lund, 1960.

65. Keller, M. On defining alcoholism: with comment on some other relevant words. In *Alcohol, Science and Society Revisited.* Ann Arbor: Univ. of Michigan Press, 1982.

66. Keller, M., McCormick, M., and Efron, V. *A Dictionary of Words About Alcohol,* 2d ed. New Brunswick, N.J.: Rutgers Univ. Center of Alcohol Studies, 1982.

67. Klatsky. A. L., Armstrong, M. A., and Friedman, G. D. Relations of alcoholic beverage use to subsequent coronary artery disease hospitalization. Am. J. Cardiol. *58*:710–714, 1986.

68. Kline, N. S., Wren, J. C., Cooper, T. B., Varga, E., and Canal, O. Evaluation of lithium therapy in chronic and periodic alcoholism. Am. J. Med. Sci. *268*:15–22, 1974.

69. Kumar, R., Mac, D. S., Gabrielli, W. F., and Goodwin, D. W. Anxiolytics and memory: a comparison of lorazepam and alprazolam. J. Clin. Psychiat. *48*:158–160, 1987.

70. Leevy, C. M., Frank, O., Leevy, C. B., and Baker, H. Nutritional factors in liver disease of the alcoholic. Acta Med. Scand. Suppl. *703*:67–79, 1985.

71. Lemoine, P., Harousseau, H., Borteyru, J. P., et al. Les Enfants de parents alcooliques: anomalies observees. Quest. Med. *25*:476–482, 1968.

72. Lieber, C. S. Metabolic effects produced by alcohol in the liver and other tisues. Adv. Intern. Med. *14*:151–199, 1968.

73. Lieber, C. S., and DeCarli, L. M. An experimental model of alcohol feeding and liver injury in the baboon. J. Med. Primatol. *3*:153–163, 1974.

74. Lieber, C. Biochemical factors in alcoholic liver disease. Semin. Liver Dis., *13*:2, 136–153, 1993.

75. Ludwig, A. M. On and off the wagon. Q. J. Stud. Alcohol *33*:91–96, 1972.

76. MacAndrew, C., and Edgerton, R. B. *Drunken Comportment: A Social Explanation.* Chicago: Aldine, 1969.

77. MacMahon, S. Alcohol consumption and hypertension. Hypertension *9*:111–121, 1987.

78. Mandell, W., Eaton, W., Anthony, J., and Garrison R. Alcoholism and occupations: a review and analysis of 104 occupations. Alcohol. Clin. Exp. Res. *16*:4, 734–746, 1992.

79. Marinacci, A. A. Electroencephalography in alcoholism. In *Alcoholism,* 484–536, Springfield, Ill.: C. C. Thomas, 1956.

80. McCord, W., and McCord, J. A longitudinal study of the personality of alcoholics. In *Society, Culture, and Drinking Patterns.* New York: Wiley, 1962.

81. Mendelson, J. H. Biologic concomitants of alcoholism. N. Engl. J. Med. *283*:24–32, 1970.

82. Merry, J., Reynolds, C. M., Bailey, J., and Coppen, A. Prophylactic treatment of alcoholism by lithium carbonate. Lancet *2*:481–482, 1976.

83. Miller, W. R., and Joyce, M. A. Prediction of abstinence, controlled drinking, and heavy drinking outcomes following behavioral self-control training. J. Consult. Clin. Psychol. *47*:773–775, 1979.

84. Morris, H. H., and Estes, M. L. Traveler's amnesia. JAMA *258*:945–946, 1987.

85. Morse, R., and Flavin, D. The definition of alcoholism. JAMA *268*:1012–1014, 1992.

86. Murray, R. M., Clifford, C., and Gurlin, H. M. Twin and alcoholism studies.

In *Recent Developments in Alcoholism*, vol. 1, chap. 5, Galanter, M. (ed.). New York: Gardner Press, 1983.

87. National Institute on Alcohol Abuse and Alcoholism. *Epidemiologic Report.* August–December 1992.

88. Nielsen, D., Goldman, D., Virkkunen, M., Tokola, R., Rawlings, R., and Linnoila, M. Suicidality and 5-hydroxyindoleacetic acid concentration associated with a tryptophan hydroxylase polymorphism. Arch. Gen. Psychiat. *51*:1, 34–38, 1994.

89. Ogata, M., Mendelson, J., and Mello, N. Electrolytes and osmolality in alcoholics during experimental intoxication. Psychosom. Med. *30*:463–488, 1968.

90. Partanen, J., Bruun, K., and Markkanen, T. Inheritance of drinking behavior: a study of intelligence, personality, and use of alcohol of adult twins. In *Emerging Concepts of Alcohol Dependence*, chap. 10, Pattison, E. M., Sobell, M. B., Sobell, L. C. (eds.). New York: Springer, 1977.

91. Peck, C. C., Pond, S. M., Becker, C. E., and Lee, K. An evaluation of the effects of lithium in the treatment of chronic alcoholism. II. Assessment of the two-period crossover design. Alcohol. Clin. Exp. Res. *5*:252, 1981.

92. Pemberton, D. A. A comparison of the outcome of treatment in female and male alcoholics. Brit. J. Psychiat. *113*:367–373, 1967.

93. Penick, E., Read, M., Crowley, P., and Powell, B. Differentiation of alcoholics by family history. J. Stud. Alcohol *39*:1944–1948, 1978.

94. Pfefferbaum. A., Lim, K., Zipursky, R., Mathalon, D., Rosenbloom, M., Lane, B., Ha, C., and Sullivan, E. Brain gray and white matter volume loss accelerates with aging in chronic alcoholics: a quantitative MRI study. Alcohol. Clin. Exp. Res. *16*:6, 1078–1089, 1992.

95. Randall, C., Taylor, W., and Walker, D. Ethanol-induced malformations in mice. Alcohol. Clin. Exp. Res. *1*:219–223, 1977.

96. Reed, R., Grant, I., and Rourke, S. Long-term abstinent alcoholics have normal memory. Alcohol. Clin. Exp. Res. *16*:4, 677–683, 1992.

97. Robins, L. N., Bates, W. M., and O'Neil, P. Adult drinking patterns of former problem children. In *Society, Culture, and Drinking Patterns*. New York: Wiley, 1962.

98. Roe, A. The adult adjustment of children of alcoholic parents raised in foster homes. Q. J. Stud. Alcohol *5*:378–393, 1944.

99. Romano, J., Michael, Jr., M., and Merritt, H. H. Alcoholic cerebellar degeneration. Arch. Neurol. Psychiat. *44*:1230–1236, 1940.

100. Roueché, B. *Alcohol.* New York: Grove Press, 1960.

101. Rush, B. *An Inquiry into the Effects of Ardent Spirits upon the Human Body and Mind*, 6th ed. New York: 1811.

102. Ryback, R. S., Eckardt, M. J., and Felsher, B. Biochemical and hematological correlates of alcoholism and liver disease. JAMA *248*:2261–2265, 1982.

103. Schuckit, M., Pitts, Jr., F. N., Reich, T., King, L. J., and Winokur, G. Alcohol. Arch. Environ. Health *18*:301–306, 1969.

104. Schuckit, M. A., Goodwin, D. W., and Winokur, G. A half-sibling study of alcoholism. Am. J. Psychiat. *128*:1132–1136, 1972.

105. Schuckit, M. Low level of response to alcohol as a predictor of future alcoholism. Am. J. Psychiat. *151*:2, 184–189, 1994.

106. Sigerist, H. E. *The History of Medicine.* New York: M.D. Publications, 1960.

107. *Sixth Special Report to the United States Congress on Alcohol and Health.* Rockville, Md.: National Institute on Alcohol Abuse and Alcoholism, 1987.

108. Tamerin, J. S., Weiner, S., Poppen, R., Steinglass, P., and Mendelson, J. H. Alcohol and memory: amnesia and short-term memory function during experimentally induced intoxication. Am. J. Psychiat. *127*:1659–1664, 1971.

109. Tarter, R. Minimal brain dsyfunction as an etiological predisposition in alcoholism. In *Evaluation of the Alcoholic: Implications for Research, Theory and Practice,* chap. 12. Res. Monog., Meyer, R., Glueck, J., Babor, T., Jaffe, J., and Stabenau, J. (eds.). Washington, D.C.: U.S. DHHS, 1981.

110. Taylor, M. E., and St. Pierre, S. Women and alcohol research: a review of current literature. J. Drug Issues *16*:621–634, 1986.

111. Turner, T. B., Bennett, V. L., and Hernandez, H. The beneficial side of moderate alcohol use. Johns Hopkins Med. J. *148*:53, 1981.

112. Vaillant, G. E. *The Natural History of Alcoholism.* Cambridge: Harvard Univ. Press, 1983.

113. Velleman, R., and Orford, J. The adult adjustment of offspring of parents with drinking problems. Brit. J. Psychiat. *162*:503–516, 1993.

114. Victor, M., and Adams, R. D. The effect of alcohol on the nervous system. In *Proceedings of the Association for Research in Nervous and Mental Disease.* Baltimore: Williams & Wilkins, 1953.

115. Victor, M., Adams, R. D., and Collins, G. H. *The Wernicke-Korsakoff Syndrome.* Philadelphia: F. A. Davis, 1971.

116. Victor, M., and Hope, J. M. The phenomenon of auditory hallucinations in chronic alcoholism. J. Nerv. Ment. Dis. *126*:451, 1958.

117. Virkkunen, M., Kallio, E., Rawlings, R., Tokola, R., Poland, R., Guidotti, A., Nemeroff, C., Bissette, G., Kalogeras, K., Karonen, S., and Linnoila, M. Personality profiles and state aggressiveness in Finnish alcoholic, violent offenders, fire setters, and healthy volunteers. Arch. Gen, Psychiat. *51*:1, 28–33, 1994.

118. Virkkunen, M., Rawlings, R., Tokola, R., Poland, R., Guidotti, A., Nemeroff, C., Bissette, G., Kalogeras, K., Karonen, S., and Linnoila, M. CSF biochemistries, glucose metabolism, and diurnal activity rhythms in alcoholic, violent offenders, fire setters, and healthy volunteers. Arch. Gen. Psychiat. *51*:1, 20–27, 1994.

119. Vitols, M. M. Culture patterns of drinking in negro and white alcoholics. Dis. Nerv. Syst. *29*:344–391, 1968.

120. Voegtlin, W. L. The treatment of alcoholism by establishing a conditioned reflex. Am. J. Med. Sci., *199*:802–809, 1940.

121. Volkow, N., Wang, G., Hitzemann, R., Fowler, J., Overall, J., Burr, G., and Wolf, A. Recovery of brain glucose metabolism in detoxified alcoholics. Am. J. Psychiat. *151*:2, 178–183, 1994.

122. Wallgren, H., and Barry, H., III. *Actions of Alcohol*, vol. I. Amsterdam: Elsevier, 1970.
123. Whitefield, J. B. Alcohol-related biochemical changes in heavy drinkers. Aust. N.Z. J. Med. *11*:132, 1981.
124. Willett, W. C., Stampfer, M. J., Colditz, G. A., Rosner, B. A., Hennekens, C. H., and Speizer, F. E. Moderate alcohol consumption and the risk of breast cancer. N. Engl. J. Med. *316*:1174–1180, 1987.
125. Woodruff, Jr., R. A., Guze, S. B., and Clayton, P. J. Divorce among psychiatric out-patients. Brit. J. Psychiat. *121*:289–292, 1972.
126. Yellowlees, P. M. Thiamin deficiency and prevention of the Wernicke-Korsakoff syndrome. Med. J. Aust. *145*:216–219, 1986.

8

DRUG DEPENDENCE

DEFINITION

Drug dependence refers to the repeated use of a psychoactive drug, causing harm to the user or to others. The World Health Organization recommends this term instead of "addiction" or "habituation" (24). Both these words are still widely used in the literature, however, and require definition.

Addiction is used in two senses, physical and psychological. *Physical addiction* refers to a drug-produced condition characterized by tolerance and physical dependence. *Tolerance* refers to an adaptive biological process in which "increasingly larger doses of a drug must be administered to obtain the effect observed with the original dose." *Physical dependence* refers to "the physiological state produced by the repeated administration of the drug which necessitates the continued administration of the drug to prevent the appearance of the stereotyped syndrome, the withdrawal or abstinence syndrome, characteristic for the particular drug" (28).

Psychological addiction refers to a "behavioral pattern of compulsive drug use, characterized by overwhelming involvement with the use of a drug, the securing of its supply, and a high tendency to relapse after withdrawal" (36). Physical and psychological addiction may overlap but do not necessarily occur together. For example, a person physically addicted to morphine

218

administered for pain in a hospital may have none of the characteristics of psychological addiction. On the other hand, individuals may be psychologically addicted to drugs with little or no tolerance or physical dependence. Except for the opiates and to a lesser extent the barbiturates, no drugs produce striking degrees of both tolerance and physical dependence and therefore meet the two pharmacological criteria for addiction (28).

Habituation refers to dependence on a drug for an "optimal state of well-being, ranging from a mild desire to a craving or compulsion (a compelling urge) to use the drug" (28).

DSM-IV lists nine symptoms of *psychoactive substance dependence* (Table 8.1). It also includes a category called *psychoactive*

Table 8.1 Diagnostic criteria for Psychoactive Substance Dependence (*DSM-IV*)

A maladaptive pattern of substance use, leading to clinically significant impairment or distress, as manifested by three (or more) of the following, occurring at any time in the same 12-month period:

(1) Tolerance, as defined by either of the following:

    (*a*) a need for markedly increased amounts of the substance to achieve intoxication or desired effect

    (*b*) markedly diminished effect with continued use of the same amount of the substance

(2) Withdrawal, as manifested by either of the following:

    (*a*) The characteristic withdrawal syndrome for the substance (refer to criteria A and B of the criteria sets for Withdrawal from the specific substances)

    (*b*) The same (or a closely related) substance is taken to relieve or avoid withdrawal symptoms

(3) The substance is often taken in larger amounts or over a longer period than was intended

(4) There is a persistent desire or unsuccessful efforts to cut down or control substance use

(5) A great deal of time is spent in activities necessary to obtain the substance (e.g., visiting multiple doctors or driving long distances), use the substance (e.g., chain-smoking), or recover from its effects

(Continued)

Table 8.1 Diagnostic criteria for Psychoactive Substance Dependence (*DSM-IV*) (*Continued*)

---

(6) Important social, occupational, or recreational activities are given up or reduced because of substance use

(7) The substance use is continued despite knowledge of having a persistent or recurrent physical or psychological problem that is likely to have been caused or exacerbated by the substance (e.g., current cocaine use despite recognition of cocaine-induced depression, or continued drinking despite recognition that an ulcer was made worse by alcohol consumption)

Specify if:
WITH PHYSIOLOGICAL DEPENDENCE: evidence of tolerance or withdrawal (i.e., either item 1 or 2 is present)
WITHOUT PHYSIOLOGICAL DEPENDENCE: no evidence of tolerance or withdrawal (i.e., neither item 1 nor 2 is present)

---

substance abuse. Individuals fitting this category do not fulfill the criteria for dependence but repeatedly use drugs despite (a) social, occupational, psychological, or physical harm from the substance or (b) a risk of drug-related accidents. Examples are persons with hepatitis who drink despite warnings from their physicians, or persons who drive while intoxicated. Alcoholism, included by *DSM-IV* as a psychoactive substance use disorder, is discussed in chapter 7.

HISTORICAL BACKGROUND

The basic needs of the human race . . . are food, clothing, and shelter. To that fundamental trinity most modern authorities would add, as equally compelling, security and love. There are, however, many other needs whose satisfaction, though somewhat less essential, can seldom be comfortably denied. One of these, and perhaps the most insistent, is an occasional release from the intolerable clutch of reality. All men throughout recorded history have known this tyranny of memory and mind, and all have sought . . . some reliable means of briefly loosening its grip.

BERTON ROUECHÉ(82)

Whether or not this fully explains the motivation behind the use of intoxicating substances, it is true they have been used by humankind for thousands of years in nearly every part of the world. Except in a few primitive cultures, humans have discovered plants whose juices and powders that on being properly prepared and consumed have caused desirable alterations of consciousness. In ancient times, these substances were widely used in religious ceremonies (as wine is still used in the Catholic mass and peyote by the North American Church), but they also have been used for recreational purposes. As the sciences of medicine and chemistry progressed, the variety of drugs increased and for many years drugs have been diverted from medical use into "illicit" channels as they are today.

The analgesic drugs derived from the poppy plant were particularly susceptible to abuse because they produced euphoria as well as analgesia. Drug "epidemics" have occurred periodically in recent centuries. The introduction of opium into England, commercially promoted as part of the Chinese opium trade, led to widespread abuse of the drug in the nineteenth century. With the introduction of the hypodermic needle during the American Civil War period, the use of morphine for nonmedicinal purposes became widespread, and by the turn of the century large numbers of people were apparently dependent on the drug, taken intravenously or more often as an ingredient of patent medicines. Heroin, the diethylated form of morphine, was introduced around the turn of the century as a "heroic" solution for the opiate problem (a form of substitution therapy, just as methadone is used today).

Another development of the mid-nineteenth century was the introduction of bromides as sedatives. There was an enormous demand for these compounds and a steady increase in their use. With use came misuse, which often resulted in intoxication and psychotic reactions. The bromide problem began to abate in the 1930s as barbiturates and other sedatives became available. The first barbiturate, Veronal, was introduced in 1903 and others appeared in quick succession. The short-acting barbiturates such as pentobarbital and amobarbital became popular in the 1930s and 1940s, their dependence-producing qualities not having been immediately recognized (28).

During the late nineteenth century individuals in the West discovered botanicals used for mind-altering purposes elsewhere, such as cocaine and hashish (the most potent form of cannabis). Cocaine was found to be useful medically (by Freud, among others), and a number of well-known physicians and surgeons became cocaine addicts.

Ether, also discovered in the nineteenth century, was used recreationally, again often by medical people, as were nitrous oxide and other volatile solvents. Doctors and nurses, presumably because of their access to these drugs and their familiarity with them, were particularly prone to take them, although reliable data regarding drug abuse by physicians at any time in history, including today, are not available. Meperidine, introduced in the 1940s as a "nonaddictive" synthetic narcotic, led to a mild epidemic of abuse among physicians before its addictive potential was appreciated.

In postwar Japan, thousands of young people turned to amphetamines. Drastic measures were required to control the problem, including the establishment of special psychiatric facilities and stringent legal controls.

The most recent epidemic of drug abuse began in the early 1960s when hallucinogens became part of the American middle-class youth culture. It originated with Hofmann's discovery in 1953 that lysergic acid diethylamide (LSD) produced perceptual distortions and other aberrant mental phenomena. Again, physicians were involved in the introduction of the drug (48). It was first used on the U.S. east and west coasts experimentally because it produced symptoms resembling those seen in psychosis. It was also used therapeutically, usually by psychoanalysts who felt the drug would dissolve "repressions." Because LSD is easy to synthesize, it became widely available and has been used, at least experimentally, by several million people, the majority of them of young age and from the middle or upper-middle class.

As mind-altering drugs became widely publicized in the 1960s, more and more young people experimented with them. In the early adolescent group, glue-sniffing and inhalation of other volatile solvents were apparently widely practiced, whereas persons in late adolescence and then early twenties, particularly on college campuses, experimented with LSD and other synthetic hallucinogens such as dimethlytryptamine (DMT) and other derivatives of the indole and catecholamines that produced psychedelic effects. Starting in the mid-1970s, the use of LSD and other psychedelics began to decline and has continued to decline since then (30), with a slight trend toward increased use in the 1990s. Meanwhile, increase in the use of amphetamines produced a generation of speed freaks who injected methamphetamine intravenously. Downers such as barbiturates and other sedative-hypnotics also became popular among young people in the late 1960s. Cocaine became available in suuburbia and on college campuses, although, as in the case of other street drugs, often the "cocaine" people thought they were obtaining was either adulterated or completely absent. This was also the case with mescaline, the active principal of peyote (61).

Apparently because marihuana also enhances sensory processes (62) and also is abundantly available, it became the most widely used illicit LSD-like drug in America during the 1960s and 1970s. Marihuana, the "tobacco" of the hemp plant, has grown wild in America since colonial times or before, but until the past decade was used recreationally only by small minorities such as jazz musicians in the 1930s and Mexican immigrant workers (13). Widely condemned in the 1930s as a dangerous drug, marihuana has been increasingly accepted in Western countries as a benign if not completely innocuous substance, and there has been increasing pressure to "decriminalize" the drug if not acutally make it legally available. Marihuana and its potent relative, hashish, are still, however, illegal in most countries, many of which are signatories to a U.N. treaty prohibiting its sale. Moreover, between 1974 and 1994, U.S. teenagers using marihuana fell from 23% to 17% (*Wall Street Journal*, March 29, 1995).

Although marihuana and the hallucinogens were being widely used in middle- and upper-middle-class America in the 1960s, heroin—the fast-acting, potent form of morphine—became a serious medical and legal problem, involving mainly lower-class black urban men. In the early 1990s it was estimated that New York City alone had more than 100,000 opiate addicts. Because of the expense of heroin, its use led to widespread criminal activities, including corruption of police authorities. Deaths resulted from overdosage, allergic responses, or medical complications following unsterile intravenous injection. The heroin "epidemic" was limited somewhat by the high price of the drug and its relative unavailability in noncoastal cities.

Nicotine addiction is not discussed in this chapter although, according to the U.S. surgeon general, it is the most addictive substance used by humans. A few years ago, half of the adult population in the US smoked nicotine cigarettes. The figure has now fallen to 25% and will probably drop even further as antismoking sentiment becomes even greater. The idea that nicotine was addictive—more addictive than cocaine or heroin—is a view that has become officially sanctioned only in recent years. The government now maintains that hundreds of thousands of Americans die every year of nicotine-related illnesses, particularly heart disease and lung cancer. Even secondhand smoke is dangerous, according to the surgeon general and the Environmental Protection Agency. A brief history of tobacco use therefore seems justified.

In 1492 Columbus recorded in his diary the gift of "strange dry leaves" from a native of San Salvador. Within a few years tobacco had crossed the Atlantic to Europe and became popular for recreational and medical uses. In 1560 Jean Nicot, French Ambassador to Portugal, touted tobacco's curative powers. The word "nicotine" comes from *nicot*. The first commercial tobacco crop was grown in Jamestown in 1612. Within a short time tobacco cultivation spread throughout the colonies. Britain wanted control of tobacco exports, increasing anti-British sentiment. Large plantations sprang up, an impetus for the use of slaves.

In 1881 a cigarette-making machine, capable of making 120,000 cigarettes a day, was invented. Cigarettes became immensely popular; this was met by an enthusiastic antismoking movement, including laws against smoking, that died out in World War I. In 1918 the United States War Department included tobacco in soldier's rations. By war's end cigarettes sales had reached one billion a year. During World War II and afterwards American cigarettes were accepted as currency around the world.

In 1964 the surgeon general linked tobacco to cancer, heart disease, and other serious ailments. Warning labels were required on packs. A ban on radio and TV advertising of cigarettes took effect. More and more of the workplaces in the country became smoke-free.

Nonsmokers became increasingly intolerant of cigarette smoke in their environment and many of the remaining smokers tried to stop but had difficulty. Teenage girls became the last remaining major group of new smokers.

EPIDEMIOLOGY

Epidemiological surveys of drug use involve not only the usual unreliability expected in prevalence studies but also problems peculiar to drug studies, especially the rapidly changing patterns of use. It is generally agreed, for example, that use of marihuana and cocaine has increased vastly since 1970, but data from earlier periods are lacking for comparative purposes.

One fact is certain: Leaving aside caffeine-containing beverages, alcohol and tobacco dominated the recreational drug scene in the United States until the 1960s (3). Opposition to the Vietnam War and the sexual revolution in the 1960s were accompanied by an explosion of illicit drug use, ranging from a rediscovery of the products of the poppy and cannabis plants to new "designer" drugs that could be synthesized in basements by people with a modicum of technical knowledge—drugs not even illegal until laws could be passed to make them so (21). The use of these drugs, singly and in combination, has produced a huge public health problem in western countries. Among young people in particular, polydrug use has led to a spectrum of bizarre reactions as confusing to physicians as to worried parents.

It now appears that drug abuse in general is leveling off and that there is a modest decline in alcohol use and a more dramatic reduction in smoking. A great many people, however, have been exposed to a wide variety of illicit drugs. More than $1 billion is spent on illicit drugs. Another $60 billion is lost in drug-related crime, health problems, and lowered productivity. Intravenous drug users are second only to homosexuals as a risk group for acquired immune deficiency syndrome (AIDS).

The image of drug abusers has changed. Socialites, athletes, and Hollywood celebrities have been arrested in increasing numbers for possession of cocaine. Marihuana has been partially decriminalized in some states: selling it is still a crime, but possession of small amounts is not. Nevertheless, law enforcement devotes heavy resources to combating marihuana use. The popularity of crack—a hazardous derivative of cocaine—in affluent suburbia as well as urban ghettoes seems one of the most serious perils in this very rapidly changing drug scene, whereas LSD and the other hallucinogens have declined greatly in use since the 1970s.

DRUG COMPARISONS

Table 8.2, based on an interview published in the *New York Times* (August 2, 1994), shows how two experts rate the six most commonly used "recreational" drugs in America. The ratings agree so closely as to indicate that a consensus has emerged from the conflicting views of the 1960s. Both experts regard cocaine as the most "reinforcing" of the substances reviewed and see alcohol as only moderately reinforcing, Reinforcement is a measure of the substance's capacity, in human and animal tests, to prompt users

Table 8.2 How experts rate problem substances*

Substance	Withdrawal	Reinforcement	Tolerance	Dependence	Intoxication
Henningfield rating					
Nicotine	3	4	2	1	5
Heroin	2	2	1	2	2
Cocaine	4	1	4	3	3
Alcohol	1	3	3	4	1
Caffeine	5	6	5	5	6
Marihuana	6	5	6	6	4
Benowitz ratings					
Nicotine	3	4	4	1	6
Heroin	2	2	2	2	2
Cocaine	3	1	1	3	3
Alcohol	1	3	4	4	1
Caffeine	4	5	3	5	5
Marihuana	5	6	5	6	4

* 1 = most serious; 6 = least serious

Dr. Jack E. Henningfield of the National Institute on Drug Abuse and Dr. Neal L. Benowitz of the University of California at San Francisco ranked six substances in five problem areas

to take it again, in preference to other substances. Addictiveness is closely linked to reinforcement. (Withdrawal, tolerance, and dependence were defined earlier. "Intoxication," though not usually counted as a measure of addiction in itself, is associated with addiction: The level of intoxication possible with a drug increases the personal and social damage a substance may do.)

DRUG CATEGORIES

Opioids

Opioids are derivatives of plant substances (opiates) that occur naturally and have morphine-like effects or opiate-like substances synthesized or semisynthesized in the laboratory. Other opiates include heroin, hydromorphone (Dilaudid), codeine, oxycodone and paregoric. Meperidine (Demerol) is a synthetic analgesic structurally dissimilar to morphine but pharmaco-logically similar. Heroin is the only one of these substances not available for medical use in the United States.

In usual therapeutic doses, opioids produced analgesia, drowsi-ness, and a change in mood described as a sense of well-being. Opioids also function as respiratory depressants (often the cause of death in cases of overdose); they produce constriction of the pupils, constipation, and occasionally nausea and vomiting.

Most heroin and morphine addicts take opiates intravenously, which produces flushing and a sensation described as similar to orgasm, known as a "rush." Initial increased activity is followed by a period of drowsiness and inactivity, which has been called "being on the nod" or "nodding out." During this time opium dreams occur.

Tolerance develops to most opioid effects, including euphoria. Libido declines; menstruation may cease. Some addicts who are able to obtain an adequate supply of opiates dress properly, main-tain nutrition, and discharge social and occupational obligations without gross impairment. Other addicts become socially dis-abled, often because the expense of drugs may lead to theft, forg-ery, prostitution, and the sale of drugs to other users.

The first symptoms of opioid withdrawal usually appear eight to twelve hours after the last dose once a habit has been established (Table 8.3). These include lacrimation, rhinorrhea, sweating, and yawning. Thereafter, the addict may fall into a fitful sleep known as "the yen" from which he or she awakens after several hours, restless and miserable. Additional signs and symptoms appear, reaching a peak between forty-eight and seventy-two hours after drug discontinuation. These include dilated pupils, anorexia, restlessness, insomnia, irritability, gooseflesh, nausea, vomiting, diarrhea, chills, and abdominal cramps. These manifestations subside gradually. After seven to ten days, most signs of withdrawal have disappeared, although the patient may continue to experience insomnia, weakness, and nervousness.

In addition to acute withdrawal symptoms, opioids may pro-duce a protracted abstinent syndrome lasting several months (20).

Body temperature and respiratory rate may be below normal. The patient may have trouble sleeping. More important, the craving for opiates may persist for several months after the last dose. This probably contributes to the high recidivism rate in opiate users. Recidivism has also been attributed to a phenomenon called the "conditioned abstinent syndrome" (20). Detoxified patients who return to the environment in which they use drugs may experience craving for the drug as well as physical manifestations of abstinence because of conditioned stimuli (seeing old friends, familiar places, and so forth).

To ameliorate withdrawal symptoms, oral methadone or LAAM (a long-acting form of methadone) can be substituted for any opioid. Methadone can be discontinued gradually over a period of one or two weeks. Clonidine, an alpha-adrenergic agonist given for hypertension, also alleviates the opiate withdrawal syndrome, suggesting that catecholamines are involved in opiate withdrawal. Clonidine has one advantage over methadone: It allows the patient to become narcotic-free (54). The disadvantages of clonidine include sedation, insomnia and hypotension (9).

The course of opiate addiction varies depending on the population studied. In Vaillant's twelve-year follow-up of opiate addicts originally treated at the federal addiction treatment center at Lexington, 98 percent had returned to the use of opiates within twelve months after release (97). On the other hand, a study of Vietnam veterans who used opium and its products extensively during their tour in Vietnam revealed that less than 10 percent continued using the drug in the year after their return to the United States (19). This suggests that circumstances of exposure and availability are important factors in maintaining use.

In America, most heroin addicts are men and, at least in inner cities on the two coasts, a majority are nonwhite. The male:female ratio is about three or four to one. Medical prescriptions of opioids increase with age. There is some evidence that heroin users from this population who do not die as a result of drugs or criminal activities may spontaneously stop using the drug after

Table 8.3 Abstinence signs in sequential appearance after last dose of opiate in patients with well-established parenteral habits*

		Hours After Last Dose					
Grades of Abstinence	Signs (Observed in Cool Room, Patient Uncovered or Under Only a Sheet)	Morphine	Heroin	Meperidine	Dihydro-Morphinone	Codeine
Grade 0	Craving for drug Anxiety	6	4	2–3	2–3	8
Grade 1	Yawning Perspiration Lacrimation Rhinorrhea Yen sleep	14	8	4–6	4–5	24
Grade 2	Increase in above signs plus: Mydriasis Gooseflesh (piloerection) Tremors (muscle twitches) Hot and cold flashes Aching bones and muscles Anorexia	16	12	8–12	7	48

| Grade 3 | Increased intensity of above plus:
Insomnia
Increased blood pressure
Increased temperature (1–2)
Increased respiratory rate and depth
Increased pulse rate
Restlessness
Nausea | 24–36 | 18–24 | 16 | 12 | — |
| Grade 4 | Increased intensity of above plus:
Febrile facies
Position—curled up on hard surface
Vomiting
Diarrhea
Weight loss (5 lb daily)
Spontaneous ejaculation or orgasm
Hemoconcentration
leukocytosis, eosinopenia,
increased blood sugar | 36–48 | 24–36 | — | 16 | — |

*Not all signs are necessary to diagnose any particular grade. Racemorphan (Dromoran) and levorphanol (Levodromoran), although three times and six times as strong as morphine sulfate, show same time curve as morphine sulfate. Similarly paregoric, laudanum, and hydrochlorides of opium alkaloids (Pantopon), depending on their relative content of morphine

Adapted from Anglin et al. (5)

their mid-thirties. School problems such as delinquency and truancy frequently antedate heroin use (13).

Even in environments where addiction is common, there seems to be a sizable number of occasional or controlled users of heroin; they are sometimes referred to as "chippers." Although well known in the street, they are rarely mentioned in the professional literature, where they are generally assumed to be people in a transition stage leading to either compulsive use or abstinence. In fact, the evidence suggests that some people may use heroin occasionally and without signs of addiction for many years. In the case of any street drug, however, the purity of the substance must be taken into account. Chippers may be able to control their heroin use because the heroin is of low potency.

There is little evidence that opiate users have other diagnosable psychiatric illnesses than opiate dependence (except perhaps sociopathy), although many of them take other drugs such as alcohol and barbiturates. Multiple drug use, based on observation in methadone clinics, is considered a bad prognostic sign in heroin addicts.

The mortality from opiate withdrawal is negligible despite the unpleasantness of the withdrawal sundrome. Deaths from medical causes occurring among addicts are mainly due to infection, overdose, and apparent hypersensitivity reactions, possibly from diluents such as quinine. Unsterile injections may produce septicemia, hepatitis, subacute bacterial endocarditis, tetanus, and AIDS. Uncertain dosage is often the cause of death from opiates. The powders sold on the street are highly variable in potency. Accustomed to the normal successive dilutions of the drug as it passes through the distribution channels, addicts may unexpectedly encounter relatively pure heroin and consequently overdose. Opioid overdose may be fatal because of respiratory depression and may require ventilatory assistance in a hospital. Naloxone, an opioid antagonist, will reverse respiratory depression.

In studies in metropolitan Chicago, Hughes and his colleagues have found that heroin addiction occurs in epidemics, that heroin use spreads from peer to peer, and that newly involved cases are more "contagious" than chronic cases. Microepidemics—five to fifteen new cases over a five-year period—are seen in some locales, and macroepidemics—more than fifty new cases over a five-year period—in others. Hughes and his associates believe macroepidemics are most likely to occur in areas of high unemployment and crime, deterioration in housing, poor or absent neighborhood leadership, a large recent influx of poor people, and the many other expressions of urban blight (47, 48). Their observations parallel those of Leighton et al. (58), who found a positive correlation between social disorganization and opiate use.

Hughes has provided some evidence that an outreach effort by community action groups can be used to abort an epidemic of heroin addiction. However, the case he cites occurred in a predominantly white neighborhood and was limited to microepidemics (47).

No one treatment for opiate addiction has been established as superior to the rest. Some years ago, methadone maintenance was introduced as a long-term treatment for narcotic users (30). Methadone is given in gradually increasing doses over a period of weeks until a high degree of cross-tolerance to all opiates is established. The euphoric effects of intravenous narcotics are blocked. Some previous drug users have become stabilized as productive citizens with this treatment. Apparently methadone alone is not enough for this outcome in many addicts; a complete program of rehabilitation is necessary.

The original methadone program of Dole and Nyswander (29) was considered impressively successful but has been criticized in that multiple drug users and other presumed poor-prognosis cases were not accepted in the program. The approach also has been challenged because it involves substituting one addiction for another, and it has led to wide dissemination of methadone through illicit channels (69). The consensus at present is that high doses of methadone are usually required for the program to be effective.

Nevertheless, in many cities, methadone has been given credit for ending the criminal activity of a high percentage of heroin addicts. In a four-year follow-up of methadone clients, Dole et al. (30) found that the majority were productively employed, living as responsible citizens, and supporting families. Most no longer engaged in criminal activity to support their habit.

Self-help groups made up of former addicts have stimulated enthusiastic responses from some participants, but their efficacy in general remains unknown.

Opioid research has led to exciting findings (5, 9, 11, 15). Injecting opiate compounds labeled with radioactive tracers into rats, investigators discovered that specific opiate receptors exist on the surfaces of particular cells in the brain stem and that the attachment of opiates to these cells could be prevented by morphine antagonists. This led to the discovery of endogenous opiates (endorphins) in pituitary gland secretions.

Sedative-Hypnotics

Sedatives produce calmness; hypnotics produce sleep. Both share similar pharmacological actions, hence the term "sedative-hypnotics." In higher doses, drugs marketed as sedatives also produce sleep. Conversely, hypnotics prescribed in lower doses produce calmness. The most popular class of sedative-hypnotics is the benzodiazepines (discussed in the next section). Benzodiazepines are also called "tranquilizers" or "minor" tranquilizers, in contradistinction to "major" tranquilizers such as the antipsychotic drugs. The term "tranquilizer" originated from the observation that benzodiazepines would "tranquilize" wild animals—make them more tame and manageable—without rendering them unconscious (42). Benzodiazepines are distinguishable from barbiturates and older sedative-hypnotics such as choral hydrate in that animals and people can easily be aroused from benzodiazepine-produced sleep, whereas this is more difficult with the older drugs.

This section will confine itself to barbiturates and synthetic hypnotics that also produce dependence and withdrawal symptoms, for example, glutethimide (Doriden), methyprylon (Noludar), and ethchlorvynol (Placidyl).

In contrast to opioids, barbiturates are usually taken orally. The short- and intermediate-acting barbiturates are most frequently used for nonmedical purposes. In both acute and chronic intoxication as well as the withdrawal syndrome, the clinical picture resembles that produced by alcohol. An intoxicated patient may show lethargy, difficulty in thinking, poor memory, irritability, and self-neglect. Nystagmus, ataxia, and a positive Romberg sign are often present.

Withdrawal symptoms may occur when patients take over 400 mg of barbiturates per day. The patient becomes anxious, restless, and weak during the first twelve to sixteen hours after the usual dose has not been supplied. Tremors of the hands are prominent; deep tendon reflexes are hyperactive. During the second or third day, grand mal seizures may occur, sometimes followed by delirium. Deaths have been reported. The syndrome clears in about a week. Long-acting barbiturates such as phenobarbital rarely if ever produce major withdrawal symptoms.

Withdrawal manifestations may be prevented or treated by administering a large dose of a short-acting barbiturate such as secobarbital (800 to 1,000 mg per twenty-four hours in divided doses) and then gradually reducing the dose over a period of seven to ten days. If a patient shows evidence of intoxication with the first or second dose (200 mg each), the diagnosis of barbiturate abuse should be questioned in view of the absence of tolerance. Because of cross-tolerance between barbiturates and other sedatives and hypnotics, withdrawal from these drugs may also be accomplished with a short-acting barbiturate.

It may be unwise to prescribe barbiturates to depressed patients unless dosage is carefully controlled. Patients often accumulate large amounts of drugs by hoarding. Unintentional death may result from slow absorption rates because large quantities of barbiturates in the stomach diminish gastric and intestinal function

(103). Users not getting the desired effect in what seems a long time continue to take tablet after tablet until they are unconscious. In the process, they ingest a lethal dose.

Two members of the minor tranquilizer and sedative group appear to have a particularly high potential for abuse. One is meprobamate (Miltown), the first minor tranquilizer to become available; and the other is methaqualone (Quaalude). Both have a risk potential roughly equivalent to that of the short-acting barbiturates. Methaqualone abuse became common among adolescents—reaching almost epidemic proportions—by the early 1980s. One reason for the increase apparently was the widespread belief that methaqualone is an aphrodisiac.

Phenobarbital is useful in detoxifying sedative-hypnotic abusers. The drug is long acting and produces a gradual cessation of withdrawal symptoms: 30 mg of phenobarbital is roughly equivalent to 100 mg of the short-acting barbiturates. Often there is uncertainty about the type and quantity of the sedative-hypnotics the patient has been using. In this event, repeated doses of phenobarbital may be given in smaller amounts to prevent withdrawal (90, 96).

Benzodiazepines

Benzodiazepines are the most widely prescribed class of medication in the Western world. At least a dozen such drugs are marketed in the United States and perhaps thirty or more are sold throughout the world. Compared to the sedative-hypnotic drugs described earlier, benzodiazepines have the following advantages: (a) they relieve anxiety without necessarily reducing alertness, impairing coordination, or interfering with normal thinking processes; (b) the regularly prescribed doses provide little or no euphoria; and (c) they are good muscle relaxants; (d) they are the safest, most effective drugs for treating alcohol withdrawal and other agitated states produced by many street drugs such as LSD. Benzodiazepines can be given to intoxicated patients in an emergency room without fear of lethal reactions, although caution should always be exercised. A benzodiazepine, alprazolam (Xanax), has been approved by the Food and Drug Administration as a treatment for depression as well as anxiety. Benzodiazepines are the most effective drugs available for insomnia. Unlike barbiturates they lose little of their effectiveness over even long periods of usage, and short-acting benzodiazepine hypnotics such as triazolam (Halcion) and temazepam (Restoril) leave few after-effects the next morning. After prolonged use, patients often experience increased insomnia for a few days—possibly a rebound from the previous hypnotic effects—but the difficuly seems to be short-lived. Finally, these drugs have one great advantage over the barbiturates and other hypnotics of the past: It is almost impossible to commit suicide by taking an overdose. Very rarely, deaths are reported from overdose, but almost always only when accompanied by other sedative agents or alcohol (42).

Reports of a benzodiazepine withdrawal syndrome have appeared for many years. Although millions of people regularly use these drugs, serious withdrawal symptoms appear uncommon (32). The symptoms range from panic and hallucinations to disorientation and grand mal seizures. Benzodiazepine users often combine the drug with alcohol or other drugs, and it is usually not clear whether the benzodiazepine alone is responsible for the abstinence syndrome (29). Abstinence syndromes are associated with low doses of benzodiazepines taken over a course of years (22).

Nevertheless, in most animal and human studies designed to predict dependence liability, benzodiazepines rank low (42). In one study, subjects were given a choice between 10 mg of diazepam or placebo; they chose the placebo (52). The same subjects preferred a 5-mg dose of dextroamphetamine to placebo. Nevertheless, physicians should be cautious in prescribing the drug for long periods, even in low dosage. Inevitably, some patients will combine them with other substances. Also, abrupt withdrawal of the drugs after relatively high dosages may produce severe anxiety and psychotic symptoms. Alprazolam (Xanax), an effective drug for anxiety, has the disadvantage of producing some degree of physical dependence, even when taken in moderate dosage. Withdrawing a patient from alprazolam should be done slowly, reducing the dosage by as little as 10 percent per week (67). Withdrawal can also be accomplished by stopping alprazolam and substituting a long-acting benzodiazopine such as chlordiazepoxide (the so-called "Librium taper") (22). Geriatric patients are particularly sensitive to benzobiazepines and should be given smaller doses than younger patients.

Amphetamines

This group of stimulants includes *d*-amphetamine (Dexedrine), *dl*-amphetamine (Benzedrine), methamphetamine (Desoxyn, Methedrine), and dextromethamphetamine ("ice"). Their effects include elevated mood, increased energy and alertness, decreased appetite, and slight improvement in task performance. Amphetamines may be taken orally, injected intravenously, or smoked.

Drug-induced psychosis is common among individuals taking large doses of amphetamines (over 50 mg per day). Such psychosis may resemble paranoid schizophrenia with persecutory delusions occurring despite a clear sensorium. Hallucinations are common. Usually the psychosis subsides one or two weeks after drug use stops. When an apparent amphetamine psychosis persists, a hidden source of drugs or the diagnosis of schizophrenia should be considered.

No specific amphetamine withdrawal syndrome has been described; however, users complain of fatigue and depression after discontinuing the drug, and these have been temporally associated with a decrease in the excretion of 3-methoxy-4-hydroxphenylglycol (MHPG), a metabolite of norepinephrine (72). Tolerance may be striking. "Speed freaks" sometimes take as much as 1 or 2 g per day (the usual therapeutic dose is 5 to 15 mg per day).

Since their introduction in the early 1930s, amphetamines have been prescribed by doctors for a variety of conditions, including depression, obesity, and narcolepsy. Starting in the 1960s increasing amounts of amphetamine entered illegal distribution channels and became available on the street. Amphetamine use declined in the 1980s, partly because of doctor's reluctance to prescribe the drug, partly because of the growing popularity of cocaine.

Concern about the increased use of amphetamines and other stimulants led to a marked curtailment of their production and availability. Cocaine, considered by many in the 1970s to be a relatively benign drug, substantially replaced amphetamines as a street drug. The trade-off—for society and for individuals—didn't work (39). First, the experience of the 1980s indicates that cocaine is more dependence-producing and dangerous than the amphetamines. Second, the previous beneficial uses of amphetamines for medical purposes were virtually denied. In some countries, amphetamines were removed from the market. Yet the evidence was strong that these and similar drugs are useful for treating patients with narcolepsy, attention-deficit disorders, and depression. Supporting this point in a general way is the 1987 report by the National Institute of Drug Abuse which concluded that nonmedical use of prescription drugs as an individual's only form of drug abuse is relatively rare; only 3 percent of the total population had used prescription drugs nonmedically and not used marihuana or any other illicit drug (62).

Drug epidemics tend to wax and wane and this has been true of amphetamine abuse. With the introduction of "ice" in Hawaii in the early 1990s, reason for concern about amphetamines has re-emerged. Ice, also known as "crystal" or "rock" and chemically named dextromethamphetamine is a designer drug that can be smoked and thus will deliver methamphetamine to the brain even faster than when injected. (Designer drugs have been defined as substances created by the manipulation of molecular structure in order to avoid prosecution for the manufacture of a scheduled drug that nonetheless retain psychoactive properties.) Ice has a long duration of action—up to eighteen hours. It stimulates the brain to a greater degree than regular methamphetamine but stimulates the heart, blood vesels, and lungs less. Its effects can be devastating, sometimes leading to a severe psychosis and intense depression as the drug wears off. Users often become paranoid. Acute hypertensive crisis and violence are possible. Haloperidol can usually control the psychotic symptoms and antidepressants the withdrawal effects. One advantage of ice is that it eliminates the use of needles—reducing the risk of AIDS. A disadvantage is that the drug affects the user's judgment regarding safe sexual practices—increasing the risk of AIDS.

Cocaine

The United States has experienced two major epidemics of cocaine abuse. The first occurred in the last decades of the nineteenth century when physicians, in particular, became addicted to the drug (thinking, as did Freud at first, that it was relatively benign and nonaddictive). The second epidemic began in the mid-1970s and has continued ever since (although abating somewhat in the 1990s). Cocaine remains a major drug of abuse throughout the country. In New York deaths because of cocaine increased 46 percent between 1985 and 1986. In Philadelphia, hospital admissions for problems stemming from cocaine use exceeded those related to heroin. Among defendants charged with major offenses, urinalysis indicated that the number of persons testing positive for cocaine had more than tripled from 1984 to 1987. In some cities, cocaine had become the leading cause of drug-related emergency room visits, surpassing even those involving alcohol.

Increasing numbers of white, employed, middle-class people in their late twenties and thirties who had never before sought psychological help now sought treatment for cocaine dependence. A cocaine hot line in Washington was receiving more than 14,000 calls daily (39, 98). Many of the callers were college graduates, professionals, and business executives. Half had incomes over $25,000 per year and a cocaine habit costing $600 a week. Dependence on the drug was intense. Nearly all callers said they could not turn the drug down when available. Most said cocaine had become more important to them than food or sex. They had physical complaints: headaches, sinus infections, sexual malfunctioning. Some had seizures or became paranoid.

The demographics of the epidemic changed as the country moved into the second half of the 1980s. Use among women, minority groups, lower-income groups, and adolescents increased. Cocaine problems infiltrated the small towns of the Middle West. Once called the champagne of drugs, cocaine became less expensive, freebasing (smoking cocaine) became popular, and cheap freebase, known as "crack," invaded the slums as well as suburbia. By the mid-1980s, cocaine was universally considered a dangerous drug (75). With recognition of its danger, cocaine use plateaued and then began falling in the early 1990s. By then, however, 12% of Americans had tried the drug. More than half of all persons arrested for reckless driving in Memphis in 1994 had marihuana or cocaine in their urine. This was a higher percentage of drug-related reckless driving use than occurred with alcohol (16).

Cocaine resembles amphetamines in many ways, but whereas amphetamines are synthetic drugs, cocaine is of botanical origin, deriving from shrubs grown in the Andes. Its effects last for a shorter period than do those of amphetamines. Like amphetamines, cocaine is a powerful stimulant of the nervous system, producing euphoria, increasing alertness, and suppressing fatigue and boredom (71). After regular, heavy use of the drug, a withdrawal syndrome may occur, in which formication (sensation of bugs crawling under the skin) is frequent together with depression and lassitude (98).

Heavy use of cocaine may produce a schizophreniform psychosis resembling paranoid schizophrenia. Occasional users sometimes report a profound dysphoria, persisting for several days after they have used the drug. Cocaine may have a deleterious effect on the health of pregnant women and on fetal development. Used during pregnancy, it may cause irregularities of placental blood flow, abruptio placentae, and premature labor.

Reported effects on fetal development include low birth weight, malformations of the urogenital system, cerebral infarction and seizures, and sudden death syndrome.

Until a few years ago, the cocaine most often smoked was cocaine hypochloride, the form most widely available on the street (44). But in the mid-1970s Americans adopted a method similar to the South American practice of smoking cocoa paste (base)—a potent extract from cocoa leaves. Users "free" street cocaine from its salts and cutting agents by a chemical process—potentially hazardous because it involves heating flammable solvents. The purified cocaine base that is left, mainly cocaine alkaloid, is highly potent. It increases heart rate and blood pressure (100); produces tremors, anorexia, insomnia; sometimes causes hallucinations (87), paranoia, and depression; and even results in occasional cardiac arrest (64) and lung damage (27). Nevertheless, according to a 1985 National Household Survey, 20 percent of cocaine users were using freebase despite its known dangers. The rate of administration—IV, intranasial, or by smoking—is relevant to the dependence potential of the drug (44). About 25 percent of users still prefer the IV route—the route still most associated with dependence. The inhaled form of the free-base, crack, relatively inexpensive and enormously popular in the urban ghetto, is considered by many authorities the most dangerous of all forms of cocaine and has accounted for a number of deaths among famous people. Crack, because it is inhaled and enters the brain rapidly, is highly addictive. It is a source of a good deal of drug-related crime and murder. By the 1990s there was little evidence that its use had subsided in the urban ghetto.

Phenothiazines may be used to treat the symptoms of amphetamine and cocaine psychoses. Antidepressants may be used to treat associated depressive symptoms (8, 37). Intravenous diazepam can be used to control seizures. Treatment for control of addiction tends to be nonspecific and to rely heavily on self-help groups and behavior modification (70). Lithium carbonate has been reported to block the effects of stimulants, but its value in the treatment of stimulant addiction awaits further study.

Hallucinogens

Perceptual distortions are the primary effect of hallucinogenic drugs, which include LSD, mescaline, psilocybin, and a family of compounds resembling either LSD or the amphetamines chemically (e.g., DMT and STP [2,5-dimethoxy-4-methylamphetamine]). Except for mescaline and psilocybin, most hallucinogens are synthetic. Because LSD has been the most widely used and studied hallucinogen, our discussion will focus on it.

Together with perceptual distortions, including illusions and hallucinations, LSD "trips" produce altered time sense, disturbed judgment, and sometimes confusion and disorientation (1). Some LSD trips are unpleasant. LSD users may be brought to emergency rooms for bad trips characterized by panic and sometimes persecutory delusions. There are reports of prolonged or flashback effects (a resurgence of the drug effect days, weeks, months, or even years subsequent to the end of a trip). Although flashbacks have not been studied systematically, they are reported so commonly that some authorities believe individuals do experience them. A number of deaths have been attributed to LSD, primarily from suicide or homicide, although the causal connection remains unclear (66).

Repeated use of LSD results in marked tolerance. No withdrawal syndrome has been reported. The drug usually produces euphoria, but dysphoria may occur. No deaths have been reported from LSD overdosage.

The use of LSD peaked in the 1970s and was in steady decline until the drug had a slight increase in popularity in the mid-1990s.

Treatment for acute adverse reactions to LSD consists of reassurance and, if this fails, tranquilizers. Diazepam appears to be as effective as phenothiazines and is somewhat safer because it is less likely to produce hypotension.

Hallucinogens have complicated the problem of diagnosing psychiatric disorders among young drug users. Prolonged psychotic episodes are probably more often attributable to schizo-

phrenia or other psychiatric illness than to LSD toxicity. To determine whether a patient has a psychiatric illness that is not associated with drug abuse, the patient must be drug free for a lenghy
period.

Phencyclidine

Angel dust (PCP—phencyclidine) has become an important drug
of abuse in recent years (23). Apparently it has caused a number
of deaths (70). Though PCP is obtainable as a veterinary anesthetic (Sernylan), most of the illegal supply is manufactured in home
laboratories. The drug is available in many forms—tablet, pow-
der, leaf, rock crystal—and can be ingested, snorted, smoked, or
injected. It is often sold under false guise as THC (tetrahydrocannabinol), LSD, or mescaline. Marihuana and other street drugs
are often adulterated with PCP. It has been called the "universal
adulterant" (23).

Moderate doses of PCP may produce bizarre behavior that is
often accompanied by a blank stare. Users become confused,
combative, stuporous, or comatose. Large doses can produce seizures and very large doses respiratory depression. Myoclonic jerks
are common. Deaths are believed to be caused by hypertensive
crises (45). One way to distinguish PCP intoxication from that of
other street drugs such as LSD and mescaline is to inspect the
pupils. Patients intoxicated with most hallucinogens have dilated
pupils; with PCP the pupils are normal or small (2). Ataxia,
nystagmus, muscular rigidity, and normal or small pupils in a
combative or stuporous patient suggest the diagnosis of PCP intoxication (23).

Phencyclidine is a "dissociative" anesthetic. It induces a cata-
leptic state in which pain is not perceived; the individual's eyes
are wide open, but he or she is unconscious and amnesic for the
experience. A noteworthy feature of PCP is the behavioral dis-
control that can produce a variety of bizarre activities or violence
that, in turn, results in encounters with police, lawsuits, unusual
accidents, strange suicides, and impulsive homicides. The user is

often amnesic about these events, and may remember only the pleasant, floaty euphoria the drug produces at low doses. Some of the reports are reminiscent of LSD descriptions: slowing of time, feelings of power, loss of appetite, illusions and pseudohallucinations. Flashbacks apparently occur even more frequently with PCP than LSD. Overdose with PCP is manifested by a prolonged eyes-open coma, often accompanied by a series of convulsions (73).

If the patient recovers from the overdose, a period of agitated delirium may ensue. This is marked by paranoid delusions, hallucinatory experiences, disorientation, and restlessness. If the dose of PCP was insufficient to induce coma, then the toxic delirium may be the presenting clinical picture. It may last up to a week after the last dose.

These patients often are admitted to psychiatric hospitals with a diagnosis of acute paranoid or catatonic schizophrenia. They are seen so frequently at present that acute schizophrenics should have a routine urine test for PCP and amphetamines (35).

Phenothiazines, the usual drug class of choice for agitated and uncontrollable patients, can cause severe postural hypotension and may increase muscle rigidity in patients intoxicated with PCP. Intramuscular benzodiazepines may be a better choice. Talking down a patient intoxicated with PCP may not be as effective as with LSD and other hallucinogens and may instead overstimulate the patient (23).

Marihuana

Cannabis sativa (hemp) contains chemicals called cannabinoids, one of which, delta-9-tetrahydrocannabinol (THC), is believed to be the main psychoactive constituent of marihuana.

The effects of THC depend on dosage, and they range from mild euphoria with small doses to LSD-like effects with high doses. Most marihuana originally grown wild in the United States contains insufficient amounts of THC to produce measurable psychological effects. Cannabis imported from Mexico, South

America, and India often contains sufficient THC to produce marked euphoria and, depending on the plant preparation used, paranoid delusions and other psychotomimetic effects. But THC deteriorates at the rate of 5 percent per month at room temperature; even imported cannabis eventually loses its potency. However, cannabis in use today tends to have a much higher THC content than that available in the mid-1970s (63).

There are two generally available cannabis preparations: marihuana and hashish. The former consists of a mixture of plant products (leaves, stems, etc.). The latter consists of the resin of the female plant and is more potent.

In parts of the world where concentrated cannabis preparations have been used by millions of people for hundreds of years, constant use is said to be associated with serious medical and psychiatric illnesses.

However, studies conducted in Jamaica, Costa Rica, and Greece—countries where cannabis has been used regularly for many years—failed to reveal any serious pathology associated with the use of the drug (83). The subjects were lower-class laborers and no conclusions could be drawn about deleterious effects in other societies and in other classes. The studies did report a decrease in respiratory capacity and minor hematological abnormalities among users. The authors warned against extrapolating their findings to other societies.

Acute psychotic episodes apparently have resulted from cannabis use, but they have been infrequent. However, a Swedish study (4) published in late 1987 reported a strong correlation between cannabis use and schizophrenia, defined by *DSM-III* criteria. The study involved a cohort of nearly 50,000 Swedish military conscripts. Those who reported using cannabis on more than fifty occasions were six times more likely subsequently to receive a diagnosis of schizophrenia than were nonusers. The relative risk increased with increased consumption. The study did not demonstrate that cannabis use *caused* schizophrenia; cannabis consumption might, on the contrary, be caused by an emerging schizophrenia. Nevertheless, the association between marihuana use and schizophrenia was the strongest yet reported. Psychiatrists have also described a condition among chronic users of marihuana called "amotivational syndrome," characterized by lassitude, apathy, and lack of ambition (62, 84). The evidence of a causal relationship with cannabis remains anecdotal.

However, marihuana does have a certain abuse potential (25, 101). In a follow-up study of ninety-seven regular users, 9 percent met operational criteria for abuse similar to criteria used in alcohol studies. In other words, marihuana use was associated with a variety of social, psychological, and medical problems in these individuals. Of the abusers, two-thirds had had traffic violations they attributed *solely* to marihuana intoxication; one-third had engaged in fights, again blaming marihuana. The latter finding was particularly interesting in view of the widespread observation that marihuana typically has antiaggressive effects. This, indeed, may be the case in most instances, but "set and setting" notoriously influence the effects of drugs, and it cannot be said any longer that marihuana has exclusively "taming" effects.

The difficulty of isolating marihuana effects is compounded by the fact that many regular users of marihuana also take other drugs. Furthermore, until the 1980s most marihuana available in this country contained small amounts of THC. Therefore, even though marihuana has been widely used in the United States, it is impossible to predict the consequences of prolonged use of high-potency canabis by large numbers of people.

American attitudes toward marihuana have changed. Experimenters with the drug in the 1960s and 1970s commonly reported mild effects, probably because of the low potency of the drug mainly available at that time. As the THC content of available marihuana increased, there was a corresponding increase in the awareness of risks in using the drug. In 1986, for example, 71 percent of high school seniors believe that regular marihuana use involved risk, more than double the rate who believed this in 1978 (68).

Evidence accumulated over the past 30 years suggests that regular use of marihuana is associated with the following hazards (19):

1. Bronchial and pulmonary irritation. Marihuana, because of its relatively poor combustibility, has up to 50 percent more polyaromatic hydrocarbons in its smoke than tobacco does (46). Cigarette for cigarette, the difference between tobacco and marihuana may be even more significant because of the way marihuana typically is smoked—down to a minuscule butt—and because the smoke itself is retained in the lung for a longer period than tobacco smoke. In one of the few human studies comparing adverse effects of cannabis and tobacco, measurements of bronchial constriction revealed that smoking less than one marihuana cigarette per day diminished vital capacity of the lungs as much as smoking sixteen tobacco cigarettes (91, 92).

2. Marihuana causes tachycardia. Smoking just one marihuana cigarette can significantly reduce exercise tolerance in heart patients with anginal syndrome (6). This would militate against marihuana use by persons who have cardiac disorders.

3. Studies consistently show short-term adverse effects of marihuana on cognition and immediate memory (63).

4. Marihuana intoxication impairs reaction time, motor coordination, and visual perception (63). Studies under simulated conditions and in traffic have confirmed that the ability to operate a motor vehicle is adversely affected by marihuana use (56).

Immunoassays for cannabinoids have been available since the early 1980s. There are technical problems with the urine immunoassay currently being used and gas chromatography–mass spectrometry assays for TCH and its metabolites in blood and urine specimens are required for confirmation. One problem is that cannabinoids are detectable in the urine for at least one or two days after smoking and for weeks in some instances (57). For these reasons it has been difficult to estimate how many traffic accidents are associated with use of marihuana. Most marihuana users sometimes drive when they are high, according to an NIDA report (63).

REFERENCES

1. *Adverse Reactions to Hallucinogenic Drugs.* Prepared by R. E. Meyer, p. 111, Washington, D.C.: U.S. GPO, NIMH, 1967.
2. Acute drug abuse reactions. Med. Lett. *27*:77–80, 1985.
3. Anderson, P., and Scott, E. The effect of general practitioners' advice to heavy drinking men. Brit. J. Addict. *87*:891–900, 1992.
4. Andréasson, S., Allebeck, P., and Engström, A. Cannabis and schizophrenia. Lancet 2, 1987.
5. Anglin, M. D., Brecht, M. L., Woodward, J. A., and Bonett, D. G. An empirical study of maturing out: conditional factors. Int. J. Addict. *21*(2):233–246, 1986.
6. Aranow, W. S., and Cassidy, J. Effects of smoking marihuana and of a high-nicotine cigarette on angina pectoris. Clin. Pharmacol. Therapy *17*:549–554, 1975.
7. Aranow, R., and Done, A. Phencyclidine overdose: an emergency concept of management. J. Amer. Coll. Emergency Physicians *7*:56–59, 1978.
8. Arndt, I., Dorozynsky, L., Woody, G., McLellan, A. T., and O'Brien, C. P. Desipramine treatment of cocaine abuse in methadone-maintained patients. In *Problems of Drug Dependence*, National Institute on Drug Abuse Research Monograph 95, Harris, L. (ed.), Rockville, M.d.: NIDAR, 1990.
9. Ausubel, D. P. Methadone maintenance treatment: the other side of the coin. Int. J. Addict. *18*(6):851–862, 1983.
10. Bakker, C. B. The clinical picture in hallucinogen intoxication. Hosp. Med. 102–114, 1969.
11. Ball, J. C., Lange, W. R., Myers, C. P., and Friedman, S. R. Reducing the risk of AIDS through methadone maintenance treatment. J. Health Social Behav. *29*:214–226, 1988.
12. Blachly, P. H. Management of the opiate abstinence syndrome. Am. J. Psychiat. *122*:742–744, 1966.
13. Bloomquist, E. R. *Marijuana.* Toronto: Glencoe Press, 1968.
14. Blum, R. H., et al. *The Utopiates: The Use and Users of LSD-25*, p. 304. New York: Atherton Press, 1964.
15. Bouckoms, A. J., Masand, P., Murray, G. B., Cassem, E. H., Stern, T. A., and Tesar, G. E. Chronic nonmalignant pain treated with long-term oral narcotic analgesics. Ann. Clin. Psychiat. *4*:185–192, 1992.
16. Brookoff, D., Cook, C. S., Williams, C., and Mann, C. S. Testing reckless drivers for cocaine and marijuana. N. Engl. J. Med. *331*:518–522, 1994.
17. Brower, K. J., Hierholzer, R. and Maddahian, E. Recent trends in cocaine abuse in a VA psychiatric population. Hosp. Community Psychiat. *37*:1229–1234, 1986.
18. Bucky, S. F. The relationship between background and extent of heroin use. Am. J. Psychiat. *130*:707–708, 1973.
19. Busto, U., Sellers, E. M., Naranjo, C. A., Cappell, H., Sanchez-Craig, M., and Sykora, K. Withdrawal reaction after long-term therapeutic use of benzodiazepines. N. Engl. M. Med. *315*:854–859, 1986.

20. Childress, A. R., McLellan, A. T., and O'Brien, C. P. Abstinent opiate abusers exhibit conditioned craving, conditioned withdrawal and reductions in both through extinction. Brit. J. Addict. *81*:655–660, 1986.

21. Climko, R. B., Roehrich, H., Sweeney, D. R., and Al-Razi, J. Ecstasy: a review of MDMA and MDA. Int. J. Psychiat. Med. *16*:359–364, 1986.

22. Closser, M. H. and Brower, K. J. Treatment of alprazolam withdrawal with chlordiazepoxide substitution and taper. J. Substance Abuse Treatment *11(4)*:319–323, 1994.

23. Cohen, S. Angel dust. JAMA *238*:515–516, 1977.

24. Cohen, S., and Edwards, A. E. LSD and organic brain impairment. Drug Depend. 1–4, 1968.

25. Committee to study the health-related effects of cannabis and its derivatives, National Academy of Sciences, Institute of Medicine. *Marijuana and Health.* Washington, D.C.: National Academy Press, 1982.

26. Council on Scientific Affairs. Marijuana, its health hazards and therapeutic potentials. JAMA *246*:1823–1827, 1981.

27. Cregler, L. L., and Mark, H. Medical complications of cocaine abuse. N. Engl. J. Med. *315*:1495–1450, 1986.

28. Dependence on barbiturates and other sedative drugs. JAMA *193*:107–111, 1965.

29. Dole, V. P., Nyswander, M. E., and Warner, A. Successful treatment of 750 criminal addicts. JAMA *206*:2708–2711, 1968.

30. Dole, V. Research on methadone maintenance treatment. Proceedings of the 2d National Conference on Methadone Maintenance, pp. 359–370, 1969.

31. Eddy, N. B., Halback, H., Isbell, H., and Seevers, M. H. Drug dependence: its significance and characteristics. Bull. WHO *32*:721–733, 1965.

32. Fleischhacker, W. W., Bamas, C., and Hackenberg, B. Epidemiology of benzodiazepine dependence. Acta Psychiat. Scand. *74*:80–85, 1986.

33. *Follow-up of Vietnam Drug Users* (Robins, L. N., principal investigator), Washington, D.C.: National Institute of Drug Abuse, Special Action Office Monogr., Series A, no. 1, 1973.

34. Fraser, H. F., Wikler, A., Essig, C. F., and Isbell, H. Degree of physical dependence induced by secobarbital or pentobarbital. JAMA *166*:126–129, 1958.

35. Garey, R. E., Daul, G. C., Samuels, M. S., Ragan, F. A., and Hite, S. A. PCP abuse in New Orleans: a six-year study. Am. J. Drug Alcohol Abuse *13*:135–140, 1987.

36. Garvey, M. J., and Tollefson, G. D. Prevalence of misuse of prescribed benzodiazepines in patients with primary anxiety disorder or major depression. Am. J. Psychiat. *143*:1601–1606, 1986.

37. Gawin, F. H. New uses of antidepressants in cocaine abuse. Psychosomatics *27*:24–29, 1986.

38. Ghodse, A. H. Cannabis psychosis. Brit. J. Addict. *81*:473–478, 1986.

39. Gold, M. S., and Galanter, M. In *Cocaine: Pharmacology, Addiction and Therapy*, Stimmel, B. (ed.), New York: Haworth Press, 1987.

40. Goodman, L. S., and Gilman, A. *The Pharmacological Basis of Therapeutics.* New York: Macmillan, 1965.

41. Goodwin, D. W. Alcoholism. In *Clinical Psychopharmacology*, vol. 1. Hippius, H., and Winokur, G. (eds.), Amsterdam: Excerpta Medica, 1983.

42. Goodwin, D. W. *Anxiety.* New York: Ballantine Books, 1986.

43. Gossop, M., Bradley, B. and Phillips, G. T. An investigation of withdrawal symptoms shown by opiate addicts during and subsequent to a 21-day inpatient methadone detoxification procedure. Addict. Behav. *12*:1–5, 1987.

44. Gossop, M., Griffiths, P., Powis, B., and Strang, J. Cocaine: patterns of use, route of administration, and severity of dependence. Brit. J. Psychiat. *164*:660–664, 1994.

45. Grinspoon, L., and Bakalar, J. B. *Psychedelic Drugs Reconsidered.* New York: Basic Books, 1979.

46. Hoffman, D., Brunnemann, K. D., Gori, G. B., et al. Carcinogenicity of marihuana smoke. In *Recent Advances of Phytochemistry*, Vol. 9, Runeckles, V. C. (ed.), New York: Plenum, 1975.

47. Hughes, P. H., et al. The social structure of a heroin coping community. Am. J. Psychiat. *128*:551–558, 1971.

48. Hughes, P. H., Senay, E. C., and Parker, R. The medical management of a heroin epidemic. Arch. Gen. Psychiat. *27*:585–593, 1972.

49. Inaba, D. S., Gay, G. R., Newmeyer, J. A., and Whitehead, C. Methaqualone abuse "luding out." JAMA *224*:1505–1514, 1973.

50. Jaffe, J. H. Drug addiction and drug abuse. In *The Pharmacological Basis of Therapeutics*, Goodman, L S., and Gilman, A. (eds.), New York: Macmillan, 1965.

51. Jain, N. C., Budd, R. D., and Budd, B. S. Growing abuse of phencyclidine: California "angel dust." N. Engl. J. Med. *297*:673, 1977.

52. Johanson, C. E., and Uhlenhuth, E. H. Drug preferences in humans. Fed. Proc. *41*:228–233, 1982.

53. Kessler, R. C., McGonable, K. A., Zhao, S., Nelson, C. B., Hughes, M., Eshleman, S., Wittchen, H., and Kendler, K. S. Lifetime and 12-month prevalence of *DSM-III-R* psychiatric disorders in the United States. Arch. Gen. Psychiat. *51*:8–19, 1994.

54. Kieber, H. D., Topazian, M., Gaspari, J., Riordan, C. E., and Kosten, T. Clonidine and naltrexone in the outpatient treatment of heroin withdrawal. Am. J. Drug Alcohol Abuse *13*:1–5, 1987.

55. Klepfisz, A., and Racy, J. Homicide and LSD. JAMA *223*:429–430, 1973.

56. Klonoff, H. Marihuana and driving in real-life situations. Science *186*:317–324, 1974.

57. Law, B., Pocock, K., and Moffat, A. C. An evaluation of homogeneous enzyme immunoassay (EMIT) for cannabinoid detection in biological fluids. J. Forensic Sci. Soc. *22*:275–281, 1982.

58. Leighton, D. C., et al. *The Character of Danger: Psychiatric Systems in Selected Communities*, *3*322–353. New York: Basic Books, 1963.

59. Lerner, P. The precise determination of tetrahydrocannabinol in marihuana and hashish. Bull. Narc. *21*:39–42, 1969.

60. Liden, C. B., Lovejoy, F. H., and Costello, C. E. Phencyclidine: nine cases of poisoning. JAMA *234*:513–516, 1975.

61. Many "street" drugs are phony. Am. Druggist, 35–44, 1971.

62. *Marihuana and Health.* 2d Annual Report to the U.S. Congress from the Secretary of HEW. Washington, D.C.: U.S. GPO, 1972.

63. *Marihuana and Health.* 8th Annual Report to the U.S. Congress from the Secretary of HEW. Washington, D.C.: U.S. GPO, 1980.

64. Mathias, D. W. Cocaine-associated myocardial ischemia. Am. J. Med. *81*:675–678, 1986.

65. McAuliffe, W. E. A test of Wikler's theory of relapse: the frequency of relapse due to conditional withdrawal sickness. Int. J. Addict. *17*:19–33, 1982.

66. McGlothlin, W. H., and Arnold, D. O. LSD revisited—a 10 year follow-up of medical LSD use. Arch. Gen. Psychiat. *24*:35, 1971.

67. Mellman, T. A., and Uhde, T. W. Withdrawal syndrome with gradual tapering of alprazolam. Am. J. Psychiat. *143*:1464–1469, 1986.

68. Millman, R. B., and Sbriglio, R. Patterns of use and psychopathology in chronic marijuana users. Psychiat. Clin. North Am. *9*:533–538, 1986.

69. Newman, R. G. Methadone treatment: defining and evaluating success. N. Engl. J. Med. *317*:447–452, 1987.

70. Newman, R. G. Frustrations among professionals working in drug treatment programs. Brit. J. Addict. *82*:115–120, 1987.

71. Noble, E. P., Blum, K., Khalsa, E., Ritchie, T., Montgomery, A., Wood, R. C., Fitch, R. J., Ozkaragoz, T., Sheridan, P. J., Anglin, M. D., Paredes, A., Treiman, L. J., and Sparkes, R. S. Allelic association of the D_2 dopamine receptor gene with cocaine dependence. Alcohol Drug Depend., in press.

72. Paul, S. M., Hulihan-Giblin, B., and Skolnick, P. (+)-Amphetamine binding to rat hypothalamus: relation to anorexic potency of phenylethylamines. Science *218*:487–489, 1982.

73. *Phencyclidine (PCP) Abuse: An Appraisal,* NIDA Res. Monogr. 21. Rockville, Md.: NIDA, 1978.

74. Phillips, G. T., Gossop, M., and Bradley, B. The influence of psychological factors on the opiate withdrawal syndrome. Brit. J. Psychiat. *149*:235–240, 1986.

75. Position statement on psychoactive substance use and dependence: up-date on marijuana and cocaine. Am. J. Psychiat. *144*:5, 1987.

76. Post, R. M. Cocaine psychoses: a continuum model. Am. J. Psychiat. *132*:225–231, 1975.

77. Rainey, Jr., J. M., and Crowder, M. K. Prevalence of phencyclidine in street drug preparations. N. Engl. J. Med. *290*:466–467, 1974.

78. Reed, D., Cravey, R. H., and Sedgwick, P. R. A fatal case involving phencyclidine. Int. Assn. Forensic Toxicol. Bull. *7*:7, 1972.

79. Rickels, K., Case, W. G., Schweizer, E. E., Swenson, C., and Fridman, R. B. Low-dose dependence in chronic benzodiazepine users: a preliminary report on 119 patients. Psychopharmacol. Bull. *22*:407–412, 1986.

80. Ritson, B., and Chick, J. Comparison of two benzodiazepines in the treatment of alcohol withdrawal: effects on symptoms and cognitive recovery. Drug Alcohol Depend. *18*:329–334, 1986.

81. Rosser, W. W., Simms, J. G., Patten, D. W., and Forster, J. Improving benzodiazepine prescribing in family practice through review and education. Can. Med. Assoc. J. *124*:147, 1981.

82. Roueché, B. *Alcohol.* New York: Grove Press, 1962.

83. Rubin, V., and Comitas, L. *Ganja in Jamaica.* The Hague and Paris: Mouton, 1975.

84. Scher, J. The marihuana habit. JAMA *214*:1120, 1970.

85. Sharma, T. D. Clinical observations of patients who used tetrahydrocannabinol (THC) intravenously. Behav. Neuropsychiat. *4*, 1972.

86. Showalter, C. V., and Thornton, W. E. The increasing abuse of phencyclidine. Ill. Med. J. *151*:387–389, 1977.

87. Siegel, R. K. Cocaine hallucinations. Am. J. Psychiat. *135*:3, 1978.

88. Siegel, R. Cocaine freebase. J. Psychoactive Drugs, December (special issue): 1982.

89. Smart, R. G., and Bateman, K. Unfavorable reactions to LSD: a review and analysis of available case reports. Can. Med. Assoc. J. *97*:1214–1221, 1967.

90. Smith, D. E., and Wesson, D. R. A new method for treatment of barbiturate dependence. JAMA *213*:294–295, 1970.

91. Tashkin, D. P., Shapiro, B. J., and Frank, I. M. Acute effects of marihuana on airway dynamics in spontaneous and experimentally induced bronchial asthma. Pharmacol. Marihuana 785–802, 1976.

92. Tashkin, D. P., Calvarese, B., and Simmons, M. Respiratory status of 75 chronic marihuana smokers. Am. Rev. Respir. Dis. 117–261, 1978.

93. Tinklenberg, J. R., and Woodrow, K. M. Drug use among youthful assaultive and sexual offenders. In *Human Aggression*, Frazier, S. H. (ed.), Baltimore: Williams & Wilkins, 1974.

94. Tjio, J., Pahnke, W. N., and Kurland, A. A. LSD and chromosomes. JAMA *210*:849–856, 1969.

95. Tong, T. G., Benowitz, N. L., Becker, C. E., et al. Phencyclidine poisoning. JAMA *234*:512–513, 1975.

96. Treatment of acute drug abuse reactions. Med. Lett. *29*:83–86, 1987.

97. Vaillant, G. E. A 12-year follow-up of New York narcotic addicts. Arch. Gen. Psychiat. *15*:599, 1966.

98. Washton, A. M., and Gold, M. S. *Cocaine: A Clinician's Handbook.* New York: Guilford Press, 1987.

99. Watson, R., Hartmann, E., and Schildkraut, J. J. Amphetamine withdrawal: affective state, sleep patterns, and MHPG excretion. Am. J. Psychiat. *129*:263–269, 1972.

100. Weinstein, S. P., Gottheil, E., Smith, R. H., and Migrala, K. A. Cocaine users seen in medical practice. Am. J. Drug Alcohol Abuse *12*:341–346, 1986.

101. Weller, R. A., and Halikas, J. A. Objective criteria for the diagnosis of marihuana abuse. J. Nerv. Ment. Dis. *168*:98–103, 1980.

102. Wetli, C. V. Changing patterns of methaqualone abuse. JAMA *249*:621–626, 1983.

103. Wikler, A. Diagnosis and treatment of drug dependence of the barbiturate type. Am. J. Psychiat. *125*:6, 1968.

104. Winokur, A., Rickels, K., Greenblatt, D. J., Snyder, P. J., and Schatz, N. J. Withdrawal reaction from long-term, low-dosage administration of diazepam: a double-blind, placebo-controlled case study. Arch. Gen. Psychiat. *37*:101, 1980.

105. Zinberg, N. E., and Jacobson, R. C. The natural history of "chipping." Am. J. Psychiat. *133*:37–40, 1976.

9

ANTISOCIAL
PERSONALITY
(SOCIOPATHY)

DEFINITION

Antisocial personality (sociopathy or sociopathic personality) refers to a pattern of recurrent antisocial, delinquent, and criminal behavior that begins in childhood or early adolescence and is manifested by disturbances in many areas of life: family relations, schooling, work, military service, and marriage.

HISTORICAL BACKGROUND

Prichard's 1835 monograph, *A Treatise on Insanity and Other Disorders Affecting the Mind,* is often cited as furnishing the first description of what is now called antisocial or sociopathic personality (66). Under the label "moral insanity" he defined the disorder in this way:

The intellectual faculties appear to have sustained little or no injury, while the disorder is manifested principally or alone in the state of the feelings, temper, or habits. In cases of this description the moral and active principles of the mind are strongly perverted and depraved, the power of self government is lost or impaired and the individual is found to be incapable . . . of conducting himself with decency and propriety, having "undergone a morbid change." As Craft makes clear (17), Prichard included under this rubric many examples of "temporary mental illness," and most of his cases were probably patients with affective disorder. Craft quotes Clouston's 1883 volume (15): "Prichard . . . vividly described the disease, but I should place most of his cases in my category of simple mania."

Clouston referred also to children "so constituted that they cannot be educated in morality on account of an innate brain deficiency . . . incapable of knowing . . . right and wrong. . . . Such moral idiots I, like others, have met with frequently . . . and persons with this want of development we may label under moral insanity."

Craft points out that Prichard used "moral" in three ways: first, in referring to "moral" treatment, meaning psychological treatment; second, in referring to emotional or affective responses in contrast to intellectual ones; and third, in an ethical sense of right or wrong. Most of the time, Prichard used the term in the first two ways and only incidentally in the last way.

As Craft also notes, Benjamin Rush in 1812 described "derangement of the moral faculties" as follows (73):

The moral faculty, conscience, and sense of deity are sometimes totally deranged. The Duke of Sully has given us a striking instance of this universal moral derangement in the character of a young man who belonged to his suite, of the name of Servin, who, after a life uncommonly distinguished by every possible vice, died, cursing and denying his God. Mr. Haslam has described two cases of it in the Bethlem Hospital, one of whom, a boy of 13 years of age, was perfectly sensible of his depravity, and often asked "why God had not made him like other men." . . . In the course of my life, I have been consulted in three cases of the total perversion of the moral faculties. One of them was in a young man, the second in a young woman, both of Virginia, and the third was in the daughter of a citizen of Philadelphia. The last was addicted to every kind of mischief. Her mischief and wickedness had no intervals while she was awake, except when she was kept busy in some steady and difficult employment. In all of these cases of innate, preternatural moral depravity, there is probably an original defective organization in those parts of the body which are occupied by the moral faculties of the mind.

It is Craft's conclusion that "Rush appears to give the first description of those with sound reason and good intellect who have an innate or lifelong irresponsibility without shame, being unchanged in affect, or by the consequences or by regard for others." Thus Craft challenges the appropriateness of crediting Prichard with the first description.

Controversy over the concept of "moral insanity" developed partly in regard to the question of whether the "morally insane" should be committed to mental hospitals or should be considered mentally ill in a court of law. The terms gradually fell into disuse as interest in the whole range of personality disorders grew.

In 1889 Koch (43) introduced the term "psychopathic inferiority" to imply a constitutional predisposition for many deviations of personality, including at least some that are now classified as anxiety disorders. Kraepelin (45), Kahn (41), and Schneider (76) proposed various classifications of personality disorders. Schneider's definition of psychopathic personalities as "all those abnormal personalities who suffer from their abnormalities or cause society to suffer" clearly included much more than "moral imbecility."

The term "psychopathic personality" was used inconsistently, sometimes to refer to the whole spectrum of deviant personalities and sometimes to a subgroup of antisocial or aggressive "psychopaths." Finally, to reduce confusion, the term "sociopathic personality disturbance" was introduced for the latter group and was adopted in 1952 by the American Psychiatric Association's *DSM-I*. Nevertheless, many went on using the terms "psychopathy" and "sociopathy" interchangeabaly, whereas others continued to regard sociopathy as only one form of psychopathy. In a further attempt to reduce confusion, "antisocial personality" was adopted as the official diagnosis for the aggressive or antisocial psychopath or sociopath in later revisions of the *DSM* and the International Classification of Disease. Sir Aubrey Lewis summarized the history of the concept (48). Because of evidence in the recent past in other countries that psychiatric diagnoses have been applied to political dissenters, some psychiatrists have been reluctant to use this diagnosis, despite the recognition that individuals with the clinical picture of antisocial personality are found all over the world and that only a few are political dissenters.

EPIDEMIOLOGY

Completely satisfactory data on the prevalence of antisocial personality are lacking. This partly reflects the failure to reach a general agreement about a definition. In the Epidemiologic Catchment Area Study, the prevalence varied between 2.6 and 5.1 percent, depending upon variation in diagnostic criteria (72). The ratio of males to females in this study varied between 1.62%/1.25% and 9.4%/1.5%. In general, we do not know what proportion of sociopaths comes to the attention of physicians. Nevertheless, sociopathy is seen frequently in psychiatric facilities, usually because of associated alcoholism, other drug abuse, and depression or because psychiatric care is made a condition of parole. In one series, 15 percent of male and 3 percent of female psychiatric outpatients were sociopaths (85).

Indirect estimates of population frequency, based on figures for juvenile delinquency and police trouble of all kinds, suggest that sociopathy is common, probably increasingly so; much more frequent in males than females, and in urban than rural environments; and most common in low socioeconomic groups (51, 70).

Sociopaths usually come from grossly disturbed families. Parental separation or divorce, early death, desertion, alcoholism and criminality are characteristic. Only a small minority of sociopaths, in fact, come from families that are not characterized by one or more of these phenomena (16, 22, 32, 40, 44).

CLINICAL PICTURE

Sociopathy begins in childhood or early adolescence (3, 59). The first manifestations may be those of the hyperactive child syndrome (22, 53, 58, 60, 74, 75, 84). A recent adoption study found evidence for a genetic factor associated with *some* cases of childhood hyperactivity/attention deficit disorder and adult antisocial personality (9). Other investigators have demonstrated, however, that when early hyperactivity is not accompanied by delinquent or antisocial behavior, it leads to antisocial personality patterns much less often. At the same time, delinquency associated with hyperactivity tends to be more severe than delinquency alone, with a worse prognosis for adult adjustment (62, 83). Restlessness, a short attention span, and unresponsiveness to discipline are common. Frequent fighting, often leading to conflicts with adults, and a history of being a general neighborhood nuisance are also common (12, 69).

A disturbed school history is characteristic of early sociopathy. In fact, a history of satisfactory school adjustment through high school is so unusual among sociopaths that either the diagnosis or the history should be questioned if it is present. Disruption of classes by talking out of turn, failure to pay attention to the teacher, fighting with clasmates, arguing with the teacher, and even fighting with the teacher occur. Academic failures, truancy, and suspension often lead to school dropout or permanent expulsion (12, 33, 69).

Running away from home is also common, though it may be limited to a few one-night episodes. Occasionally, adolescent sociopaths will disappear for weeks or months. During such absences, they may wander over the country, hitchhiking, doing odd jobs, bumming around (69).

The sociopath's job history is characterized by poor performance. Undependability (being late, missing work, quitting without warning), inability to accept criticism and advice, frequent job changes without advancement, and being fired are typical (12, 69). Poor job performance coupled with limited and incomplete education result in low socioeconomic status, low income, and frequent need for financial assistance from family or society.

Sociopaths begin heterosexual experiences earlier than others and are much more likely to be promiscuous and indiscriminate in their sexual behavior. Homosexual behavior may be more common among sociopaths than in the general population (13). Prostitution is frequent among female sociopaths, and homosexual prostitution is common among male sociopaths.

Early marriage is typical, especially among women. Very few sociopathic women, in fact, fail to marry. Their marriages are marked by infidelity, separation, and divorce. Male sociopaths have similar marital difficulties. Sociopaths tend to marry sociopaths; this is particularly true of women (13, 30).

Judges used to handle male delinquents by suspending punishment if the delinquent enlisted in the armed services. Generally, however, sociopaths do not do well in military service. Undependable and unable to conform to military discipline, they go AWOL, have difficulty with their superiors, are subjected to court-martials, and receive various nonhonorable discharges. The type of discharge is usually determined by the nature of the offenses, the philosophy of the commanding officer, and general military policy at the time.

Sooner or later most sociopaths have trouble with the police. Some investigators, in fact, have required police trouble for the diagnosis of sociopathy (29). Stealing money from mother's purse or father's wallet or from a schoolmate may be an early sign of a budding criminal career. Shoplifting, peace disturbance (usually associated with drunkenness and fighting), various traffic offenses, auto theft, burglary, larceny, rape, robbery, and homicide may all occur. A sociopathic pattern of behavior is found in many convicted male felons (29, 31, 36) as well as in convicted female felons (13).

Many sociopaths engage in lying and the use of aliases, usually as understandable responses to social or legal difficulties, but sometimes without any obvious need to avoid punishment or retaliation. Such behavior has been called "pathological lying." Elaborate stories may be told to confuse or impress relatives. This behavior can take extreme forms such as masquerading as a physician, military officer, or businessperson. In time, relatives, friends, parole officers, and physicians learn to discount a good deal of what they are told by sociopaths.

Conversion symptoms (unexplained neurological symptoms) are common among sociopaths; in fact, sociopathy is second only to hysteria in producing such symptoms (34). Among sociopaths, conversion symptoms are characteristically associated with obvious social stresses such as police trouble. The full Briquet's syndrome (hysteria) may also be seen in association with sociopathy. Many female hysterics give a history of previous or concurrent sociopathy (13); many young delinquent and antisocial girls become hysterics as adults (13, 52, 69).

Most studies of delinquents and sociopaths indicate that their average IQ is below normal, but only a minority of delinquents and sociopaths suffer from significant mental deficiency, with an IQ less than 70 (17, 51). These studies have not all been adequately controlled for socioeconomic status, sibship size, and other variables correlated with intelligence. Low intelligence probably is not an important factor in the etiology of sociopathy.

Some studies have attempted to assess "constitutional" factors in sociopathy (79). Nonspecifically disordered electroencephalograms (EEGs) have been reported more frequently among sociopaths than controls, but many, if not most, sociopaths do not have abnormal EEGs (2, 26). Some authors have reported an association between delinquency, learning disability, and neurological impairment, but this has not been a completely consistent finding (82). Many studies have explored psychophysiological response patterns in sociopaths, and a theory of low autonomic and cortical arousal has been formulated to account for a persistent "stimulus hunger" or for the inability to learn socially approved behavior. The theory is thought to explain the sociopath's impulsive, excitement-seeking, and antisocial behavior (35, 57, 67, 74). More recent studies have suggested that lowered cerebrospinal fluid 5-hydroxyindoleacetic acid levels, pointing to some alteration in serontonin metabolism, may predict antisocial behavior, alone or in combination with various measures of autonomic arousal (47). The research findings have not been entirely consistent (57), and some authors (56) have emphasized "a wider degree of variability in arousal levels and reactivity than [in] normal individuals." An association between criminal behavior and chromosomal abnormalities has been reported. In particular, XYY karyotype, unusual height, and impulsive crimes have been associated, but not all studies are consistent (1, 20, 39, 61). On the other hand, more cases of the XXY karyotype (Klinefelter's syndrome) than of the XYY karyotype were found in a large Finnish series of male criminals referred for psychiatric evaluation (77). Studies of hormone levels, including androgens and adrenal steroids, have shown inconsistent differences between sociopathic and nonsociopathic subjects (21, 46, 55).

A charming manner, lack of guilt or remorse, absence of anxiety, and a failure to learn by experience are said to be characteristic of sociopathy. The easygoing, open, and winning style, when present, presumably accounts for the sociopath's success as a confidence man. At best, however, the charm and appeal are superficial; often they are entirely absent.

When seen by psychiatrists, many sociopaths report anxiety symptoms, depression, and guilt (10, 85). These frequently occur with alcoholism. The guilt and remorse do not seem to lead to reduction of sociopathic behavior, however. This persistence of sociopathic behavior, despite repeated failure and punishment, is the basis for the statement that sociopaths "do not learn from experience." Suicide attempts are not rare, but completed suicide, in the absence of alcoholism or drug dependence, is infrequent (23).

Many people occasionally manifest antisocial or delinquent behavior. But only a minority demonstrate a consistent pattern of recurrent and repeated antisocial, delinquent, and criminal behavior beginning in childhood and lasting well into adulthood. The following case provides a vivid example of such persistent and pervasive behavior, justifying the diagnosis of antisocial personality.

A twenty-eight-year-old white man was seen in a hospital's emergency room because of repeated "spells" or "fits" while in jail; he had been arrested for driving while intoxicated, disturbing the peace, and resisting arrest. The patient's problem behavior began at about age seven or eight when his parents reported to the local school that they could not handle their son because he was "wild" and "couldn't sit still." Similar behavior had been noted by the school and the parents had been requested to meet with the teacher. From that time forward, a recurrent pattern became evident of fighting in school, other discipline troubles, poor academic performance, several periods of suspension, and several periods of truancy.

At the same time, the parents noted that the patient stole money from them and began to stay out late at night, presumably running around with a neighborhood gang. At about age fourteen, the boy had his first police contact. Several members of the gang were arrested for stealing from a number of neighborhood stores. Nothing came of this, but at age seventeen the patient was arrested for driving a stolen vehicle; he received a suspended sentence. Soon thereafter, he dropped out of school and started to work. His work record was most unsatisfactory, however, because of frequently missing days of work and because he was considered to be a troublemaker by his supervisors. As a result of this pattern, he failed at several jobs. He then enlisted in the army, where his inability to conform to expectations and accept military discipline resulted in a discharge "without honor" after about ten months.

Soon after leaving the army, he got married, but, as soon as his wife became pregnant, he deserted her and, at the same time, his parents became aware that he was drinking excessively on repeated occasions and that he was experimenting with a variety of illicit street drugs. He and his wife had a stormy marriage with frequent separations and reconciliations, though, after the birth of three children, they separated permanently. His wife accused him of physical abuse and repeated infidelity and also reported that he was physically aggressive toward the children, beating them without justification.

His work record continued to be erratic, and he was a frequent visitor to local medical clinics and emergency rooms with a variety of physical complaints. On one occasion, he was admitted briefly to a psychiatric unit because of taking an overdose of sleeping pills and some of the other drugs he was using.

In short, this patient's history is typical for antisocial personality. It includes all sorts of interpersonal and social difficulties, including problems and conflicts at school, with parents, on the job, in the army, with his wife and children, and with the police.

The diagnostic criteria from *DSM-IV* are presented in Table 9.1.

Table 9.1 Diagnostic criteria for Antisocial Personality Disorder (*DSM-IV*)

A. There is a pervasive pattern of disregard for and violation of the rights of others occurring since age 15 years, as indicated by three (or more) of the following:

  (1) Failure to conform to social norms with respect to lawful behaviors as indicated by repeatedly performing acts that are grounds for arrest

  (2) Deceitfulness, as indicated by repeated lying, use of aliases, or conning others for personal profit or pleasure

  (3) Impulsivity or failure to plan ahead

  (4) Irritability and aggressiveness, as indicated by repeated physical fights or assaults

  (5) Reckless disregard for safety of self or others

  (6) Consistent irresponsibility, as indicated by repeated failure to sustain consistent work behavior or honor financial obligations

  (7) Lack of remorse, as indicated by being indifferent to or rationalizing having hurt, mistreated, or stolen from another

B. The individual is at least age 18 years

C. There is evidence of Conduct Disorder with onset before age 15 years

D. The occurrence of antisocial behavior is not exclusively during the course of Schizophrenia or a Manic Episode

---

NATURAL HISTORY

Sociopathy begins early in life (70). In some cases it may begin before the child starts attending school. Few sociopaths get through high school without recurrent difficulties. If the antisocial and delinquent pattern has not begun by age fifteen or sixteen, it is unlikely to occur. The prognosis may be better when the juvenile delinquency is "socialized," that is, when it occurs in a setting of close group involvement or loyalty (37). Lower social class, being female, and relative youth may adversely affect the clinical picture, but this is not a consistent finding (4).

The disorder is recurrent and varies in severity. Some sociopaths, generally milder cases, may remit during the late teens or early or mid-twenties (42). In other instances, sociopathic behavior persists into early middle age and then remits. Some sociopaths never improve. Attempts to explain remission have been based on hypothetical maturing or burning-out.

Remission, when it occurs, usually comes only after years of sociopathic behavior, during which education and work achievement have been severely compromised. Sociopaths rarely recover sufficiently to compensate for the "lost years." Thus "remission" usually means no more than a marginal social adjustment. Among many sociopaths, even if sociopathic behavior subsides, alcoholism and drug abuse persist and influence long-term adjustment (54).

COMPLICATIONS

The complications of sociopathy explain why the disorder is legitimately a medical concern. High rates of venereal disease, out-of-wedlock pregnancies, injuries from fights and accidents, alcoholism and drug dependence (8, 24, 38, 49, 50), and various medical complications of these conditions mean that sociopaths often come to the attention of doctors. Furthermore, increased mortality from accidents and homicide contributes to a reduced life expectancy, particularly in early adulthood (29, 71).

FAMILY STUDIES

As noted, sociopaths generally come from families that show severe social disturbances and disruption. Much of this family pathology consists of sociopathy and alcoholism (63–65).

In a study of male felons, most of whom were sociopaths, one-fifth of the first-degree male relatives were sociopaths and one-third were alcoholics (32). In a study of female felons, half of whom were sociopaths, one-third of the male relatives were sociopaths and one-half were alcoholics (14). In a study of children seen in a child guidance clinic (69), one-third of the fathers and one-tenth of the mothers of sociopaths were either sociopathic or alcoholic.

Among the attempts to determine whether this familial pattern reflects genetic factors have been investigations of twins and adoptees. Twin studies generally have focused on antisocial behavior, delinquency, or criminality, without distinguishing between sociopaths and others who show these behavior patterns. Nevertheless, as most criminals apparently are sociopaths (29), this approach appears somewhat justified. In twin studies, the concordance rates with regard to behavior difficulties, delinquency, and criminality have nearly always been higher for monozygotic than dizygotic twins (57, 80). However, the differences have not been as great as those seen in other psychiatric illnesses where a genetic predisposition is suspected. Furthermore, all of the series have been small and the monozygotic–dizygotic difference in some does not reach statistical significance.

Twin studies of psychiatric illness may involve bias in ascertainment of cases because concordant cases may come to the attention of physicians more often than discordant cases. Population twin registries have been proposed as more suitable for unbiased ascertainment. Christiansen, having access to a register of all Danish twin births, was able to obtain a presumably unselected series of criminal twins (11). He found that monozygotic twins had a significantly higher concordance rate than dizygotic twins (36 percent versus 12 percent).

Several follow-up studies of children of criminals and "psychopaths" indicate that these children, when adopted early in life by nonrelatives, are more likely to reveal psychopathic and criminal behavior as adults than are adopted children whose biological parents were not criminals or psychopaths (5–7, 18, 19, 78).

The association between sociopathy and somatization disorder (hysteria) within families and in the same individual (discussed in chapter 4) has been confirmed in other studies (81).

In summary, twin and adoptee studies at least suggest a genetic predisposition in some cases of sociopathy.

DIFFERENTIAL DIAGNOSIS

The differential diagnosis of sociopathy includes alcoholism, drug dependence, hysteria, schizophrenia, mania, and organic brain syndrome.

Alcoholism and drug abuse are frequent complications of sociopathy, and they aggravate antisocial and criminal patterns. In addition, however, some alcoholics and drug abusers who did not show sociopathic behavior in childhood or adolescence before the onset of alcoholism or drug dependence do show such behavior as a manifestation of the alcoholism or drug dependence. In these cases, the crucial diagnostic feature is the age of onset of antisocial and delinquent behavior; it is usually after age fifteen and coincident with, or following, the onset of the alcohol and drug abuse. When sociopathic behavior and alcohol or drug abuse all begin about the same time and before age fifteen, only follow-up may clarify the diagnosis, and often it is not possible to separate the sociopathy from the alcoholism or drug dependence.

The familial and clinical associations between sociopathy and somatization disorder (hysteria) have already been noted. Many female sociopaths and an occasional male sociopath develop the picture of somatization disorder (hysteria) (33, 52). Moreover, there is an increased frequency of antisocial behavior and delinquency in the past histories and family histories of hysterics who are not sociopaths (33). Finally, somatization disorder (hysteria) and sociopathy cluster in the same families. All these observations suggest that the differential diagnosis between the two conditions may involve the recognition of overlapping manifestations of similar etiologic factors (28).

A small minority of male schizophrenics give a history of sociopathic patterns in adolescence, and a small number of young sociopaths, at follow-up, turn out to be schizophrenics (69), but the prevalence of antisocial personality is not increased in the biological relatives of schizophrenics compared to the relatives of controls (68). If evidence of schizophrenia has not appeared by the early twenties, however, it is unlikely to develop.

The behavior of some early onset manics may mimic that of sociopaths, especially in women. Occasionally it will be difficult to distinguish mania from sociopathy when the latter is complicated by amphetamine or other drug abuse. Follow-up should clarify the issue. Because mania before age fifteen is rare, a history of antisocial and delinquent behavior before that age would suggest sociopathy rather than mania.

Although antisocial and criminal behavior may accompany an organic brain syndrome, the latter rarely develops in childhood or early adolescence.

CLINICAL MANAGEMENT

A major problem in treating sociopathy is the patient's lack of motivation for change. Few sociopaths volunteer for treatment. They are nearly always brought to the physician's attention by pressure from schools, parents, or judges. Moreover, the commonly disturbed family situation and poor socioeconomic circumstances provide little support for any treatment program. Many therapists believe that early institutional therapy offers the only hope for success, but there is no consensus about this (27). Psychotherapy has not achieved impressive results (86).

It is particularly difficult to carry out treatment if associated alcoholism or drug dependence cannot be controlled. In many cases, remission of the alcoholism or drug abuse is accompanied by a reduction in antisocial and criminal behavior (29). Since sociopathy begins early and individuals at high risk can be readily recognized (25, 69), early case finding and treatment may ultimately offer hope of prevention.

REFERENCES

1. Akesson, H. O., Forssman, H., Wahlstrom, J., and Wallin, L. Sex chromosome aneuploidy among men in three Swedish hospitals for the mentally retarded and maladjusted. Brit. J. Psychiat. *125*:386–389, 1974.
2. Arthurs, R., and Cahoon, E. A clinical and electroencephalographic survey of psychopathic personality. Am. J. Psychiat. *120*:875–877, 1964.
3. Behar, D., and Stewart, M. A. Aggressive conduct disorder of children. The clinical history and direct observations. Acta Psychiat. Scand. *65*:210–220, 1982.
4. Behar, D., and Stewart, M. A. Aggressive conduct disorder: the influence of social class, sex and age on the clinical picture. J. Child. Psychol. Psychiat. *25*:119–124, 1984.
5. Cadoret, R. J. Psychopathology in adopted-away offspring of biologic parents with antisocial behavior. Arch. Gen. Psychiat. *35*:176–184, 1978.
6. Cadoret, R. J., Cunningham, L., Loftus, R., and Edwards, J. Studies of adoptees from psychiatrically disturbed biological parents. II. Temperament, hyperactive, antisocial and developmental variables. J. Pediatr. *87*:301–306, 1975.
7. Cadoret, R. J., and Cain, C. Sex differences in predictors of antisocial behavior in adoptees. Arch. Gen. Psychiat. *37*:1171–1175, 1980.
8. Cadoret, R. J., O'Gorman, T. W., Troughton, E., and Heywood, E. Alcoholism and antisocial personality. Arch. Gen. Psychiat. *42*:161–167, 1985.
9. Cadoret, R. J., and Stewart, M. A. An adoption study of attention deficit/hyperactivity/aggression and their relationship to adult antisocial personality. Compr. Psychiat. *32*:73–82, 1991.
10. Chiles, J. A., Miller, M. L., and Cox, C. B. Depression in an adolescent delinquent population. Arch. Gen. Psychiat. *37*:1179–1184, 1980.

11. Christiansen, K. O. Crime in a Danish twin population. Acta Genet. Med. Gemellol. *19*:323–326, 1970.

12. Cleckley, H. *The Mask of Sanity.* St. Louis: C. V. Mosby, 1950.

13. Cloninger, C. R., and Guze, S. B. Psychiatric illness and female criminality: the role of sociopathy and hysteria in the antisocial woman. Am. J. Psychiat. *127*:303–311, 1970.

14. Cloninger, C. R., and Guze, S. B. Psychiatric illness in the families of female criminals: a study of 288 first-degree relatives. Brit. J. Psychiat. *122*:697–703, 1973.

15. Clouston, T. S. *Clinical Lectures on Mental Diseases.* London: Churchill, 1883.

16. Cowie, J., Cowie, V., and Slater, E. *Delinquency in Girls.* London: Humanities Press, 1968.

17. Craft, M. *Ten Studies into Psychopathic Personality.* Bristol: John Wright & Sons, 1965.

18. Crowe, R. R. The adopted offspring of women criminal offenders. Arch. Gen. Psychiat. *27*:600–603, 1972.

19. Crowe, R. R. An adoption study of antisocial personality. Arch. Gen. Psychiat. *31*:785–791, 1974.

20. Editorial. What becomes of the XYY male? Lancet *2*:1297–1298, 1974.

21. Ehrenkranz, J., Bliss, E., and Sheard, M. H. Plasma testosterone: correlation with aggressive behavior and social dominance in man. Psychosom. Med. *36*:469–475, 1974.

22. Farrington, D. P. Childhood origins of teenage antisocial behaviour and adult social dysfunction. J. R. Soc. Med. *86*:13–17, 1993.

23. Garvey, M. J., and Spoden, F. Suicide attempts in antisocial personality disorder. Compr. Psychiat. *21*:146–149, 1980.

24. Gerstley, L. J., Alterman, A. I., McLellan, A. T., and Woody, G. E. Antisocial personality disorder in patients with substance abuse disorders: a problematic diagnosis? Am. J. Psychiat. *147*:173–178, 1990.

25. Glueck, S., and Glueck, E. *Predicting Delinquency and Crime.* Cambridge: Harvard Univ. Press, 1959.

26. Gottlieb, J. S., Ashby, M. C., and Knott, J. R. Primary behavior disorders and psychopathic personality. Arch. Neurol. Psychiat. *56*:381–400, 1946.

27. Gralnick, A. Management of character disorders in a hospital setting. Am. J. Psychotherapy *33*:54–66, 1979.

28. Guze, S. B. The role of follow-up studies: their contribution to diagnostic classification as applied to hysteria. Semin. Psychiat. *2*:392–402, 1970.

29. Guze, S. B., Goodwin, D. W., and Crane, J. B. Criminality and psychiatric disorders. Arch. Gen. Psychiat. *20*:583–591, 1969.

30. Guze, S. B., Goodwin, D. W., and Crane, J. B. A psychiatric study of the wives of convicted felons: an example of assortative mating. Am. J. Psychiat. *126*:1773–1776, 1970.

31. Guze, S. B., Goodwin, D. W., and Crane, J. B. Criminal recidivism and psychiatric illness. Am. J. Psychiat. *127*:832–835, 1970.

32. Guze, S. B., Wolfgram, E. D., McKinney, J. K., and Cantwell, D. P. Psychi-

atric illness in the families of convicted criminals. A study of 519 first-degree relatives. Dis. Nerv. Syst. *28*:651–659, 1967.

33. Guze, S. B., Woodruff, Jr., R. A., and Clayton, P. J. Hysteria and antisocial behavior: further evidence of an association. Am. J. Psychiat. *127*:957–960, 1971.

34. Guze, S. B., Woodruff, R. A., and Clayton, P. J. A study of conversion symptoms in psychiatric outpatients. Am. J. Psychiat. *128*:643–646, 1971.

35. Hare, R. D. *Psychopathy: Theory and Research.* New York: John Wiley & Sons, 1970.

36. Hare, R. D. Diagnosis of antisocial personality disorder in two prison populations. Am. J. Psychiat. *140*:887–890, 1983.

37. Henn, F. A., Bardwell, R., and Jenkins, R. L. Juvenile delinquents re-visited. Adult criminal activity. Arch. Gen. Psychiat. *37*:1160–1163, 1980.

38. Hesselbrock, V., Meyer, R., and Hesselbrock, M. Psychopathology and addictive disorders. In *Addictive States*, O'Brien, C. P., and Jaffe, J. H. (eds.), 179–191. New York: Raven Press, Ltd., 1992.

39. Hook, E. B. Behavioral implications of the human XYY genotype. Science *179*:139–150, 1973.

40. Jonsson, G. Delinquent boys, their parents and grandparents. Acta Psychiat. Scand. Suppl. *195*:43, 1967.

41. Kahn, E. *Psychopathic Personalities.* New Haven, Conn.: Yale Univ. Press, 1931.

42. Kelso, J., and Stewart, M. A. Factors which predict the persistence of aggressive conduct disorder. J. Child Psychol. Psychiat. *27*:77–86, 1986.

43. Koch, J. L. A. *Leitfaden der Psychiatrie*, 2d ed. Ravensburg, Germany: Dorn, 1889.

44. Koller, K. M., and Castanos, J. N. Family background in prison groups: a comparative study of parental deprivation. Brit. J. Psychiat. *117*:371–380, 1970.

45. Kraepelin, E. *Psychiatrie.* Leipzig: J. A. Banth, 1909.

46. Kreuz, L. E., and Rose, R. M. Assessment of aggressive behavior and plasma testosterone in a young criminal population. Psychosom. Med. *34*:321–332, 1972.

47. Kruesi, M. J. P., Hibbs, E. D., Zahn, T. P., Keysor, C. S., Hamburger, S. D., Bartko, J. J., and Rapoport, J. L. A 2-year prospective follow-up study of children and adolescents with disruptive behavior disorders. Arch. Gen. Psychiat. *49*:429–435, 1992.

48. Lewis, A. Psychopathic personality: a most elusive category. Psychol. Med. *4*:133–140, 1974.

49. Lewis, C. E. Alcoholism, antisocial personality, narcotic addiction: an integrative approach. Psychiat. Dev. *3*:223–235, 1984.

50. Lucker, G. W., Kruzich, D. J., Holt, M. T., and Gold, J. D. The prevalence of antisocial behavior among U.S. Army DWI offenders. J. Stud. Alcohol *52*:318–320, 1991.

51. Lunden, W. A. *Statistics on Delinquents and Delinquency.* Springfield, Ill.; C. C. Thomas, 1964.

52. Maddocks, P. D. A five-year follow-up of untreated psychopaths. Brit. J. Psychiat. *116*:511–515, 1970.

53. Mannuzza, S., Klein, R. G., Bessler, A., Malloy, P., and LaPadula, M. Adult outcome of hyperactive boys. Arch. Gen. Psychiat. *50*:565–576, 1993.

54. Martin, R. L., Cloninger, C. R., and Guze, S. B. The evaluation of diagnostic concordance in follow-up studies: II. A blind, prospective follow-up of female criminals. J. Psychiat. Res. *15*:107–125, 1979.

55. Mattsson, A., Schalling, D., Olweus, D., Löw, H., and Svensson, J. Plasma testosterone, aggressive behavior, and personality dimensions in young male delinquents. J. Am. Acad. Child Psychiat. *19*:476–490, 1980.

56. Mawson, A. R., and Mawson, C. D. Psychopathy and arousal: a new interpretation of the psychophysiological literature. Biol. Psychiat. *12*:49–74, 1977.

57. Mednick, S., and Christiansen, K. O. (eds.). *Biosocial Bases of Criminal Behavior.* New York: Gardner Press, 1977.

58. Mendelson, W., Johnson, N., and Stewart, M. A. Hyperactive children as teenagers: a follow-up study. J. Nerv. Ment. Dis. *153*:273–279, 1971.

59. Mitchell, S., and Rosa, P. Boyhood behaviour problems as precursors of criminality: a fifteen-year follow-up study. J. Child Psychol. Psychiat. *22*:19–33, 1981.

60. Morrison, J. Adult psychiatric disorders in parents of hyperactive children. Am J. Psychiat. *137*:825–827, 1980.

61. Nielsen, J., and Henriksen, F. Incidence of chromosome aberrations among males in a Danish youth prison. Acta Psychiat. Scand. *48*:87–102, 1972.

62. Offord, D. R., Sullivan, K., Allen, N., and Abrams, N. Delinquency and hyperactivity. J. Nerv. Ment. Dis. *167*:734–741, 1979.

63. Oliver, J. E. Successive generations of child maltreatment. Brit. J. Psychiat. *147*:484–490, 1985.

64. Oliver, J. E. Successive generations of child maltreatment. The children. Brit. J. Psychiat. *153*:543–553, 1988.

65. Oliver, J. E. Intergenerational transmission of child abuse: rates, research, and clinical implications. Am. J. Psychiat. *150*:1315–1324, 1993.

66. Prichard, J. C. *A Treatise on Insanity and Other Disorders Affecting the Mind.* London: Sherwood, Gilbert, and Piper, 1835.

67. Raine, A., Venables, P. H., and Williams, M. Relationships between central and autonomic measures of arousal at age 15 years and criminality at age 24 years. Arch. Gen. Psychiat. *47*:1003–1007, 1990.

68. Rimmer, J., and Jacobsen, B. Antisocial personality in the biological relatives of schizophrenics. Compr. Psychiat. *21*:258–262, 1980.

69. Robins, L. N. *Deviant Children Grown Up.* Baltimore: Williams & Wilkins, 1966.

70. Robins, L. N. *The Consequences of Conduct Disorder in Girls. Development of Antisocial and Prosocial Behavior.* New York: Academic Press, 1986.

71. Robins, L., and O'Neal, P. Mortality, mobility, and crime: problem children thirty years later. Am. Sociol. Rev. *23*:162–171, 1958.

72. Robins, L. N., and Regier, D. A. (eds.). *Psychiatric Disorders in America. The Epidemiologic Catchment Area Study.* New York: The Free Press, 1991.
73. Rush, B. *Medical Inquiries and Observations upon the Diseases of the Mind.* New York: Hafner, 1962.
74. Satterfield, J. H. The hyperactive child syndrome: a precursor of adult psychopathy. Proceedings of the NATO Advanced Study Institute on Psychopathic Behavior, Les Arcs, France, September 1975. In *Psychopathic Behavior,* Hare, R. D., and Schalling, D. (eds.), 329–346, New York: John Wiley & Sons, 1978.
75. Satterfield, J. H., Hoppe, C. M., and Schell, A. M. A prospective study of delinquency in 110 adolescent boys with attention deficit disorder and 88 normal adolescent boys. Am. J. Psychiat. *139*:795–798, 1982.
76. Schneider, K. *Psychopathic Personalities.* London: Cassell, 1958.
77. Schröder, J., de la Chapelle, A., Hakola, P., and Virkkunen, M. The frequency of XYY and XXY men among criminal offenders. Acta Psychiat. Scand. *63*:272–276, 1981.
78. Schulsinger, F. Psychopathy, heredity, and environment. Int. J. Ment. Health *1*:190–206, 1972.
79. Shah, S. A., and Roth, L. H. Biological and psychophysiological factors in criminality. In *Handbook of Criminology,* Glaser, D. (ed.), 101–173, Chicago: Rand McNally, 1974.
80. Slater, E., and Cowie, V. *The Genetics of Mental Disorders.* London: Oxford Univ. Press, 1971.
81. Spalt, L. Hysteria and antisocial personality. A single disorder: J. Nerv. Ment. Dis. *168*:456–464, 1980.
82. Spreen, O. The relationship between learning disability, neurological impairment, and delinquency. Results of a follow-up study. J. Nerv. Ment. Dis. *169*:791–799, 1981.
83. Stewart, M. A., Cummings, C., Singer, S., and deBlois, C. S. The overlap between hyperactive and unsocialized aggressive children. J. Child. Psychol. Psychiat. *22*:35–45, 1981.
84. Weiss, G., Hechtman, L., Milroy, T., and Perlman, T. Psychiatric status of hyperactives as adults: a controlled prospective 15-year follow-up of 63 hyperactive children. J. Am. Acad. Child Psychiat. *24*:211–220, 1985.
85. Woodruff, Jr., R. A., Guze, S. B., and Clayton, P. J. The medical and psychiatric implications of antisocial personality (sociopathy). Dis. Nerv. Syst. *32*:712–714, 1971.
86. Woody, G. E., McLellan, A. T., Luborsky, L., and O'Brien, C. P. Sociopathy and psychotherapy outcome. Arch. Gen. Psychiat. *42*:1081–1086, 1985.

10

DELIRIUM, CONFUSIONAL STATES, AND DEMENTIA (BRAIN SYNDROME)

DEFINITION

Delirium, confusional states, and dementia are often referred to as organic brain syndrome, or simply brain syndrome. This clinical diagnosis is based primarily on the mental status examination and usually is applied to patients with recognizable medical and neurological disorders affecting brain structure and function. In *DSM-IV*, these conditions are described as "Delirium, Dementia, and Other Cognitive Disorders." The older term, "brain syndrome," will be used in this chapter for simplicity. The diagnosis depends on finding impairment of orientation, memory, and other intellectual or cognitive functions. Additional psychiatric symptoms may occur, including hallucinations, delusions, depression, obsessions, and personality change. Judgment is impaired. Patients may or may not be aware of having the disorder.

Brain syndromes may be divided into acute and chronic forms. An acute brain syndrome is brief and presumably reversible. Delirium is an acute brain syndrome associated with excitement and agitation, and often with hallucinations and delusions as well. A chronic brain syndrome, or dementia, is often progressive and chances of recovery are limited.

HISTORICAL BACKGROUND

It is not known with any certainty when the clinical picture of brain syndrome was first recognized as distinct from other psychiatric disorders. On this subject, much interesting material is presented in an annotated anthology of selected medical texts (62).

One of the earliest descriptions in English was provided in 1615 by a clergyman, Thomas Adams, in his treatise *Mystical Bedlam, the World of Mad-Men* (2). He referred to "some mad, that can rightly judge of the things they see, as touching imagination and phantasie: but for cogitation and reason, they swarve from naturale judgment."

In 1694 William Salmon (93) described in detail a case of dementia and noted that the patient was "not mad, or distracted like a man in Bedlam [but] decayed in his Intellectuals."

In 1761 Giovanni Battista Morgagni, the great Italian pioneer in morphologic pathology, who first systematically correlated clinical features and course with postmortem findings, described certain areas of "hardness" in the brains of former mental patients (81). He emphasized, however, that the correlation between clinical picture and anatomical findings was not consistent.

Morgagni's work set the stage for Antoine Laurant Jesse Bayle who, in 1822, published the first systematic clinicopathologic study of paresis. In this study the clinical symptoms, including progressive dementia, were correlated with changes in brain parenchyma and meninges (11). Bayle's findings were confirmed in 1826 by Louis Florentin Calmeil (23).

Another milestone in the understanding of brain syndrome was Korsakoff's investigation of the disorder that bears his name (104). His observations, reported between 1887 and 1891, correlated a particular form of dementia manifested by extreme amnesia with lesions of the brain stem.

Over the years the accumulation of case reports and clinical experience indicated that disorientation and memory impairment were the hallmarks of a clinical syndrome seen frequently in the presence of demonstrable brain damage, systemic infections, or intoxications. But systematic investigations were infrequent. Two modern studies based on autopsy results indicate that brain syndromes are associated with brain pathology in the majority of cases (26, 50).

EPIDEMIOLOGY

There have been few epidemiologic studies of acute brain syndrome. It occurs commonly in the presence of pneumonia, systemic infections, congestive heart failure, high fever, fluid and electrolyte imbalance, stroke, the postoperative state, and intoxication with alcohol or other drugs, but the exact frequency is unknown. Reports have dealt with cases referred for psychiatric consultation because of disturbed behavior rather than with the frequency of the syndrome as determined by systematic study.

It is known that dementia of the Alzheimer's type and vascular disease of the brain are two of the most common causes of chronic brain syndromes and that their prevalence increases with age. But epidemiologic studies of chronic brain syndrome have serious flaws. Most have been based on hospitalization rates. Different rates have been reported related to urban versus rural status, sex, race, educational achievement, and marital status. Many authors, however, emphasize the need for caution in extrapolating from hospitalization rates to true prevalence (32, 73, 74). A review of recent field surveys indicates inconsistent findings in regard to these same social and economic factors (32, 37), making it clear that most such correlations can only be regarded as tentative.

CLINICAL PICTURE (Tables 10.1, 10.2, and 10.3)

The acute brain syndrome is nearly always associated with medical, surgical, or neurological disorders, or with drug intoxications. This association is so consistent that an unexplained acute brain syndrome should alert the physician to the likelihood that such a disorder exists or is developing. A patient with pneumonia, for example, will sometimes present with an acute brain syndrome hours before the other clinical findings appear.

An acute brain syndrome may vary clinically, but two features are of special diagnostic importance: disorientation and impairment of recent memory. Without at least one of these, the diagnosis can only be suspected.

Patients may complain that they do not understand where they are and that they cannot find the bathroom; or they may bitterly insist that no one has fed them, even though the remains of the last meal are on the tray next to their bed. Other common clinical features include a depressed or fearful mood, apathy, irritability, impaired judgment, suspiciousness, delusions, hallucinations, and combative, uncooperative, or frightened behavior.

A labile, shifting affect with sudden crying spells; an argumentative, demanding manner ("I've called and called and no one pays any attention to me"); visual hallucinations of frightening or threatening faces ("They're grinning at me all the time, . . . they know something bad will happen"); unreasonable pressure for changes in room, personnel, or food; inappropriate efforts to get dressed and leave the hospital or to "escape" other patients who "want to hurt me" are examples of such clinical features.

The combination of disorientation, impaired memory, suspiciousness, hallucinations, and combative or frightened behavior constitutes delirium. This is the most dramatic, clinically severe form of acute brain syndrome. It may develop rapidly without any preceding manifestations or gradually in a patient who has been quietly confused and apathetic for many hours or days. Sometimes it may complicate a chronic state of dementia. The diagnostic criteria for delirium, according to *DSM-IV*, are presented in Table 10.1.

Acute brain syndrome may fluctuate strikingly from day to day and even from hour to hour. Some patients show a diurnal pattern with the most obvious and severe manifestations at night. They may appear normal in the morning except for haziness about the night before and yet be frankly disoriented, confused, and hallucinating that night. In some cases, the patient's mental status must be checked repeatedly to elicit disorientation or recent memory difficulty.

Disorientation may relate to time, place, or person. The first is the most common, the last the least common. Minor errors by patients who have been sick or hospitalized for some time should not receive undue emphasis. But persistent inability to recall the month or year correctly, especially if the correct answers have been offered recently, recurrent failure to identify where the patient is, or repeated inability to recall recent events correctly, is diagnostic. Because the manifestations are often more definite at night, the first indication of acute brain syndrome may be recorded in the nurse's notes. A report of the patient mistaking the nurse for someone else—such as a neighbor or relative ("What is

Table 10.1 Diagnostic criteria for Delirium due to . . .
[*Indicate the General Medical Condition*]

A. Disturbance of consciousness (i.e., reduced clarity of awarenss of the environment) with reduced ability to focus, sustain, or shift attention

B. A change in cognition (such as memory deficit, disorientation, language disturbance) or the development of a perceptual disturbance that is not better accounted for by a preexisting, established, or evolving dementia

C. The disturbance develops over a short period of time (usually hours to days) and tends to fluctuate during the course of the day

D. There is evidence from the history, physical examination, or laboratory findings that the disturbance is caused by the direct physiological consequences of a general medical condition my sister doing here?'') or experiencing hallucinations—is sometimes ignored until the patient is frankly disoriented and combative.

Acute brain syndrome seen in a general hospital usually indicates that the patient is seriously ill physically. Available evidence suggests that when the condition interferes with nursing care or treatment or when it disturbs other patients, the prognosis is poorer than is the case for patients with similar medical illnesses matched for age, sex, and race who do not have acute brain syndrome (25, 42, 50, 51, 86).

Diagnostic criteria for dementia, according to *DSM-IV*, are presented in Table 10.2. Many patients with dementia may present with depressive symptoms (69) or somatic complaints such as headache, abdominal pain, and constipation. Others are brought to physicians by relatives because of temper outbursts, socially

Table 10.2   Diagnostic criteria for Dementia due to other general medical conditions

A. The development of multiple cognitive deficits manifested by both

   (1) Memory impairment (impaired ability to learn new information or to recall previously learned information)
   (2) One (or more) of the following cognitive disturbances:
       (*a*) aphasia (language disturbance)
       (*b*) apraxia (impaired ability to carry out motor activities despite intact motor function)
       (*c*) agnosia (failure to recognize or identify objects despite intact sensory function)
       (*d*) disturbance in executive functioning (i.e., planning, organizing, sequencing, abstracting)

B. The cognitive deficits in criteria A1 and A2 each cause signficant impairment in social or occupational functioning and represent a significant decline from a previous level of functioning

C. There is evidence from the history, physical examination, or laboratory findings that the disturbance is the direct physiological consequence of one of the general medical conditions listed below.

D. The deficits do not occur exclusively during the course of a delirium.

embarrassing behavior, or suspiciousness. The cognitive and memory impairment may become evident only as the patient's history is elicited. *DSM-IV* provides additional diagnostic criteria for subtypes with prominent delusions or prominent disturbances of mood; it remains to be seen whether such subdivisions will prove useful.

Depressed patients may complain of poor memory and some studies have revealed impairment of short-term memory in many. The memory difficulty improves with remission of the depression (98). Sometimes, however, it is important to distinguish between complaints of memory difficulty (pseudodementia) and actual impairment of memory. Some have argued that the term "pseudodementia" can be misleading since depression may also include significant cognitive impairment as part of the clinical picture, especially in older patients.

It has therefore been suggested that a more appropriate name for this condition might be *cognitive impairment of depression*. In some middle-aged and older patients suffering from depression, the complaint of memory impairment is disproportionately greater than the degree of memory impairment noted on systematic testing, and the perceived memory difficulty subsides as the depression improves (24, 55, 64, 78, 108). Clearly the relationship between depression and cognitive impairment may sometimes be puzzling. It is important to recognize that some patients with depression, especially older ones, may present with enough cognitive difficulty to raise differential diagnostic problems. In such cases physicians should be cautious about making a firm diagnosis and be prepared to change their diagnosis as the clinical picture unfolds.

In dementia, the patient's insight may vary greatly. Sometimes, especially earlier in the illness, the patient may volunteer that, "I keep losing things. I don't know where I left them. I occasionally can't remember the directions when I drive home." Often, however, and especially as the illness progresses, the patient may deny any memory difficulty and insist that he was preoccupied or distracted by worries or interruptions. Inability to follow directions and confusion about what others intend may lead to irritability and anger: "Nobody tries to explain things to me. Nobody cares about how I feel—I'll show them." Frustration at being unable to accomplish specific tasks, including specific cognitive tests, frequently leads to suspicion and resistance: "That's a silly thing to do. I could do it if I really wanted to, but I don't see a good reason for it. You're trying to trip me up and fool me."

Inattention to cleanliness and grooming, deterioration in table manners, the use of abusive and foul language, social withdrawal and a generally inconsiderate manner, sudden and seemingly unprovoked outbursts of anger and even physical violence present increasingly heavy burdens to the family as the disorder worsens, and may require institutionalization.

The most important point about dementia is that in some cases the underlying illness is treatable (27, 55, 105, 106). These cases should be recognized as early as possible because recovery may be related to the duration of the dementia. Drug intoxication (13, 85, 96, 102, 103), liver failure (95), hypothyroidism (36, 97), pernicious anemia (99), paresis (44), subdural hematomas and benign brain tumors (6), and normal-pressure hydrocephalus (63, 70, 88) are infrequent but recognizable causes of dementia, though debate continues about the diagnosis and validity of the last entity (4). Recurrent hypoglycemia because of insulin treatment of diabetes, pancreatic islet-cell tumors, or the too-rapid alimentary absorption of glucose in patients who have undergone subtotal gastric resection may also lead to severe dementia (7, 8, 21). All these disorders may be correctable. Chronic alcohol abuse has been associated with a memory impairment (12, 71, 77, 90) that is distinct from the Wernicke-Korsakoff syndrome and that, if recognized early, often can be reversed by abstention from further drinking; however, debate continues about the validity of an alcohol-induced dementia separate from Wernicke's encephalopathy or hepatic encephalopathy (101). Recent work has suggested that the dementia frequently associated with chronic renal dialysis may be caused by aluminum intoxication from the water used in such great quantities during dialysis (3, 5, 79, 87).

Although probably not readily reversible, this syndrome may now be preventable.

Most cases of dementia, however, are the result of intrinsic brain disease or arteriosclerotic changes in the blood vessels supplying the brain (1). Studies by Roth (92) suggest that in both groups of patients there is "a fairly strict quantitative relationship . . . between the amount of intellectual deterioration and the amount of cerebral damage at postmortem. In each group of disorders there are . . . threshold effects, suggesting that up to a certain limit the destruction wrought by degenerative changes can be accommodated within the reserve capacity of the brain."

Recent usage indicates a preference for the term "multi-infarct dementia" rather than "arteriosclerotic dementia." This change reflects the recognition that the dementia results from loss of brain tissue, typically with a deterioration in intellecual function proportionate to the amount lost.

Other causes of dementia, still untreatable, are a variety of presenile brain degenerations and traumatic injuries to the brain (10, 38, 47, 53, 61, 65, 75, 94, 110) (Tables 10.4 and 10.5).

For many years a distinction was made between Alzheimer's disease, a presenile dementia, and senile brain disease or dementia, despite the fact that the anatomical findings (senile plaques, neurofibrillary tangles, and granulovacuolar degenerative changes) in the two groups of patients are similar. In current practice the two conditions are viewed as identical (91, 107).

Recent work indicates that dementia of the Alzheimer type, whether presenile or senile, is associated with a variety of pathological and biochemical changes involving many brain areas and systems (67). Finally, there is evidence that the neurofibrillary tangles characteristic of Alzheimer's originate from neurotubules and that plaques originate from amyloid deposits (48, 67).

The genetic defect in most cases of *familial* Alzheimer's disease is located on chromosome 14, 19, or 21 (54). The last chromosome is involved in Down's syndrome (45, 60, 100). This finding is of special interest in view of the observation that changes similar to those seen in Alzheimer's disease are also found in patients

Table 10.3   Diagnostic criteria for Dementia of the Alzheimer's Type

A. The development of multiple cognitive deficits manifested by both

  (1) Memory impairment (impaired ability to learn new information or to recall previously learned information)
  (2) One (or more) of the following cognitive disturbances:
    (*a*) Aphasia (language disturbance)
    (*b*) Apraxia (impaired ability to carry out motor activities despite intact motor function)
    (*c*) Agnosia (failure to recognize or identify objects despite intact sensory function)
    (*d*) Disturbance in executive functioning (i.e., planning, organizing, sequencing, abstracting)

B. The cognitive deficits in Criteria A1 and A2 each cause significant impairment in social or occupational functioning and represent a significant decline from a previous level of functioning

C. The course is characterized by gradual onset and continuing cognitive decline

D. The cognitive deficits in Criteria A1 and A2 are not due to any of the following:

  (1) Other central nervous system conditions that cause progressive deficits in memory and cognition (e.g., cerebrovascular disease, Parkinson's disease, Huntington's disease, subdural hematoma, normal-pressure hydrocephalus, brain tumor)
  (2) Systemic conditions that are known to cause dementia (e.g., hypothyroidism, vitamin B_{12} or folic acid deficiency, niacin deficiency, hypercalcemia, neurosyphilis, HIV infection)
  (3) Substance-induced conditions

E. The deficits do not occur exclusively during the course of a delirium

F. The disturbance is not better accounted for by another Axis I disorder (e.g., Major Depressive Disorder, Schizophrenia)

---

with Down's syndrome who survive until early middle age (28, 39, 59).

Related to the findings concerning the role of impaired cholinergic function in dementia of the Alzheimer's type is work suggesting that age-related memory disturbances in animals and humans may also be associated with cholinergic dysfunction (9, 30, 83). Whether the problem in Alzheimer patients is simply a more rapid progression of age-related changes or whether it involves certain more specific factors is not yet clear. There is also growing evidence that lipoprotein E4 genotype is involved in the risk for Alzheimer's disease (67).

Huntington's disease, another form of severe dementia, long known to be caused by a dominant gene, is now clearly linked to chromosome 4 (49, 76). The gene contains an unstable DNA triplet (CAG) that is repeated more frequently in Huntington's disease patients than in normals. At the same time, several investigators have emphasized an association between Huntington's disease and affective disorder, noting that the affective disorder often may be an early manifestation of the Huntington's disease (22, 40, 41). This association may help account for clinical obser-

Table 10.4   Diagnostic criteria for Dementia due to Multiple Etiologies

A. The development of multiple cognitive deficits manifested by both

   (1) Memory impairment (impaired ability to learn new information or to recall previously learned information)

   (2) One (or more) of the following cognitive disturbances:

      (*a*) Aphasia (language disturbance)

      (*b*) Apraxia (impaired ability to carry out motor activities despite intact motor function)

      (*c*) Agnosia (failure to recognize or identify objects despite intact sensory function)

      (*d*) Disturbance in executive functioning (i.e., planning, organizating, sequencing, abstracting)

B. The cognitive deficits in Criteria A1 and A2 each cause significant impairment in social or occupational functioning and represent a significant decline from a previous level of functioning.

C. There is evidence from the history, physical examination, or laboratory findings that the disturbance has more than one etiology (e.g., head trauma plus chronic alcohol use, Dementia of the Alzheimer's Type with the subsequent development of Vascular Dementia).

D. The deficits do not occur exclusively during the course of a delirium.

Table 10.5   Diagnostic criteria for 290.4x Vascular Dementia

A. The development of multiple cognitive deficits manifested by both

  (1) Memory impairment (impaired ability to learn new information or to recall previously learned information)

  (2) One (or more) of the following cognitive disturbances:

   (*a*) Aphasia (language disturbance)

   (*b*) Apraxia (impaired ability to carry out motor activities despite intact motor function)

   (*c*) Agnosia (failure to recognize or identify objects despite intact sensory function)

   (*d*) Disturbance in executive functioning (i.e., planning, organizing, sequencing, abstracting)

B. The cognitive deficits in Criteria A1 and A2 each cause significant impairment in social or occupational functioning and represent a significant decline from a previous level of functioning

C. Focal neurological signs and symptoms (e.g., exaggeration of deep tendon reflexes, extensor plantar response, pseudobulbar palsy, gait abnormalities, weakness of an extremity) or laboratory evidence indicative of cerebrovascular disease (e.g., multiple infarctions involving cortex and underlying white matter) that are judged to be etiologically related to the disturbance

D. The deficits do not occur exclusively during the course of a delirium

vations that suggest suicide is a frequent complication of Huntington's disease, even when little or no dementia is present. The possibility of testing presymptomatically for the disorder by using a deoxyribonucleic acid (DNA) marker raises obvious and difficult ethical and legal concerns (14) about testing for a serious illness for which there is no known treatment or prevention.

Another form of dementia has been associated with the central nervous system (CNS) involvement in acquired immune deficiency syndrome (AIDS). Indeed, dementia may be an early or even the first clinical manifestation of human immunodeficiency virus (HIV) infection (46).

The use of computerized tomography (CT) may contribute valuable information for the diagnosis of dementia, but it is important to remember that the correlation between cognitive impairment and the radiological findings is sometimes poor. It is likely, however, that refinements in CT will improve such correlations in the future (18).

NATURAL HISTORY

As noted, acute brain syndrome may occur in the course of various medical illnesses. Often it is impossible to determine the most crucial factor in a patient with simultaneous heart failure, infection, fever, and dehydration who is also receiving a variety of medications. Generally, the brain syndrome subsides as the underlying abnormalities are corrected. Sometimes, when patients have been very sick and have had a prolonged brain syndrome, many days pass after medical abnormalities are controlled before the mental picture clears. Acute brain syndromes resulting from drug intoxication or drug withdrawal (e.g., alcohol, barbiturates, or benzodiazepines) nearly always subside within a few days after discontinuing the drug.

Chronic brain syndromes usually develop insidiously. The early manifestations may be subtle, and only in retrospect does their significance become evident. Fatigability, moodiness, distractibility, depression, irritability, and carelessness may be present long before memory difficulty, intellectual deterioration, and disorientation can be clearly and easily detected. Depending on the underlying brain disease, the dementia may either progress to total incapacity and death or stabilize for long periods (17, 55, 72, 91, 107). As in acute brain syndrome associated with delirium, chronic brain syndrome also appears to be associated with an excess mortality (15).

COMPLICATIONS

Faulty judgment in important decisions, inability to care for oneself, accidents, and suicide are the principal complications of brain syndromes.

One of the more difficult decisions physicians must make concerns patients with chronic brain syndromes whose behavior raises questions about their mental competence. At some point in the course of many chronic brain syndromes, the patients' confusion, forgetfulness, temper outbursts, and questionable financial dealings will lead relatives and friends to question whether they are still competent to handle their affairs and care for themselves properly. Losing or giving away large sums of money, writing bad checks, extreme carelessness of dress, unprecedented sexual behavior (e.g., molesting children or displaying genitals), wandering away from home and getting lost, and unpredictable temper displays may require legal action to protect patients from their own acts and to permit extended institutionalization.

Chronic brain syndrome, complicated by secondary depression, is one of the psychiatric disorders associated with suicide risk, though it accounts for only a small portion of suicides (89).

In some cases of delirium it is not possible to tell whether the patient jumped from a window with the intention of committing suicide or fell because of confusion and fear.

The role of dementia—especially that of Alzheimer's disease—as an important risk factor for serious falls has only recently gained recognition (82).

FAMILY STUDIES

Investigations of the familial prevalence of organic brain syndromes have been concerned primarily with specific disorders that lead to dementia such as Huntington's chorea. As noted earlier, the genetic basis of Huntington's chorea, which is carried by an autosomal dominant gene, is established (84), and senile dementia is apparently increased, perhaps fourfold, among the relatives of index cases (19, 20, 68, 80). Similarly, the familial, often genetic, basis of certain rare neurological disorders leading to dementia is clear (84). Yet there is no evidence of any general familial predisposition to brain syndromes.

Of considerable theoretical interest, however, is the observation that Alzheimer's disease, Down's syndrome, and myeloproliferative disorder cluster in the same families. Changes in the brain characteristic of Alzheimer's disease and associated with a dementing illness are seen in most persons with trisomy 21 (Down's syndrome) who die as they approach middle age. These observations, taken together, have led to the suggestion that an important common denominator may be a genetically determined defect in neuronal microtubules (29, 56–58), though another study failed to find such association (109).

Individuals suffering from Wernicke-Korsakoff syndrome may have a genetic predisposition to thiamine deficiency that becomes clinically significant when they are exposed to a poor diet: This is one possible explanation why only some chronic alcoholics develop the syndrome (16).

DIFFERENTIAL DIAGNOSIS

Other psychiatric conditions may be mimicked by brain syndromes: Patients' anxiety attacks may suggest a primary anxiety disorder; low mood and apathy, an affective disorder; hallucinations and delusions, schizophrenia. The crucial question in each case is whether the patient exhibits definite disorientation or memory impairment. These mental status abnormalities, when they are clearly present, are pathognomonic of a brain syndrome; they are not manifestations of an uncomplicated, so-called "functional," disorder. If a patient with another psychiatric illness develops disorientation or memory impairment, one should suspect that something else has developed: a drug reaction or medical or neurologic illness.

When a patient is unable or unwilling to cooperate in the mental status examination, an acute brain syndrome may be suspected. If there has been a sudden change in his or her behavior, speech, or manner and if the behavioral change develops in a clinical situation that frequently predisposes to an acute brain syndrome, the diagnosis of brain syndrome should be considered.

A definitive diagnosis must await evidence of disorientation or memory impairment; these will usually become apparent as the patient is observed carefully.

CLINICAL MANAGEMENT

Correction of the underlying medical or neurological condition, whenever possible, is the principal aim of therapy for patients with brain syndromes. At the same time, certain measures often help in the management of the brain syndrome itself. Good nursing care is very important. A calm, sympathetic, reassuring approach can turn a frightened, combative patient into a quiet, cooperative one. A patient with an acute brain syndrome often misinterprets stimuli and has unpredictable emotional responses. It is important, therefore, to provide a familiar, stable, unambiguous environment for such patients. Repeated simple explanations and frequent reassurance from familiar nurses, attendants, or relatives may be helpful. Patients do better with constant light; shadows or the dark easily frighten them.

Only the smallest effective doses of drugs acting on the CNS should be used because patients with brain syndromes are frequently sensitive to these agents. Brain syndromes are, in fact, often precipitated by sedatives or hypnotics and may subside when such drugs are discontinued. No drug is entirely safe. Careful attention to dosage and mental status is more important than the particular sedative or hypnotic used.

Some patients need to be kept from harming themselves. Usually, a relative, friend, or attendant who is able to be with the patient constantly—talking to him, explaining things, reassuring him—can calm him enough to permit appropriate care without restraints on a general hospital service. When this does not work or is not possible, rather than risk having a confused and frightened patient fall out of bed or jump out a window, transfer to the psychiatric service or physical restraint may be necessary.

If a psychiatric unit is not available or if the patient's medical condition and treatment require bed rest, a body restraint may be necessary. Obviously, a restrained patient should be watched carefully, and the previously described measures should be continued with the hope of calming him quickly, making any period of restraint brief.

Organized groups for relatives of demented patients can be very helpful in providing emotional support and practical suggestions for handling the wide range of problems that dementia presents to families (43). Too often the impact on family members is overwhelming, and this must be considered by the physician so that appropriate steps can be taken to reduce the burden, at least intermittently (33–35). Similarly, the introduction of systematic genetic counseling and family support for relatives of patients with Huntington's disease can offer much needed assistance to those who are at high risk for developing the disorder (52).

It should be noted that a number of new drugs are being developed to treat Alzheimer's dementia. Some reports of the use of tacrine, a "potent, centrally active, reversible acetylcholinesterase inhibitor," suggest that positive results may be achievable in some patients (31, 66).

REFERENCES

1. Adams, R. D., and Victor, M. *Principles of Neurology*, 5th ed. New York: McGraw Hill, 1993.
2. Adams, T. *Mystical Bedlam, the World of Mad-Men.* London, 1615.
3. Alfrey, A. C., LeGendre, G. R., and Kachny, W. D. The dialysis encephalopathy syndrome. N. Engl. J. Med. *294*:184–188, 1976.
4. Anderson, M. Normal pressure hydrocephalus. Brit. Med. J. *293*:837–838, 1986.
5. Arieff, A. I., Cooper, J. D., Armstrong, D., and Lazarowitz, V. C. Dementia, renal failure, and brain aluminum. Ann. Intern. Med. *90*:741–747, 1979.
6. Avery, T. L. Seven cases of frontal tumour with psychiatric presentation. Brit. J. Psychiat. *119*:19–23, 1971.
7. Bale, R. N. Brain damage in diabetes mellitus. Brit. J. Psychiat. *122*:337–342, 1973.
8. Banerji, N. K., and Hurwitz, L. J. Nervous system manifestations after gastric surgery. Acta Neurol. Scand. *47*:485–513, 1971.

9. Bartus, R. T., Dean, R. L., III, Beer, B., and Lippa, A. S. The cholinergic hypothesis of geriatric memory dysfunction. Science *217*:408–417, 1982.

10. Baxter, L. R., Mazziotta, J. C., Pahl, J. J., Grafton, S. T., St. George-Hyslop, P., Haines, J. L., Gusella, J. F., Szuba, M. P., Selin, C. E., Guze, B. H., and Phelps, M. E. Psychiatric, genetic, and positron emission tomographic evaluation of persons at risk for Huntington's disease. Arch. Gen. Psychiat. *49*:148–154, 1992.

11. Bayle, A. L. J. *Recherches sur l'arachnitis chronique*. Paris: M.D. thesis, 1822.

12. Berglund, M., Gustafson, L., Hagberg, B., Ingvar, D. H., Nilsson, L., Risberg, J., and Sonesson, B. Cerebral dysfunction in alcoholism and presenile dementia. Acta Psychiat. Scand. *55*:391–398, 1977.

13. Bergman, H., Borg, S., and Holm, L. Neuropsychological impairment and exclusive abuse of sedatives or hypnotics. Am. J. Psychiat. *137*:215–217, 1980.

14. Bird, S. J. Presymptomatic testing for Huntington's disease. JAMA *253*:3286–3291, 1985.

15. Black, D. W., Warrack, G., and Winokur, G. The Iowa record-linkage study. II. Excess mortality among patients with organic mental disorders. Arch. Gen. Psychiat. *42*:71–81, 1985.

16. Blass, J. P., and Gibson, G. E. Abnormality of a thiamine-requiring enzyme in patients with Wernicke-Korsakoff syndrome. N. Engl. J. Med. *297*:1367–1370, 1977.

17. Blessed, G., and Wilson, I. D. The contemporary natural history of mental disorder in old age. Brit. J. Psychiat. *141*:59–67, 1982.

18. Bondareff, W., Baldy, R., and Levy, R. Quantitative computed tomography in senile dementia. Arch. Gen. Psychiat. *38*:1365–1368, 1981.

19. Breitner, J. C. S., Folstein, M. F., and Murphy, E. A. Familial aggregation in Alzheimer dementia: I. A model for the age-dependent expression of an autosomal dominant gene. J. Psychiat. Res. *20*:31–43, 1986.

20. Breitner, J. C. S., Murphy, E. A., and Folstein, M. F. Familial aggregation in Alzheimer dementia: II. Clinical genetic implications of age-dependent onset. J. Psychiat. Res. *20*:45–55, 1986.

21. Burton, R. A., and Raskin, N. H. Alimentary (post gastrectomy) hypoglycemia. Arch. Neurol. *23*:14–17, 1970.

22. Caine, E. D., and Shoulson, I. Psychiatric syndromes in Huntington's disease. Am. J. Psychiat. *140*:728–733, 1983.

23. Calmeil, L. F. *De la paralysie considérée chez les aliénés*. Paris, 1826.

24. Cavenar, Jr., J. O., Maltbie, A. A., and Austin, L. Depression simulating organic brain disease. Am. J. Psychiat. *136*:521–523, 1979.

25. Cole, M. G., and Primeau, F. J. Prognosis of delirium in elderly hospital patients. Can. Med. Assoc. J. *149*:41–46, 1993.

26. Corsellis, J. A. N. *Mental Illness in the Aging Brain*. London: Oxford Univ. Press, 1962.

27. Cummings, J., Benson, D. F., and LoVerme, Jr., S., Reversible dementia. Illustrative cases, definition, and review. JAMA *243*:2434–2439, 1980.

28. Cutler, N. R., Heston, L. L., Davies, P., Haxby, J. V., and Schapiro, M. B.

Alzheimer's disease and Down's syndrome: new insights. Ann. Intern. Med. *103*:566–578, 1985.

29. Dahl, D., Selkoe, D. J., Pero, R. T., and Bignami, A. Immunostaining of neurofibrillary tangles in Alzheimer's senile dementia with a neurofilament antiserum. J. Neurosci. *2*:113–119, 1982.

30. Davis, K. L., Mohs, R. C., and Tinklenberg, J. R. Enhancement of memory by physostigmine (letter to the editor). N. Engl. J. Med. *301*:946, 1979.

31. Davis, K. L., Thal, L. J., Gamzu, E. R., et al. A double-blind, placebo-controlled multicenter study of tacrine for Alzheimer's disease. N. Engl. J. Med. *327*:1253–1259, 1992.

32. de Alarcón, J. Social causes and social consequences of mental illness in old age. In *Recent Developments in Psychogeriatrics*, Kay, D. W. K., and Walk, A. (eds.). Ashford, Kent: Headley Brothers, 1971.

33. Eagles, J. M., Craig, A., Rawlinson, F., Restall, D. B., Beattie, J. A. G., and Besson, J. A. O. The psychological well-being of supporters of the demented elderly. Brit. J. Psychiat. *150*:293–298, 1987.

34. Eagles, J. M., Beattie, J. A. G., Blackwood, G. W., Restall, D. B., and Ashcroft, G. W. The mental health of elderly couples. 1. The effects of a cognitively impaired spouse. Brit. J. Psychiat. *150*:299–303, 1987.

35. Eagles, J. M., Walker, L. G., Blackwood, G. W., Beattie, J. A. G., and Restall, F. B. The mental health of elderly couples: II. Concordance for psychiatric morbidity in spouses. Brit. J. Psychiat. *150*:303–308, 1987.

36. Easson, W. Myzedema with psychosis. Arch. Gen. Psychiat. *14*:277–283, 1966.

37. Eastwood, M. R., Rifat, S. L., and Roberts, D. The epidemiology of dementia in North America. Eur. Arch. Psychiat. Clin. Neurosci. *240*:207–211, 1991.

38. Enna, S. J., Bird, E. D. Bennett, J. P. Bylund, D. B., Yamamura, H. I., Iversen, L. L., and Snyder, S. H. Huntington's chorea: changes in neurotransmitter receptors in the brain. N. Engl. J. Med. *294*:1305–1309, 1976.

39. Evenhuis, H. M. The natural history of dementia in Down's syndrome. Arch. Neurol. *47*:263–267, 1990.

40. Folstein, S. E., Franz, M. L., Jensen, B. A., Chase, G. A., and Folstein, M. F. Conduct disorder and affective disorder among the offspring of patients with Huntington's disease. Psychol. Med. *13*:45–52, 1983.

41. Folstein, S. E., Abbott, M. H., Chase, G. A., Jensen, B. A., and Folstein, M. F. The association of affective disorder with Huntington's disease in a case series and in families. Psychol. Med. *13*:537–542, 1983.

42. Francis, J., Martin, D., and Kapoor, W. N. A prospective study of delirium in hospitalized elderly. JAMA *263*:1097–1101, 1990.

43. Fuller, J., Ward, E., Evans, A., Massam, K., and Gardner, A. Dementia: supportive groups for relatives. Brit. Med. J. *1*:1684–1685, 1979.

44. Gjestland, T. The Oslo study of untreated syphilis. Acta Derm. Venereol. Suppl. 34, 1955.

45. Goldgaber, D., Lerman, M. I., McBride, O. W., Saffiotti, U., and Gajdusek, D. C. Characterization and chromosomal localization of a cDNA encoding brain amyloid of Alzheimer's disease. Science *235*:877–880, 1987.

46. Grant, I., and Martin, A. *Neuropsychology of HIV Infection.* New York: Oxford University Press, 1994.

47. Gronwall, D., and Wrightson, P. Cumulative effect of concussion. Lancet 2:995–997, 1975.

48. Grundke-Iqbal, I., Johnson, A. B., Wisniewski, H. M., Terry, R. D., and Iqbal, K. Evidence that Alzheimer neurofibrillary tangles originate from neurotubules. Lancet *1*:578–580, 1979.

49. Gusella, J. F., Wexler, N. S., Conneally, P. M., Naylor, S. L., Anderson, M. A., Tanzi, R. E., Watkins, P. C., Ottina, K., Wallace, M. R., Sakaguchi, A. Y., Young, A. B., Shoulson, I., Bonilla, E., and Martin, J. B. A polymorphic DNA marker genetically linked to Huntington's disease. Nature *306*:234–238, 1983.

50. Guze, S. B., and Cantwell, D. P. The prognosis in "organic brain" syndromes. Am. J. Psychiat. *120*:878–881, 1964.

51. Guze, S. B., and Daengsurisri, S. Organic brain syndromes. Prognostic significance in general medical patients. Arch. Gen. Psychiat. *17*:365–366, 1967.

52. Harper, P. S., Tyler, A., Smith, S., Jones, P., Newcombe, R. G., and McBroom, V. Decline in the predicted incidence of Huntington's chorea associated with systematic genetic counselling and family support. Lancet 2:411–413, 1981.

53. Harrison, P. J., and Roberts, G. W. "Life, Jim, but not as we know it"? Brit. J. Psychiat. *158*:457–470, 1991.

54. Harrison, P. Alzheimer's disease and chromosome 14. Different gene, same process? Brit. J. Psychiat. *163*:2–5, 1993.

55. Hendrie, H. C. (ed.). *Brain Disorders: Clinical Diagnosis and Management.* Psychiat. Clin. North Am. *1*, 1978.

56. Heston, L. L., and Mastri, A. R. The genetics of Alzheimer's disease. Arch. Gen. Psychiat. *34*:976–981, 1977.

57. Heston, L. L. Alzheimer's disease, trisomy 21, and myeloproliferative disorders: associations suggesting a genetic diathesis. Science *1966*:322–323, 1977.

58. Heston, L. L., Mastri, A. R., Anderson, V. E., and White, J. Dementia of the Alzheimer type. Arch. Gen. Psychiat. *38*:1085–1090, 1981.

59. Heston, L. L. Down's syndrome and Alzheimer's dementia: defining an association. Psychiat. Dev. *4*:287–294, 1984.

60. Heston, L. L., Orr, H. T., Rich, S. S., and White, J. A. Linkage of an Alzheimer disease susceptibility locus to markers on human chromosome 21. Am. J. Med. Genet. *40*:449–453, 1991.

61. Hudson, A. J. Amyotrophic lateral sclerosis and its association with dementia, parkinsonism and other neurological disorders: a review. Brain *104*:217–247, 1981.

62. Hunter, R., and Macalpine, I. *Three Hundred Years of Psychiatry. 1535–1860.* London: Oxford Univ. Press, 1963.

63. Jacobs, L., Conti, D., Kinkel, W. R., and Manning, E. J. "Normal pressure" hydrocephalus: relationship of clinical and radiographic findings to improvement following shunt surgery. JAMA *235*:510–512, 1976.

64. Kahn, R. L., Zarit, S. H., Hilbert, N. M., and Niederehe, G. Memory complaint and impairment in the aged. Arch. Gen. Psychiat. *32*:1569–1573, 1975.

65. Kim, R. C., Collins, G. H., Parisi, J. E., Wright, A. W., and Chu, Y. B. Familial dementia of adult onset with pathological findings of a "nonspecific" nature. Brain *104*:61–78, 1981.

66. Knapp, M. J., Knopman, D. S., Solomon, P. R., Pendlebury, W. W., Davis, C. S., and Gracon, S. I. A 30-week randomized controlled trial of high-dose tacrine in patients with Alzheimer's disease. JAMA *271*:985–991, 1994.

67. Kosik, K. S. Alzheimer's disease: a cell biological perspective. Science *256*:780–783, 1992.

68. Larsson, T., Sjogren, T., and Jacobson, G. Senile dementia. Acta Psychiat. Suppl. 167, 1963.

69. Lazarus, L. W., Newton, N., Cohler, B., Lesser, J., and Schweon, C. Frequency and presentation of depressive symptoms in patients with primary degenerative dementia. Am. J. Psychiat. *144*:41–45, 1987.

70. Leading Article. Communicating hydrocephalus. Lancet 2:1011–1012, 1977.

71. Lishman, W. A. Cerebral disorder in alcoholism. Syndromes of impairment. Brain *104*:1–20, 1981.

72. Liston, E. H. Clinical findings in presenile dementia. A report of 50 cases. J. Nerv. Ment. Dis. *167*:337–342, 1979.

73. Liston, E. H. The clinical phenomenology of presenile dementia. A critical review of the literature. J. Nerv. Ment. Dis. *167*:329–336, 1979.

74. Locke, B. Z., Kramer, M., and Pasamanick, B. Mental disorders of the senium at mid-century: first admissions to Ohio State public mental hospitals. Am. J. Public Health. *50*:998–1012, 1960.

75. Lyle, O. E., and Gottesman, I. I. Subtle cognitive deficits as 15- to 20-year precursors of Huntington's disease. In *Advances in Neurology*, Chase, T. N. et al. (eds.), 23:227–238. New York: Raven Press, 1979.

76. Martin, J. B., and Gusella, J. F. Huntington's disease. Pathogenesis and management. N. Engl. J. Med. *315*:1267–1276, 1986.

77. Martin, P. R., McCool, B. A., and Singleton, C. K. Genetic sensitivity to thiamine deficiency and development of alcoholic organic brain disease. Alcohol. Clin. Exp. Res. *17*:31–37, 1993.

78. McAllister, R. W., and Price, T. R. P. Severe depressive pseudodementia with and without dementia. Am. J. Psychiat. *139*:626–629, 1982.

79. McDermott, J. R., Smith, A. I., Ward, M. K., Parkinson, I. S., and Kerr, D. N. S. Brain-aluminium concentration in dialysis encephalopaty. Lancet *1*:901–904, 1978.

80. Mohs, R. C., Breitner, J. C. S., Silverman, J. M., and Davis, K. L. Alzheimer's disease. Morbid risk among first-degree relatives approximates 50% by 90 years of age. Arch. Gen. Psychiat. *44*:405–408, 1987.

81. Morgagni, G. B. *The Seats and Causes of Diseases Investigated by Anatomy* (Alexander, B., trans.). Venice, 1761. London: Millar et al., 1769.

82. Morris, J. C., Rubin, E. H., Morris, E. J., and Mandel, S. A. Senile dementia

of the Alzheimer's type: an important risk factor for serious falls. J. Gerontol. *42*:412–417, 1987.

83. Potamianos, G., and Kellett, J. M. Anti-cholinergic drugs and memory: the effects of benzhexol on memory in a group of geriatric patients. Brit. J. Psychiat. *140*:470–472, 1982.

84. Pratt, R. T. C. *The Genetics of Neurological Disorders.* New York: Oxford Univ. Press, 1967.

85. Preskorn, S. H., and Simpson, S. Tricyclic-antidepressant-induced delirium and plasma drug concentration. Am. J. Psychiat. *139*:822–823, 1982.

86. Rabins, P. V., and Folstein, M. F. Delirium and dementia: diagnostic criteria and fatality rates. Brit. J. Psychiat. *140*:149–153, 1982.

87. Report from the Registration Committee of the European Dialysis and Transplant Association. Dialysis dementia in Europe. Lancet *2*:190–192, 1980.

88. Rice, E., and Gendelman, S. Psychiatric aspects of normal pressure hydrocephalus. JAMA *223*:409–412, 1973.

89. Robins, E., Murphy, G. E., Wilkinson, Jr., R. H., Gassner, S., and Kayes, J. Some clinical considerations in the prevention of suicide based on a study of 134 successful suicides. Am. J. Public Health *49*:888–899, 1959.

90. Ron, M. A. Brain damage in chronic alcoholism: a neuropathological, neuroradiological and psychological review. Psychol. Med. *7*:103–112, 1977.

91. Ron, M. A., Toone, B. K., Garralda, M. E., and Lishman, W. A. Diagnostic accuracy in presenile dementia. Brit. J. Psychiat. *134*:161–168, 1979.

92. Roth, M. Classification and etiology in mental disorders of old age. In *Recent Developments in Psychogeriatrics*, Kay, D. W. K., and Walk, A. (eds.). Ashford, Kent: Headley Brothers, 1971.

93. Salmon, W. *Iatrica: Sen Praxis Medendi. The Practice of Curing Disease*, 3d ed. London: Rolls, 1964.

94. Sapolsky, R. M., Uno, H., Rebert, C. S., and Finch, C. E. Hippocampal damage associated with prolonged glucocorticoid exposure in primates. J. Neurosci. *10*:2897–2902, 1990.

95. Schafer, D. F., and Jones, E. A. Hepatic encephalopathy and the gamma amino-butyric-acid neurotransmitter system. Lancet *1*:18–20, 1982.

96. Schentag, J. J., Cerra, F. B., Calleri, G., DeGlopper, E., Rose, J. Q., and Bernhard, H. Pharmacokinetic and clinical studies in patients with cimetidine-associated mental confusion. Lancet *1*:177–181, 1979.

97. Smith, C. K., Barish, J., Correa, J., and Williams, R. H. Psychiatric disturbance in endocrinologic disease. Psychosom. Med. *34*:69–86, 1972.

98. Sternberg, D. E., and Jarvik, M. E. Memory functions in depression. Arch. Gen. Psychiat. *33*:219–224, 1976.

99. Strachan, R., and Henderson, J. Psychiatric syndromes due to avitaminosis B12 with normal blood and marrow. Q. J. Med. *34*:303–317, 1965.

100. Tanzi, R. E., Gusella, J. F., Watkins, P. C., Bruns, G. A. P., St. George-Hyslop, P., Vam Keuren, M. L., Patterson, D., Pagan, S., Kurnit, D. M., and Neve, R. L. Amyloid β protein gene: cDNA, mRNA distribution, and genetic linkage near the Alzheimer locus. Science *235*:880–884, 1987.

101. Thomas, P. K. Brain atrophy and alcoholism. Brit. Med. J. *292*:787, 1986.
102. Trimble, M. R., and Reynolds, E. H. Anticonvulsant drugs and mental symptoms: a review. Psychol. Med. *6*:169–178, 1976.
103. Tune, L. E., Damlouji, N. F., Holland, A., Gardner, T. J., Folstein, M. F., and Coyle, J. T. Association of postoperative delirium with raised serum levels of anticholinergic drugs. Lancet *2*:651–653, 1981.
104. Victor, M., Adams, R. D., and Collins, G. H. *The Wernicke-Korsakoff Syndrome*. Philadelphia: F. A. Davis, 1971.
105. Victoratos, G. C., Lenman, J. A. R., and Herzberg, L. Neurological investigation of dementia. Brit. J. Psychiat. *130*:131–133, 1977.
106. Winberger, D. R. Brain disease and psychiatric illness: when should a psychiatrist order a CAT scan? Am. J. Psychiat. *141*:1521–1527, 1984.
107. Well, C. E. Chronic brain disease: an overview. Am. J. Psychiat. *135*:1–12, 1978.
108. Wells, C. E. Pseudodementia. Am. J. Psychiat. *136*:895–900, 1979.
109. Whalley, L. J., Carothers, A. D., Collyer, S., DeMay, R., and Frackiewicz, A. A study of familial factors in Alzheimer's disease. Brit. J. Psychiat. *140*:249–256, 1982.
110. Wolkowitz, O. M., Reus, V. I., Weingartner, H., Thompson, K., Breier, A., Doran, A., Rubinow, D., and Pickar, D. Cognitive effects of corticosteroids. Am. J. Psychiat. *147*:1297–1303, 1990.

11

EATING
DISORDERS

DEFINITION

The major eating disorders are anorexia nervosa and bulimia. Anorexia nervosa is characterized by peculiar attitudes toward eating and weight that lead to obsessive refusal to eat, profound weight loss, and, when the disorder occurs among girls, persistent amenorrhea. Bulimia refers to the gorging of food, typically followed by induced vomiting or purging. It is seen in many patients with anorexia nervosa and also may occur alone or as the predominant clinical feature (34).

HISTORICAL BACKGROUND

In 1689 Richard Morton published a monograph entitled *Phthisiologia or a Treatise of Consumptions*. One of its early chapters, "Nervous Phthisis," contains case histories of the illness we recognize today as anorexia nervosa. An example follows:

Mr. Duke's Daughter is S. Mary Axe, in the Year 1684 and the Eighteenth Year of her Age, in the Month of July fell into a total Suppression of her Monthly Courses from a multitude of Cares and Passions of her Mind, but without any Symptoms of the Green-Sickness following upon it. From which time her Appetite began to abate, and her Digestion to be bad; her Flesh also began to be flaccid and loose, and her Looks pale, with other symptoms usual in Universal Consumption of the Habit of the Body and by the extreme and memorable cold weather which happened the Winter following, this Consumption did seem to be not a little improved; for that she was wont by her studying at Night, and continual poring upon Books, to expose herself both Day and Night to the Injuries of the Air, which was at that time extremely cold, not without some manifest Prejudice to the System of her Nerves. The Spring following, by the Prescription of some Empirik, she took a Vomit, and after that I know not what Steel Medicine, but without any Advantage. So from that time loathing all sorts of Medicaments, she wholly neglected the care of herself for two full Years, till at last being brought to the last degree of Marasmus, or Consumption, and thereupon subject to frequent Fainting-Fitts, she apply'd herself to me for Advice.

I do not remember that I did ever in all my practice see one, that was conversant with the Living so much wasted with the greatest degree of Consumption, (like a Skeleton only clad with Skin) yet there was no Fever, but on the contrary a Coldness of the whole Body; no cough, or Difficulty of Breathing nor an appearnace of any other distemper of the Lungs, or of any other Entrail; No Looseness, or any other sign of a Colliquation, or Preternatural Expence of the Nutritious Juices. Only her Appetite was diminished, and her Digestion uneasy, with Fainting-Fitts, which did frequently return upon her. Which symptoms I did endeavor to relieve by the outward Application of Aromatick Bags made to the Region of the Stomach, and by Stomach-Plaisters, as also by the internal use of bitter Medicines, Chalybeates, and Juleps made of Cephalick and Antihysterick Waters, sufficiently impregnated with Spirit of Salt Armoniack, and Tincture of Castor, and other things of that Nature. Upon the use of which she seemed to be much better; but being quickly tired with Medicines, she beg'd that the whole Affair might be committed again to Nature, whereupon, consuming every day more and more, she was after three Months taken with a Fainting-Fitt, and died.

Another vivid and accurate description was presented in 1908 by Dejerine and Gauckler (20):

It sometimes happens that a physician has patients—they are more apt to be women—whose appearance is truly shocking. Their eyes are brilliant. Their cheeks are hollow, and their cheek bones seem to protrude through the skin. Their withered breasts hang from the walls of their chest. Every rib stands out. Their shoulder blades appear to be loosened from their frame. Every vertebra shows through the skin. The abdominal wall sinks in below the floating ribs and forms a hollow like a basin. The thighs and the calves of their legs are reduced to a skeleton. One would say it was the picture of an immured nun, such as the old masters have portrayed. These women appear to be fifty or sixty years old. Sometimes they seem to be sustained by some unknown miracle of energy; their voices are strong and their steps firm. On the other hand, they often seem almost at the point of death, and ready to draw their last breath.

Are they tuberculous or cancerous patients, or muscular atrophies in the last stages, these women whom misery and hunger have reduced to this frightful gauntness? Nothing of the kind. Their lungs are healthy, there is no sign of any organic affection. Although they look so old they are young women, girls, sometimes children. They may belong to good families, and be surrounded by every care. These patients are what are known as mental anorexics, who, without having any physical lesions, but by the association of various troubles, all having a psychic origin, have lost a quarter, a third, and sometimes a half of their weight. The affection which has driven them to this point may have lasted months, sometimes years. Let it go on too long and death will occur, either from inanition or from secondary tuberculosis. However, it is a case of nothing but a purely psychic affection of which the mechanisms are of many kinds.

Gull and Lasègue described the syndrome independently in 1873 (33, 62). The English term for the illness has been "anorexia nervosa," the French *l'anorexie hysterique,* and the German *Pubertaetsmagersucht.* Of these, the last is probably most precise; its literal meaning is "adolescent pursuit of thinness." It is this relentless pursuit of thinness that especially distinguishes anorexia nervosa from other illnesses associated with loss of weight.

Older historical accounts of patients wasting to the point of death do not usually provide enough information to permit distinguishing between cases of anorexia nervosa, tuberculosis, or panhypopituitarism. Until relatively recently it was not possible to make the distinction with confidence. Some early photographs of alleged pituitary disease, illustrating markedly wasted patients, probably represent cases of anorexia nervosa (see Differential Diagnosis).

The cause of the illness is not known, though hypotheses

involving endocrine, hypothalamic, and psychosocial factors abound (18, 37, 44, 70). One frequently invoked hypothesis is that the syndrome represents a rejection of adult sexuality with associated fears of oral impregnation. A wide spectrum of sexual knowledge, attitudes, and behavior was found in one study of patients with anorexia nervosa, though many believed that their illnesses had been precipitated by some sexual experience (4).

EPIDEMIOLOGY

Anorexia nervosa is not a common illness. On the basis of data from three community psychiatric case registers, in Scotland, England, and the United States, the average annual incidence appears to be low, in the range of one case per 100,000 population (17, 58). The Maudsley Hospital in London admitted thirty-eight patients over a twenty-year period (57). Most large teaching hospitals admit several cases each year. Recent evidence suggests, however, that the incidence of anorexia nervosa may be increasing (54, 63), particularly the type associated with bulimia, gorging of food followed by self-induced vomiting (26, 40, 78, 86). Bulimia itself is probably more common than anorexia nervosa.

Anorexia nervosa occurs much more frequently in females than in males. Probably 90 percent of cases are females (43, 69). A similar female preponderance is seen in cases of bulimia (13). Obviously, if amenorrhea is required for the diagnosis, the disorder will be limited to females. Some authors believe anorexia nervosa is mainly an illness of middle-class and upper-class girls, but there are no controlled data to support this hypothesis. Anorexia nervosa appears to be rare in blacks, though there is a suggestion that such cases may be increasing (80). It is apparently overrepresented among professional dance and modeling students, usually developing after the students have begun their studies (28, 31). One report suggests that adoptees may be a high-risk group for eating disorders (47).

CLINICAL PICTURE (Tables 11.1, and 11.2)

The syndrome typically begins with concern about mild obesity, followed by negative attitudes toward eating. A disgust for food that is far stronger than hunger develops. As weight loss progresses, patients may lose their hunger. However thin, they still consider themselves fat and continue to lose weight. These patients may lose so much weight that they resemble survivors of concentration camps, but with several differences. Patients with anorexia nervosa are usually alert and cheerful. In addition, they may be hyperactive. They often engage in strenuous exercise, sometimes in an open effort to keep from gaining weight.

From the onset of the illness, odd behavior relating to food may be seen. Patients may gorge themselves (bulimia), then induce vomiting voluntarily. This feature has attracted considerable attention in recent years, and, in some patients it may be the dominant clinical problem (14, 26, 30, 40, 71). Although starving themselves, patients may hoard food secretly or throw it away. To reduce weight, they may abuse laxatives, enemas, and diuretics.

Amenorrhea may begin before, with, or after the disturbance of appetite (27). It is present in most cases. A few patients develop anorexia nervosa after they have had the experience of motherhood, indicating that an undeveloped reproductive system is not an essential feature of the illness. Other physical findings are bradycardia and lanugo (soft, downy body hair).

Physiological differences between patients with anorexia nervosa and others have been noted (1, 9, 49, 66, 72). Most investigators believe that starvation produces these abnormalities, which include an abnormal glucose tolerance curve; increased serum cholesterol; increased serum carotene levels; diminished urinary 17-ketosteroids, estrogens, and gonadotropins; and low basal metabolic rate (18, 51). A striking "immaturity" in the pattern of luteinizing hormone secretion has been described in which the patients' hormone functioning resembles that of prepubertal girls but returns to normal after remission of the anorexia nervosa (8,

Table 11.1 Diagnostic criteria for Anorexia Nervosa

A. Refusal to maintain body weight at or above a minimally normal weight for age and height (e.g., weight loss leading to maintenance of body weight less than 85% of that expected; or failure to make expected weight gain during period of growth, leading to body weight less than 85% of the expected)

B. Intense fear of gaining weight or becoming fat, even though underweight

C. Disturbance in the way in which one's body weight or shape is experienced, undue influence of body weight or shape on self-evaluation, or denial of the seriousness of the current low body weight

D. In postmenarcheal females, amenorrhea, i.e., the absence of at least three consecutive menstrual cycles. (A woman is considered to have amenorrhea if her periods occur only following hormone, e.g., estrogen, administration)

Table 11.2 Diagnostic criteria for Bulimia Nervosa

A. Recurrent episodes of binge eating. An episode of binge eating is characterized by both of the following:
   (1) Eating, in a discrete period of time (e.g., within any 2-hour period), an amount of food that is definitely larger than most people would eat during a similar period of time and under similar circumstances
   (2) a sense of lack of control over eating during the episode (e.g., a feeling that one cannot stop eating or control what or how much one is eating)

B. Recurrent inappropriate compensatory behavior in order to prevent weight gain, such as self-induced vomiting; misuse of laxatives, diuretics, enemas, or other medications; fasting; or excessive exercise

C. The binge eating and inappropriate compensatory behaviors both occur, on average, at least twice a week for 3 months

D. Self-evaluation is unduly influenced by body shape and weight

E. The disturbance does not occur exclusively during episodes of Anorexia Nervosa

55). Male anorexia nervosa patients are reported to have low testosterone levels (6).

Many reports suggest an association between anorexia nervosa and Turner's syndrome or other congenital gonadal dysgenesis (19, 21, 24, 38, 45, 60, 61), but the data are still not conclusive (84).

DSM-IV criteria for the diagnosis of anorexia nervosa and its bulimic variant are presented in Tables 11.1 and 11.2.

NATURAL HISTORY

There has been disagreement about whether anorexia nervosa is a specific illness or a manifestation of other illnesses (57). In recent years, most patients with eating disorders report high rates of depression, anxiety, and substance dependence (9). These additional disorders typically complicate the eating disorder. However, if patients who have a preexisting psychiatric illness other than anorexia nervosa are separated from those whose history begins with the symptoms of anorexia nervosa, a pure group can be isolated (59).

The age of onset ranges from prepuberty to young adulthood, with the mean in the midteens (85). Premorbidly, patients with anorexia nervosa tend to be shy and introverted (18). A history of early feeding difficulties is common, as is a history of obsessional traits (18). The onset may be abrupt. There is one recorded case of an interval of six months from onset to the time of death (57). The illness may involve one lengthy episode lasting many months or years or it may be marked by remissions and exacerbations.

Full or nearly full recovery may occur in up to half the patients. In one study from Germany (25) about half the patients, after nearly ten years of follow-up, were free of symptoms (14 percent) or only "presented slight symptoms" (39 percent). Thirty patients (14 percent) had died. A similarly high mortality rate of 15 percent was reported in a study from England (68). A review of a number of follow-up studies (75) showed generally similar results but suggested that mortality rates may be falling.

Some patients have persistent difficulties, even when the problem of initial massive weight loss has been resolved. These include menstrual dysfunction, sexual maladjustment, large weight fluctuations, and disturbed appetite (3, 15, 36, 50, 57, 77, 81, 82). When full recovery occurs, it is usually within three years of onset (18). Depressive symptoms are common (12, 23); occasionally patients describe previous periods of anorexia nervosa so as to make them sound like episodes of depression. Dexamethasone suppression of cortisol secretion is impaired in some patients with anorexia nervosa, particularly those with considerable weight loss (32). This raises the possibility that impaired dexamethasone suppression in some patients with depression may be due to the associated weight loss or that some cases of anorexia nervosa may be manifestations of an underlying affective illness.

Sometimes the illness is associated with possible precipitating events such as the death of a relative or a broken engagement (4, 57). On the other hand, many patients can give no reason for the onset of their dieting (18).

A better prognosis appears to be related to earlier age at onset, though not all have reported this finding (42), and to greater educational achievement. A poorer prognosis appears to be related to later age at onset, longer duration of illness, disturbed relationship with parents, vomiting, laxative abuse, and the severity of obsessional and depressive symptoms (5, 39, 64, 79).

Though the immediate response to treatment may be good, premature death occurs in up to 10 or 15 percent of cases hospitalized psychiatrically; sometimes patients die a few years after the onset of their illnesses. In one series there was a 5 percent mortality within four years (64). Thus, anorexia nervosa should not be regarded lightly. When death occurs, the causes are commonly starvation and its complications, but it is often not possible to determine the cause of death (67).

The course and outcome of anorexia nervosa do not appear to differ significantly in males and females (11, 83).

COMPLICATIONS

The most obvious complication of anorexia nervosa is death from starvation. Some patients develop a variety of medical complications, including cardiovascular ones, that may contribute to the increased mortality (10, 73). Patients with anorexia nervosa apparently develop psychoses no more often than do persons in the general population (18). When psychotic features do develop, they usually appear to be part of associated major affective disorders (52).

FAMILY STUDIES

Some clinicians say that anorexia patients have dominating mothers and passive fathers (59); others disagree, finding neither a single personality pattern among parents nor a single pattern of interaction among family members (18, 29, 35). Close relatives of patients with anorexia nervosa do not have an increased prevalence of schizophrenia (84), but the findings concerning familial affective disorders are contradictory, as are the data concerning the association between anorexia nervosa and affective disorder in index patients (2, 53, 56, 65). There is evidence of increased parental psychopathology (18, 57, 59), but anorexia nervosa in the families is rare, though in one study (79) an increased prevalence among sisters was found. In another study (41), an increased familial prevalence of alcoholism was noted.

Of four pairs of monozygotic twins, three were concordant for anorexia nervosa and one discordant (38, 74). A more recent series of thirty-four twin pairs and one set of triplets in which the proband had anorexia nervosa showed a striking increase in concordance among female monozygotic twins compared to dizygotic twins, but no concordance in the small number of male twins (48).

DIFFERENTIAL DIAGNOSIS

Anorexia nervosa is characterized by unceasing pursuit of thinness and should not be confused with weight loss occurring in the course of illness such as depression or schizophrenia.

Starvation, when it has causes other than anorexia nervosa, is usually accompanied by apathy and inactivity rather than by the alertness and hyperactivity characteristic of anorexia nervosa.

Patients with anorexia nervosa or panhypopituitarism may both have low levels of urinary gonadotrophins, but they are not as consistently low in the former as in the latter (57). Hypopituitarism is seldom associated with the severe cachexia of anorexia nervosa or the strikingly high level of physical activity.

CLINICAL MANAGEMENT

Treatment of patients with anorexia nervosa is far from satisfactory, and there is no agreement about the best form. Some patients require constant observation on a locked psychiatric floor and tube feeding. Others have been successfully treated with phenothiazines (16) or antidepressants (46). Techniques of behavior modification have been used with reported success (7, 22, 76).

REFERENCES*

1. Ainley, C. C., Cason, J., Carlsson, L., Thompson, R. P. H., Slavin, B. M., and Norton, K. R. W. Zinc state in anorexia nervosa. Brit. Med. J. 293:992–993, 1986.
2. Altshuler, K. Z., and Weiner, M. F. Anorexia nervosa and depression: a dissenting view. Am. J. Psychiat. 142:328–332, 1985.
3. Bassø, H. H., and Eskeland, I. A prospective study of 133 patients with anorexia nervosa. Acta Psychiat. Scand. 65:127–133, 1982.

* See also the extensive review of the field presented at an International Conference on Anorexia Nervosa and Related Disorders. J. Psychiat. Res. 19:79–521, 1985.

4. Beumont, P. J. V., Abraham, S. F., and Simson, K. G. The psychosexual histories of adolescent girls and young women with anorexia nervosa. Psychol. Med. *11*:131–140, 1981.

5. Beumont, P. J. V., George, G. C. W., and Smart, D. E. "Dieters" and "vomiters and purgers" in anorexia nervosa. Psychol. Med. *6*:617–622, 1976.

6. Beumont, P. J. V., Veardwood, C. J., and Russell, G. F. M. The occurrence of the syndrome of anorexia nervosa in male subjects. Psychol. Med. *2*:216–231, 1972.

7. Blinder, B. J., Freeman, D. M. A., and Stunkard, A. J. Behavior therapy of anorexia nervosa: effectiveness of activity as a reinforcer of weight gain. Am. J. Psychiat. *126*:1093–1099, 1970.

8. Boyar, R. M., Katz, J., Finkelstein, J. W., Kapen, S., Wiener, H., Weitzman, E. D., and Hellman, L. Anorexia nervosa: immaturity of the 24-hour luteinizing hormone secretory pattern. N. Engl. J. Med. *291*:861–865, 1974.

9. Braun, D. L., Sunday, S. R., and Halmi, K. A. Psychiatric comorbidity in patients with eating disorders. Psychol. Med. *24*:859–867, 1994.

10. Brotman, A. W., Rigotti, N., and Herzog, D. B. Medical complications of eating disorders: outpatient evaluation and management. Compr. Psychiat. *26*:258–273, 1985.

11. Burns, T., and Crisp, A. H. Outcome of anorexia nervosa in males. Brit. J. Psychiat. *145*:319–325, 1984.

12. Cantwell, D. P., Sturzenberger, S., Burroughs, J., Salkin, B., and Green, J. K. Anorexia nervosa: an affective disorder? Arch. Gen. Psychiat. *34*:1087–1093, 1973.

13. Carlat, D. J., and Camargo, C. A. Review of bulimia nervosa in males. Am. J. Psychiat. *148*:831–843, 1991.

14. Casper, R. C., Eckert, E. D., Halmi, K. A., Goldberg, S. C., and Davis, J. M. Bulimia. Its incidence and clinical importance in patients with anorexia nervosa. Arch. Gen. Psychiat. *37*:1030–1035, 1980.

15. Casper, R. C., Halmi, K. A., Goldberg, S. C., Eckert, E. D., and Davis, J. M. Disturbances in body image estimation as related to other characteristics and outcome in anorexia nervosa. Brit. J. Psychiat. *134*:60–66, 1979.

16. Crisp, A. H. A treatment regimen for anorexia nervosa. Brit. J. Psychiat. *172*:505, 1966.

17. Crisp, A. H., Palmer, R. L., and Kalucy, R. S. How common is anorexia nervosa? A prevalence study. Brit. J. Psychiat. *128*:549–554, 1976.

18. Dally, P. *Anorexia Nervosa.* New York: Grune & Stratton, 1969.

19. Darby, P. L., Garfinkel, P. E., Vale, J. M., Kirwan, P. J., and Brown, G. M. Anorexia nervosa and "Turner syndrome": cause or coincidence? Psychol. Med. *11*:141–145, 1981.

20. Dejerine, J., and Gauckler, E. Le Réeducation des faux gastropathies. Presse Méd. *16*:225, 1908.

21. Dougherty, Jr., G. G., Rockwell, W. J. K., Sutton, G., and Ellinwood, Jr., E. H. Anorexia nervosa in treated gonadal dysgenesis: case report and review. J. Clin. Psychiat. *44*219–221, 1983.

22. Eckert, E. D., Goldberg, S. C., Halmi, K. A., Casper, R. C., and Davis, J. M.

Behaviour therapy in anorexia nervosa. Brit. J. Psychiat. *134*:55–59, 1979.

23. Eckert, E. D., Goldberg, S. C., Halmi, K. A., Casper, R. C., and Davis, J. M. Depression in anorexia nervosa. Psychol. Med. *12*:115–122, 1982.

24. El-Badri, S. M., and Lewis, M. A. Anorexia nervosa associated with Klinefelter's syndrome. Compr. Psychiat. *32*:317–319, 1991.

25. Engel, K., Hentz, M., Wittern, M., and Meyer, A. E. Long-term stability of anorexia nervosa treatments: follow-up study of 218 patients. Psychiat. Dev. *4*:395–407, 1989.

26. Fairburn, C. G., and Cooper, P. J. Self-induced vomiting and bulimia nervosa: an undetected problem. Brit. Med. J. *284*:1153–1155, 1982.

27. Falk, J. R., and Halmi, K. A. Amenorrhea in anorexia nervosa: examination of the critical body weight hypothesis. Biol. Psychiat. *17*:799–806, 1982.

28. Frisch, R. E., Wyshak, G., and Vincent, L. Delayed menarche and amenorrhea in ballet dancers. N. Engl. J. Med. *303*:17–19, 1980.

29. Garfinkel, P. E., Garner, D. M., Rose, J., Darby, P. L., Brandes, J. S., O'Hanlon, J., and Walsh, N. A comparison of characteristics in the families of patients with anorexia nervosa and normal controls. Psychol. Med. *13*:821–828, 1983.

30. Garfinkel, P. E., Moldofsky, H., and Garner, D. M. The heterogeneity of anorexia nervosa. Arch. Gen. Psychiat. *37*:1036–1040, 1980.

31. Garner, D. M., and Garfinkel, P. E. Socio-cultural factors in the development of anorexia nervosa. Psychol. Med. *10*:647–656, 1980.

32. Gerner, R. H., and Gwirtsman, H. E. Abnormalities of dexamethasone suppression test and urinary MHPG in anorexia nervosa. Am. J. Psychiat. *138*:650–653, 1981.

33. Gull, W. W. Anorexia nervosa (apepsia hysterica). Brit. Med. J. *2*:527, 1873.

34. Gwirtsman, H. E. Bulimic disorders: pharmacotherapeutic and biological studies. Psychopharm. Bull. *29*:109–114, 1993.

35. Hall, A., Leibrich, J., Walkey, F. H., and Welch, G. Investigation of "weight pathology" of 58 mothers of anorexia nervosa patients and 204 mothers of schoolgirls. Psychol. Med. *16*:71–76, 1986.

36. Hall, A., Slim, E., Hawker, F., and Salmond, C. Anorexia nervosa: longterm outcome in 50 female patients. Brit. J. Psychiat. *145*:407–413, 1984.

37. Halmi, K. A. The state of research in anorexia nervosa and bulimia. Psychiat. Dev. *3*:247–262, 1983.

38. Halmi, K., and Brodland, G. Monozygotic twins concordant and discordant for anorexia nervosa. Psychol. Med. *3*:521–524, 1973.

39. Halmi, K., Brodland, G., and Loney, J. Prognosis in anorexia nervosa. Ann. Intern. Med. *78*:907–909, 1973.

40. Halmi, K. A., Falk, J. R., and Schwartz, E. Binge-eating and vomiting: a survey of a college population. Psychol. Med. *11*:697–706, 1981.

41. Halmi, K. A., and Loney, J. Familial alcoholism in anorexia nervosa. Brit. J. Psychiat. *123*:53–54, 1973.

42. Hawley, R. M. The outcome of anorexia nervosa in younger subjects. Brit. J. Psychiat. *146*:657–660, 1985.

43. Hay, G. G., and Leonard, J. C. Anorexia nervosa in males. Lancet 2:574–576, 1979.

44. Herzog, D. B., and Copeland, P. M. Eating disorders. N. Engl. J. Med. 313:295–303, 1985.

45. Hindler, C. G., and Norris, D. L. A case of anorexia nervosa with Klinefelter's syndrome. Brit. J. Psychiat. 149:659–660, 1986.

46. Hoffman, L., and Halmi, K. A. Treatment of Anorexia Nervosa. In *Current Psychiatric Therapy*, Dunner, D. L. (ed.). Philadelphia: W. B. Saunders, 1993.

47. Holden, N. L. Adoption and eating disorders: a high-risk group? Brit. J. Psychiat. 158:829–833, 1991.

48. Holland, A. J., Hall, A., Murray, R., Russell, G. F. M., and Crisp, A. H. Anorexia nervosa: a study of 34 twin pairs and one set of triplets. Brit. J. Psychiat. 145:414–419, 1984.

49. Holt, S., Ford, M. J., Grant, S., and Heading, R. C. Abnormal gastric emptying in primary anorexia nervosa. Brit. J. Psychiat. 139:550–552, 1981.

50. Hsu, L. K. G. Outcome of anorexia nervosa. Arch. Gen. Psychiat. 37:1041–1046, 1980.

51. Hudson, J. I., and Hudson, M. S. Endocrine dysfunction in anorexia nervosa and bulimia: comparison with abnormalities in other psychiatric disorders and disturbances due to metabolic factors. Psychiat. Dev. 4:237–272, 1984.

52. Hudson, J. I., Pope, Jr., H. G., and Jonas, J. M. Psychosis in anorexia nervosa and bulimia. Brit. J. Psychiat. 145:420–423, 1984.

53. Hsu, L. K. G., Holder, D., Hindmarsh, D., and Phelps, C. Bipolar illness preceded by anorexia nervosa in identical twins. J. Clin. Psychiat. 45:262–266, 1984.

54. Jones, D. J., Fox, M. M., Babigian, H. M., and Hutton, H. E. Epidemiology of anorexia nervosa in Monroe County, New York: 1960–1976. Psychosom. Med. 42:551–558, 1980.

55. Kanis, J. A., Brown, P., Fitzpatrick, K., Hibbert, D. J., Horn, D. B., Nairn, I. M., Shirling, D., Strong, J. A., and Walton, H. J. Anorexia nervosa: a clinical, psychiatric, and laboratory study. Q. J. Med. 43:321–338, 1974.

56. Katz, J. L. Eating disorder and affective disorder: relatives or merely chance acquaintances? Compr. Psychiat. 28:220–228, 1987.

57. Kay, D. W., and Leigh, D. The natural history, treatment and prognosis of anorexia nervosa based on a study of 38 patients. J. Ment. Sci. 100:411–431, 1954.

58. Kendell, R. E., Hall, D. J., Hailey, A., and Babigian, H. M. The epidemiology of anorexia nervosa. Psychol. Med. 3:200–203, 1973.

59. King, A. Primary and secondary anorexia nervosa syndromes. Brit. J. Psychiat. 109:470, 1963.

60. Kron, L., Katz, J. L., Gorznski, G., and Wiener, H. Anorexia nervosa and gonadal dysgenesis. Arch. Gen. Psychiat. 34:332–335, 1977.

61. Larocca, F. E. F. Concurrence of Turner's syndrome, anorexia nervosa, and mood disorders: case report. J. Clin. Psychiat. 46:296–297, 1985.

62. Lasègue, E. C. De l'anorexia hystérique. Arch. Gen. Med. 21:385, 1873.

63. Lucas, A. R., Beard, C. M., O'Fallon, W. M., and Kurland, L. T. 50-year trends in the incidence of anorexia nervosa in Rochester, Minn.: a population-based study. Am. J. Psychiat. 148:917–922, 1991.

64. Morgan, H. G., and Russell, G. F. M. Value of family background and clinical features as predictors of long-term outcome in anorexia nervosa: four-year follow-up study of 41 patients. Psychol. Med. 5:355–371, 1975.

65. Pope, Jr., H. G., and Hudson, J. I. Antidepressant drug therapy for bulimia: current status. J. Clin. Psychiat. 47:339–345, 1986.

66. Pops, M. A., and Schwabe, A. D. Hypercarotenemia in anorexia nervosa. JAMA 205:533–534, 1968.

67. Rajs, J., Rajs, E., and Lundman, T. Unexpected death in patients suffering from eating disorders. Acta Psychiat. Scand. 74:587–596, 1986.

68. Ratnasuriya, R. H., Eisler, I., Szmukler, G. I., and Russell, G. F. M. Anorexia nervosa: outcome and prognostic factors after 20 years. Br. J. Psychiat. 158:495–502, 1991.

69. Robinson, P. H., and Holden, N. L. Bulimia nervosa in the male: a report of nine cases. Psychol. Med. 16:895–903, 1986.

70. Russell, G. F. M. Metabolic aspects of anorexia nervosa. Proc. R. Soc. Med. 58:811–814, 1965.

71. Russell, G. Bulimia nervosa: an ominous variant of anorexia nervosa. Psychol. Med. 9:429–448, 1979.

72. Schwabe, A. D., Lippe, B. M., Chang, R. J., Pops, M. A., and Yager, J. Anorexia nervosa. Ann. Intern. Med. 94:371–381, 1981.

73. Sharp, C. W., and Freeman, C. P. L. The medical complications of anorexia nervosa. Br. J. Psychiat. 162:452–462, 1993.

74. Simmons, R. C., and Kessler, M. D. Identical twins simultaneously concordant for anorexia nervosa. J. Am. Acad. Child Psychiat. 18:527–536, 1979.

75. Steinhausen, H.-Ch., Rauss-Mason, C., and Seidel, R. Follow-up studies of anorexia nervosa: a review of four decades of outcome research. Psychol. Med. 21:447–454, 1991.

76. Stunkard, A. New therapies for the eating disorders. Arch. Gen. Psychiat. 26:391–398, 1972.

77. Swift, W. J. The long-term outcome of early onset anorexia nervosa. J. Am. Acad. Child Psychiat. 21:38–46, 1982.

78. Szmukler, G., McCance, C., McCrone, L., and Hunter, D. Anorexia nervosa: a psychiatric case register study from Aberdeen. Psychol. Med. 16:49–58, 1986.

79. Theander, S. Anorexia nervosa: a psychiatric investigation of 94 female patients. Acta. Psychiat. Scand. Suppl. 214:5–194, 1970.

80. Thomas, J. P., and Szmukler, G. I. Anorexia nervosa in patients with Afro-Caribbean extraction. Brit. J. Psychiat. 146:653–656, 1985.

81. Tolstrup, K., Brinch, M., Isager, T., Nielsen, S., Nystrup, J., Severin, B., and Olesen, N. S. Long-term outcome of 151 cases of anorexia nervosa. Acta Psychiat. Scand. 71:380–387, 1985.

82. Toner, B. B., Garfinkel, P. E., and Garner, D. M. Long-term follow-up of anorexia nervosa. Psychosom. Med. 48:520–529, 1986.

83. Vandereycken, W., and Van den Broucke, S. Anorexia nervosa in males. Acta Psychiat. Scand. *70*:447–454, 1984.

84. Wålinder, J., and Mellbin, G. Karyotyping of women with anorexia nervosa. Brit. J. Psychiat. *130*:48–49, 1977.

85. Warren, W. A study of anorexia nervosa in young girls. J. Child Psychol. Psychiat. *9*:27–40, 1968.

86. Williams, J., King, M. The "epidemic" of anorexia nervosa: another medical myth? Lancet *I*:205–207, 1987.

12

THE PSYCHIATRIC
EXAMINATION

Such is man that if he has the name for something, it ceases to be
a riddle.

ISAAC BASHEVIS SINGER

The purpose of a psychiatric examination is to evaluate psychological function and to diagnose psychiatric disorders. To elicit
enough information about the disorders in order to diagnose
them, one must know their signs and symptoms, course and complications. That is why this chapter ends the book.

There is an art to eliciting clinical information. It can be
learned in a formal way, but only in part. To establish the trust
and rapport between doctor and patient that brings out reliable
information, empathy, intuition, and common sense are essential.
These cannot be learned from books. Here we will give advice on
interviewing, provide a logical framework for organizing observations, and suggest how case histories should be presented. But
first a few words about terminology and time.

A *mental status* examination is the part of the physical examination that deals with the patient's thoughts, feelings, and behavior at a particular point in time. This term is often used as a
synonym for a *psychiatric examination*, but *mental status* refers to
one part of the psychiatric examination: the current thoughts,
feelings, and behavior of the patient. *Psychiatric examination* in-

cludes the past history of the patient as well. The distinction between the two terms is somewhat artificial. As with *liver status* or *cardiac status*, what exists now is inseparable from what came before; a certain amount of historical background is unavoidable in describing the current mental status of a patient. Still, the term "mental status" is used when the *primary* focus of the questioning is on current functioning.

Internists, family practitioners, and other nonpsychiatrists generally have little time to conduct a physical examination: often no more than fifteen or twenty minutes. If the examination is "complete," it will include some attention to the mental status of the patient. This may be limited to a few minutes.

Later we will provide some screening questions that will help nonpsychiatrists decide quickly whether the mental state of the patient is abnormal. For now, we will assume the mental status examination is being conducted by a psychiatrist, a student or a resident in psychiatry who has the luxury of being able to spend a fair amount of time with the patient, observing him or her and asking questions.

ADVICE ON INTERVIEWING

Here are four rules for conducting a psychiatric examination.

1. *Start open ended.* Unless the patient is uncooperative or incapable of free expression (perhaps because of physical disability), let the patient tell his or her story with little or no interruption during the first five to fifteen minutes. After exchanging friendly greetings with the patient and attempting to set a relaxed tone, the interviewer should ask an open-ended question such as, "What is the problem that brings you here?" "What can I do for you?"

   The patient is often tense early in the interview and this tension may indeed stimulate the information flow. A patient with a *formal thought disorder* (where the thoughts do not connect coherently) will reveal this quickly. Much of the information needed for the diagnosis is often provided in the first few minutes if the patient proceeds uninterruptedly. By steering the questions along certain lines, one may miss important material.

On the other hand, for a particularly tense patient, more structure at the beginning of the interview may lead to easier communication. With such a patient, the interviewer can ask specific questions that are emotionally neutral. Questions about the patient's background—where the patient grew up and went to school, marital status, job, other physicians seen—usually are not difficult to answer and provide a comfortable transition into asking about the presenting problems.

2. *Ask specific questions later.* One purpose of the mental status examination is to make a diagnosis, if possible. This requires specific questions if merely to rule out remote possibilities. For example, patients often avoid volunteering information about hallucinations. "Do you hear voices or see things that others do not hear or see?" or some variation on this query is often necessary to determine whether the patient is psychotic. "Do you feel in danger?" may elicit persecutory delusions. "Do you have a special mission in life?" may bring out grandiose delusions. "What are your plans after leaving the hospital?" may bring out unrealistic thinking, raising questions about judgment.

Even with the advantage of a long interview, the psychiatric examiner must ask specific questions bearing on a reasonable differential diagnosis. There is usually no point, for example, in going through a complete review of systems if the patient experiences excellent health and presents with symptoms of a psychiatric condition in which physical symptoms do not usually play a role.

Details about early life experiences rarely bear on the problem of making a differential diagnosis in adults. School and social history are often important but not always, particularly in dealing with elderly people.

3. *Establish the chronology of the illness.* Kraepelin (3) noted that the course of a psychiatric illness is as important as the symptoms. Sydenham (5) said that "true" illnesses should have common symptoms and a common course. Few, if any, pathognomonic symptoms exist in psychiatry. We agree with Kraepelin that establishing the course of an illness is as important as recognizing current symptoms.

When did the symptoms begin? Was the patient ever free of psychiatric symptoms? When? Age of onset is an important clue to diagnosis as many conditions typically begin at particular times in life. Has the illness been continual, always present with fluctuations, or episodic in the sense that symptoms sometimes go away entirely? How rapid was the onset? (Psychotic illnesses with abrupt onsets generally have a better prognosis than those with a gradual onset.) Have professional interventions (medications, psychotherapy) altered the course of illness? In general, has the patient tended to improve or get worse?

"Diagnosis is prognosis" is an old saying in medicine, and knowledge of the course of illness as well as the symptoms forms the basis for determining prognosis.

4. *Be friendly, sympathetic, respectful.* Examiners should never insult patients. They should never make fun of them. This may seem obvious, but there are subtle ways of betraying disrespect. Adult patients should be called "Mr." or "Mrs." or "Ms.," at least until the examiner knows them well.

Be sensitive to the emotional state of the patient. If certain questioning makes the patient angry, anxious, depressed, or tearful, this may offer an opportunity to enhance the patient's ability to communicate, though sometimes a return to more neutral ground is indicated so that the patient is not overwhelmed by the emotion.

A word about the uncooperative patient: To say, "I can't help you unless you help me" sometime works, but usually it does not. Asking specific questions such as "What led to your coming here?" or "Whose idea was it that you come here?" may help lower resistance. Sometimes the interview must be postponed until another time when the patient may be more helpful. Anger toward the uncooperative patient is never appropriate.

Psychiatry, probably more than any other specialty, benefits greatly from informants—friends and family who will tell what the patient will not (or cannot). Although caution should be exercised in judging the merit of such information, it can be very helpful in making a diagnosis.

THE DECISION TREE

Except for open-ended questions at the beginning and specific questions toward the end, history taking should flow easily and casually, as in a conversation. Patients should be permitted to talk about what they want to talk about, but they should be gently guided back into channels that provide information the examiner requires for a diagnosis. From the minute a patient walks into the examination room, however, the examiner's mental "computer" starts making decisions. How is the patient dressed and groomed? Does the patient have a normal gait and range of motion? Is the patient hostile or friendly? How old does the patient appear to be?

Based on these first impressions, the interviewer starts narrowing the diagnostic range. The examiner's choices about *probable* diagnoses will determine which areas to emphasize and which to skip over lightly or omit entirely. The examiner's mind, indeed, functions as a computer. By the end of the interview—if it is successful—the choices will have narrowed to one or a few.

Table 12.1 shows a highly simplified branching process for approaching the diagnosis of psychiatric disorders. The first decision concerns *memory*. If the patient has a normal memory, move to the right of the line in Table 12.1. The second decision concerns psychosis. Is the patient psychotic or nonpsychotic? Psychosis can be both broadly or narrowly defined. Broadly defined, it refers to the gravity or seriousness of the condition; a suicidal patient might be called psychotic because suicide is serious. Nar-

Table 12.1 Major branches in diagnosis making

Impaired Memory			Normal Memory	
Acute	Chronic		Psychotic	Nonpsychotic
(Delirium)	Dementia	Retardation	Schizophrenia	Anxiety disorders
			Acute	Panic
			Chronic	Obsessional
			Affective disorders	Phobic
			Depression	Somatization disorder
			Mania	Antisocial personality
			Both	Chemical dependence
			Drugs	Affective disorders
				"Personality disorders"

rowly defined, as here, psychosis means the presence of persistent hallucinations and/or delusions and/or disordered thoughts.

As shown in Table 12.1, a *psychotic* person with *a normal memory* may suffer from schizophrenia, an affective disorder, or drug intoxication. Hallucinogens, amphetamines, and phencyclidine (PCP) are commonly associated with psychosis in the presence of a normal memory.

If the patient has a normal memory and is not psychotic, diagnostic possibilities include the anxiety disorders (there are eight in *DSM-III-R*), somatization disorder (hysteria), antisocial personality, drug (chemical) dependence, affective disorders, and other personality disorders. Thus, in some conditions such as affective disorders and drug dependence, the patient may or may not be psychotic. The term "personality disorders" is included for purposes of completeness, but these conditions are still either too vaguely defined or too poorly studied to be useful diagnostic categories.

In most hospitals, about one-fifth of the patients who clearly have psychiatric abnormalities do not fit any of the categories in Table 12.1. The suitable label for these people is *undiagnosed.* One advantage of this term is that physicians who deal with the patient in the future will not be biased by having a poorly grounded diagnosis in the chart. Another advantage is the sense of modesty it correctly implies.

A disadvantage is that many insurance companies *require* a diagnosis. In this case, one can include the most likely diagnosis or diagnoses prefaced by the term "rule out." Most insurance companies will accept this practice.

Outside of hospitals, many patients who consult psychiatrists do not have a diagnosable illness. They even lack symptoms of sufficient severity to justify being called "undiagnosed." One diagnosis for these more or less normal people who see psychiatrists is "problem of living," which suggests, if nothing else, that no conventional diagnosis seems to fit them.

Left of the center line in Table 12.1 are conditions associated with impaired memory. Acute refers to those of recent onset (less than a month); chronic to those of longer duration. "Organic brain disorder" or "organic brain syndrome" are commonly used terms for patients with impaired memories. An acute brain disorder includes delirium. Dementia is a chronic brain disorder that represents a deterioration from a previous level of normal cognitive function.

As noted earlier, the first and in some ways most important decision concerns whether the patient has an impaired or normal memory. Although IQ tests measure more than memory, performance depends to a large extent on what persons have learned and how well they can recall it, that is, memory. Though memory loss may affect some functions more than others, *gross* memory disturbance usually affects intellectual functioning across the board.

To be "impaired" the patient's memory must be *really* impaired, in contradistinction to "normal forgetting." (Sometimes, admittedly, the distinction is not easy to make.) Disorientation is a form of memory impairment. Inability to do simple arithmetic reflects a bad memory, assuming the person once knew how to do arithmetic.

Diagnosing dementia is best done by estimating what the patient *should* know. If patients are interested in sports, they should be able to name sports figures. If interested in gardening, they should be able to name plants. Patients are often asked to do "serial sevens," whereby they subtract seven from one hundred and then continue subtracting sevens in a descending scale. In fact, normal people with little talent in arithmetic have trouble with serial sevens and their failure to do them may not be clinically significant. (Serial sevens tests attention and concentration as well as memory.) On the other hand, if certified public accountants cannot do serial sevens, dementia is likely, although their performance may have faltered because they were anxious or distracted.

Delirium is usually accompanied by agitation and autonomic hyperactivity as well as hallucinations and delusions (perhaps more often illusions: misinterpretation of stimuli). Sometimes delirious patients lie quietly in bed but still misidentify people and cannot remember the year or where they are. Delirious people may be dangerous. To escape their delusional persecutors they may jump out of hospital windows or attack those around them. They must be watched closely.

Poor intellectual functioning is associated with, and often indistinguishable from, bad memory. Impaired memory *produces* impaired intellectual functioning. As noted, "intelligence" encompasses more than memory, but even those skills not normally associated with memory (e.g., reasoning ability) often suffer when memory is impaired.

Depressed patients sometimes have bad memories and this is called "pseudodementia." Their memory improves as their depression improves. Stroke patients and patients with Alzheimer's disease also experience depression, but *their* memory usually does not improve as the depression improves.

Here is the important point about gross memory impairment (as distinguished from absentmindedness, normal forgetting, or "not paying attention"): Patients with organic brain disorders may display *any* psychiatric symptom associated with disorders on the right side of Table 12.1, *but organic brain disorders still take precedence as the diagnosis* unless the other disorders clearly antedated the brain disorder. Anxiety, depression, delusions, hallucinations, mania, incoherence, obsessions, phobias may all occur in organic brain disorders. Diagnosing organic brain disorders is one of the most important things a psychiatrist can do. It initiates a search for the *cause* of the disorder and the cause may be *treatable*. Physicians are uniquely qualified to identify the organic disese. Knowing anatomy, physiology, and biochemistry and aided by modern imaging and laboratory techniques, physicians can evaluate the entire range of causes of organic brain disorders, including brain tumor, endocrine and metabolic disorders, and infections.

THE MENTAL STATUS FORMAT

The purpose of the mental status format is to help the interviewer organize and communicate his or her observations about a patient. Minor deviations occur in the format from expert to expert, but *some* framework for observations is necessary to facilitate thinking and communication. The format presented here is commonly used and includes the following categories:

Appearance and behavior
Form and content of thought
Affect and mood
Memory and intellectual functioning
Insight and judgment

Appearance and Behavior

The patient's appearance is often relevant to the diagnosis. Schizophrenics, for example, are often poorly groomed and sometimes dirty. Depressives also are often negligent about their dress and grooming. A manic may wear a funny hat. Sunglasses worn indoors may suggest paranoia; tattoos often suggest antisocial personality; a puffy face and red palms are suggestive of, but not diagnostic of, alcoholism.

If the patients look older than their stated age, this may suggest depression or long-term substance abuse. If this is the case, they may begin to look younger as they recover.

The patient's attitude toward the interviewer may be significant. Paranoids are often suspicious, guarded, or hostile. Hysterics sometimes try to flatter interviewers by comparing them favorably with previous doctors; they are often dramatic, friendly—sometimes seductive. Manics may crack jokes and occasionally are quite funny—when they are not irritable or obnoxious. Sociopaths may seem like con men—and sometimes are.

The patient may be agitated—unable to sit still, moving constantly. Others are retarded, slumping in their seats, slow in movement and speech. Talking may seem an effort.

Agitation and retardation can have several causes. Neuroleptic drugs may produce a restlessness called "akathisia," in which the patient cannot sit still and feels compelled to walk. Neuroleptics also may produce Parkinson-type symptoms, including tremor and an expressionless face. Pacing and handwringing may be expressions of depression; joviality and volubility may portray mania.

Neuroleptic drugs are given so commonly that it is often impossible to determine whether abnormal movements are drug induced or are catatonic symptoms. In fact, similar involuntary movements were observed in schizophrenics years ago before drugs were introduced. It is said that catatonic symptoms are disappearing, but what previously was called catatonic may now be interpreted as drug induced without knowing whether drugs are responsible or not.

Schizophrenia also may involve psychomotor disturbances such as mannerisms, posturing, stereotypical movements, and negativism (doing the opposite of what is requested). Also seen is *echopraxia*, in which movements of another person are imitated, and *waxy flexibility*, in which awkward positions are maintained for long periods without apparent discomfort. Some patients say nothing. This is called "mutism"; it may be seen in schizophrenia, depression, brain syndrome, and drug intoxication.

Form and Content of Thought

Form refers to intelligibility related to associations: Does the patient have "loose associations" in the sense of being circumstantial, tangential, or incoherent? Elderly people are often circumstantial. They return to the subject but only after providing excessive detail. Tangentiality is a flow of thought directed away from the subject being inquired about, with no return to the point of departure. Schizophrenics are often tangential. Pressure of speech and flight of ideas are seen in mania and in drug intoxication. With pressure of speech, the patient seems compelled to talk. Manic speech flits from idea to idea, sometimes linked by only the most tenuous connections. Unlike tangentiality, however, manic speech frequently has connections that can be surmised. Manics often rhyme or pun and make "clang" associations, using one word after another because they sound similar. Manics tend to be overinclusive, including irrelevant and extraneous details.

Derailment, often seen in schizophrenia, is a form of speech in which it is impossible to follow the logic of the associations. Sometimes schizophrenics invent new words (neologisms) that presumably have a private meaning. Sometimes schizophrenics display poverty of thought, conveying little information with their words. *Echolalia* refers to occasions when the patient repeats words back to the interviewer. Other abnormal speech patterns associated with schizophrenia (as well as dementia) are perseveration, in which the patient seems incapable of changing topics, and blocking, in which the flow of thought is suddenly stopped, often followed by a new and unrelated thought.

When patients persistently display any of these symptoms (excluding poverty of thought), they are said to have a *formal thought disorder*, meaning that the structure or form of thinking is disordered.

Content of thought refers to what the patient thinks and talks about. Under this category come hallucinations, delusions, obsessions, compulsions, phobias, and preoccupations deemed relevant to the psychiatric problem.

Delusions are fixed false ideas neither amenable to logic or social pressure nor congruent with the patient's culture. They should be distinguished from *overvalued* ideas; fixed notions that most people consider false but that are not entirely unreasonable or that cannot be disproven, such as certain superstitions. Delusions occur in organic brain disorders, schizophrenia, affective disorders, and various intoxications.

Jaspers (2) believed the *subject* of the delusion had diagnostic significance. If the delusional ideas were "understandable," they more likely occurred in depressed patients. Understandable delusions included those in which persons were convinced they had a serious life-threatening illness such as cancer, were impoverished, or were being persecuted because they were bad persons. Jaspers pointed out that healthy, prosperous, and likable people often worry about their health, finances, and approval by others. Such delusions are thus understandable.

Delusions that are *not* understandable are seen in schizophrenia, according to Jaspers. Schizophrenic delusions tend to be bizarre; for example, one's acts are controlled by outside forces (delusions of control or influence) or one believes that one is Jesus or Napoleon. Schizophrenia-like delusions occur often in amphetamine psychosis and, less commonly, in other intoxicated states (e.g., from cocaine or cannabis). The delusions of schizophrenia fall outside the ordinary person's experience: The examiner finds it difficult to identify with the schizophrenic's private world; hence the term "autism," derived from "auto," is often applied to schizophrenic thinking.

Religious delusions are sometimes hard to interpret. Religious beliefs often seem delusional to those who do not accept the beliefs but normal to those who do. Among fundamentalist religious people, truly pathological delusions are usually identified without difficulty by others in the congregation.

Content also encompasses perceptual disturbances. In *illusions*, real stimuli are mistaken for something else (a belt for a snake).

Hallucinations are perceptions without an external stimulus. *Auditory hallucinations* may consist of voices or noises. They are associated primarily with schizophrenia but occur in other conditions such as chronic alcoholic hallucinosis and affective disorders (1). *Visual hallucinations* are most characteristic of organic brain disorders, especially delirious states. They also occur with psychedelic drug use and in schizophrenia. (Certain hallucinations are more common in some conditions, but no type of hallucination is found exclusively in any illness.) *Hypnagogic hallucinations* arise in the period between sleep and wakefulness, especially when falling asleep. Their occurrence is normal except when they are a symptom of narcolepsy (1).

Olfactory hallucinations are sometimes associated with complex partial seizures that involve the temporal lobes. *Haptic* (tactile) *hallucinations* occur in schizophrenia and also in cocaine intoxication and delirium tremens. The sensation of insects crawling in or under one's skin (formication) is particularly common in cocaine intoxication, but it also happens in delirium tremens.

In *extracampine hallucinations*, the patient sees objects outside the sensory field (e.g., behind his head). In *autoscopic hallucinations*, the patient visualizes himself projected into space. The patient occasionally has a *doppelgänger* (sees his double).

Other perceptual distortions include *depersonalization* (the feeling that one has changed in some bizarre way), *derealization* (the feeling that the environment has changed), and déjà vu (a sense of familiarity with a new perception).

In one study of nonpsychiatric patients, 40 percent reported hallucinations, particularly seeing dead relatives. They had no other psychiatric symptoms and the hallucinations were not judged to be clinically important. Thus a history of transient hallucinations or other perceptual disturbances, which occur occasionally during exhaustion or grief, does not necessarily signify the presence of psychosis. They must be interpreted in the context of the overall clinical picture.

Affect and Mood

Affect refers to a patient's outwardly (externally) expressed emotion, which may or may not be appropriate to her reported mood and content of thought. For example, if a person smiles happily while telling of people trying to poison her, the affect would be described as inappropriate. If one describes unbearable pain but looks as if she were discussing the weather, the affect again would be inappropriate.

Affect is sometimes referred to as "flat," meaning that the usual fine modulation in facial expression is absent. Schizophrenics sometimes have a flat affect, but so do patients taking neuroleptic drugs, and a depressed patient may show little change of expression while speaking.

"Flat affect" is probably the most overused and misused term in the psychiatric examination. It should only be used if the affect is extremely "flat" or "blunted." Inappropriate and flat affects are especially associated with schizophrenia.

Sometimes hysterics have an inappropriate affect in that they describe excruciating pain and other extreme distress with the same indifference or good cheer with which they would describe a morning of shopping. (The French call this *la belle indifférence*.)

Mood refers to what the patient says about his internal emotional state. "I am sad," "I am happy," "I am angry" are examples. Mood and affect are sometimes *labile*, meaning that there is rapid fluctuation between manifestations of happiness, sadness, anger, and so on. Labile affect is often seen in patients with organic brain disorders.

Memory and Intellectual Functioning

Subsumed under memory is orientation, meaning orientation for person, place, and time. To be disoriented for time, the patient should be more than one day off the correct day of the week and more than several days off the current date. Misidentifying people (thinking the nurse is one's aunt) is a clear case of disorientation, as is giving the wrong year or the wrong city and wrong hospital where one is currently residing. This part of the mental status is exceedingly important because, if a patient has a gross memory impairment (and is not malingering), he or she almost always has an organic brain disorder and all other psychiatric symptoms may be explainable in this context. (The pseudodementia of depression is one exception.)

There are many tests for memory and intellectual functioning. Memory can be subdivided into immediate, short-term, recent, and remote memory. Serially subtracting seven from one hundred is a test of immediate memory (assuming the person's arithmetic was ever adequate for the task) as well as a test of attention and concentration. Short-term-memory loss can be tested by asking patients to remember three easy words you have spoken or by showing them three objects and then, five to fifteen minutes later, asking them to repeat what they heard or saw. A short-term memory deficit is the sine qua non of Korsakoff's syndrome. Recent memory refers to recall of events occurring in recent days, weeks, or months; remote memory involves recall of events occurring many years before, such as the winner of a long-ago presidential election. In dementia, recent memory is usually more severely impaired than remote memory.

As noted earlier, tests of intellectual functioning should be interpreted with the patient's background, education, cooperativeness, and mood state in mind. A history major should be able to name seven presidents, but a "normal" person with a third-grade education may not be able to do so. Depressed patients may be too slowed down or distractible to concentrate. One approach is to ask patients about their interests and then test their fund of information in those areas.

Insight and Judgment

A person who has insight will know whether he is (or was) psychiatrically ill. If he says, for example, that the voices are "real," he lacks insight. If he says it was simply his imagination playing tricks on him, he has insight. If he says there is nothing wrong with him but that his evil uncle has arranged for his hospitalization because of a Communist conspiracy, he may or may not have insight. (Even paranoids, as the saying goes, sometimes have real enemies.) Psychosis and organic brain disorders are both associated with lack of insight; so-called "neurotics" usually realize they have something wrong with them.

The term "judgment" is used here in the same sense as "competence" is used in civil court: A competent person is able to understand the nature of the charges and to cooperate with counsel. It implies that a person is realistic about his limitations and life circumstances. A good question to ask is, "What are your plans when you leave the hospital?" If the patient says that he plans to start a chain of restaurants and has no money, this displays impaired judgment. Severe impairment of judgment is seen most often in dementia and psychotic disorders.

EXCLUDING PSYCHIATRIC DISORDERS

Sometimes for all physicians and often for nonpsychiatric physicians, examination of the "mind" must be accomplished quickly, lest the liver, lungs, heart, and deep tendon reflexes be slighted. For the dozen disorders described in this book, a single question may suffice to exclude the possibility the patient has a given disorder. Some disorders will be missed, but one or two questions will identify the great majority of patients who do *not* have a particular psychiatric illness:

Depression: Ask if the patient sleeps well. If she sleeps well without medication, the chances of a serious depression are slight. (Oversleeping represents "not sleeping well" as much as undersleeping.)

Mania: Ask if the patient has ever gone on a spending spree. Most manics have, even manics who cannot afford it.

Schizophrenia: Ask if the patient has ever heard or seen things that other people did not hear or see. Ask if he has ever been afraid of being poisoned or controlled by external forces. Hallucinations sometimes occur in normal people, but the presence of both hallucinations and delusions in a person with more or less normal mood suggests schizophrenia.

Panic disorder (anxiety neurosis): Has the patient ever thought she was having a heart attack that did not occur? Does she ever become intensely apprehensive for no apparent reason? Anxiety neurotics report both. At church, does she find a seat on the aisle close to the back? Anxiety neurotics almost always do. They feel the need to make a quick exit if a panic attack seems impending.

Hysteria (somatization disorder): Hysterics are mostly women. Get a menstrual history. If the woman denies having problems with her menstrual periods—if she has never missed work or school because of dysmenorrhea—hysteria is unlikely. If she has reached the age of thirty-five without having her appendix removed, plus some other elective operation, she is probably not hysteric.

Obsessive compulsive disorder: Does the patient, sitting in a waiting room, count things, such as the number of tiles on the floor? Does the patient repeatedly check a door to see if it is locked or an oven to see if it is turned off? Counting and checking are so common in this disorder that, if absent, the diagnosis should be questioned.

Phobic disorders: Does the patient avoid certain situations because they frighten him? Is the fear unreasonable?

Alcoholism: Has the patient ever stopped drinking for a period of time? If so, and the reason is not medical or a desire to lose weight, the patient probably stopped because he was worried about his drinking. At this point, the clinician can ask *why* he was worried, and this may break down the denial that is characteristic of alcoholism. Almost every alcoholic has stopped, or tried to stop, at some time in his life. This is a better approach than asking, "Do you drink too much?"

Drug dependence: "Have you ever worried about a drug habit?" is probably as good an opener as any.

Antisocial personality (sociopathy): Ask if the patient was frequently truant in grade and high school. Rare is the sociopath who did not cut classes and get in trouble with school authorities as a teenager.

Dementia: Ask if the patient forgets where she parks her car. If this happens often, there should be some concern about her memory. Or simply ask, "How is your memory?" Many people with memory problems are relieved to have the chance to talk about them.

Anorexia nervosa: If the person is intelligent, ask her (and it is usually a her) if she has ever been told she had anorexia nervosa. Anorectics usually know their diagnosis; the press is full of it. Does the patient stuff herself (or himself) with food and then induce vomiting? This practice, called "bulimia," often goes with anorexia in both sexes.

Another question: "Are you the right weight?" If the patient is five foot seven inches, weighs ninety-two pounds, is not a model, and says, "I'm too fat," the diagnosis is made.

Sexual problems: "Do you have a sex problem?" is usually sufficient. Since the Sexual Revolution, people are not as reticent about sexual matters as they once were.

These questions when answered in the negative will eliminate most people who have the above disorders. There will be few false negatives. There will be many false positives. (Many people sleep poorly and sit at the back of churches who do not have depression or anxiety disorders.) But for the physician trying to rule out disorders, false positives are unimportant. They simply mean probing is required. Probing takes time and referral to a psychiatrist may be in order.

Suggestions for Presenting Cases

There is obviously a good deal of latitude in presenting case histories for teaching purposes. Different institutions and different teachers within the institutions will have their own advice on the subject. However, discussions with these teachers reveal some agreement about certain points. Here are some general rules for presenting patients.

1. Don't read the history.
2. Don't exceed ten to fifteen minutes (allowing for interruptions).
3. Start with *identifying data:* name, age, race, marital status, vocation.
4. Provide a clue to the problem you will highlight, e.g., "This patient presents a diagnostic problem," "He has not responded to standard treatments," "She comes from an unusual family." Such clues offer a framework for your audience into which the rest of the presentation will fit.
5. Avoid dates. Open with "Patient was admitted to [hospital] _____ (days, weeks, months) ago. Do not refer to events occurring on December 3, 1937, but say, "At the age of 15, the patient _____." Instead of saying "Between November and January of 1955 and 1956," say, "For a three-month period when the patient was twenty years old, he _____." It may be easier for patients to remember events by dates, but the listener has to translate dates into ages and, for the unmathematically inclined, this may be difficult while concentrating on the presentation.
6. Begin with the *psychiatric history*. A good way to begin is, "The patient had no psychiatric problems until age _____ (or _____ days, weeks, or months ago) when he (slowly or rapidly) developed the following symptoms _____"; then list the symptoms in order of severity. Tell how long the symptoms persisted (for weeks, months, years, or to the present) and what happened as a result (hospitalization, other treatment, full or partial recovery).

Often, of course, establishing time of onset is difficult or impossible, particularly when dealing with a poor historian or a complicated case. The onset of illness in a mentally retarded person would be "from birth," which does not help much. But an *attempt* to establish onset can be of considerable help because different illnesses characteristically begin at different ages.

7. It is impotant to know whether the illness has been *chronic*, perhaps with fluctuations, or *episodic* with full remissions between episodes (4). If the patient has had more than one episode, describe subsequent episodes, briefly giving the same information that was given for the first episode. Symptoms and life events obviously are interrelated, but emphasize the symptoms rather than the life events unless the life events appear to be causally related to the symptoms.

8. A brief *family history* should include the following: whether a close blood relative of the patient had a serious psychiatric illness requiring treatment (and what the treatment was, if known), pertinent medical illnesses, and suicide, alcohol or drug problems.

9. *Social history* should include (very briefly) circumstances of upbringing, particularly whether the parents were divorced or separated or whether the patient was brought up by both parents; parental vocation; siblings; years of education and how well the patient did in school from the standpoint of grades and adjustment; military and job history; marital history; and number and ages of children.

10. Review the *medical history* only as it is pertinent to the psychiatric problems. The same applies to the review of systems, physical findings, and laboratory results.

11. Give the *mental status* as it was obtained either on admission or at the first opportunity to fully examine the patient. The mental status findings should be presented in the order provided in the previous section.

12. End the presentation with *course in hospital.* Tell how the

patient has been doing, whether he has improved, what treatment he is receiving. In other words, bring the patient up to the present moment.

13. With rare exceptions, all this can be presented in ten to fifteen minutes. The trick is to keep in mind at all times the goal of the presentation. If it is diagnostic, the differential diagnosis and the points for and against each of the reasonably likely diagnoses should be given. If you start out by saying the patient was psychiatrically well until the age of sixty, dwelling on such diagnoses as mental retardation, schizophrenia, somatization disorder, or panic disorder is unlikely to be useful. Assuming the history is correct (though, granted, this is often a dubious assumption), people who are well until the age of sixty and then develop major psychiatric problems generally have either an affective disorder or an organic brain syndrome.

14. The reasons for presenting the history and mental status according to the above sequence are to avoid leaving out important information and to make it easier for the listeners to follow the narration. There are many variations on this format, none perfect. (People's lives are much more complicated than formats.) Unlike written psychiatric histories, however, oral presentations should not attempt to be comprehensive. They should touch on the following categories, but not all with equal emphasis.

HISTORY

Identifying data
Focus of the presentation
Psychiatric history
Family history
Social history
Medical history
Review of systems
Physical findings
Laboratory results

MENTAL STATUS

Appearance and behavior
Form and content of thought
Affect and mood
Memory and intellectual functioning
Insight and judgment

REFERENCES

1. Goodwin, D. W., Alderson, P., and Rosenthal, R. Clinical significance of hallucinations in psychiatric disorders. Arch. Gen. Psychiat. *24*:76–80, 1971.
2. Jaspers, K. *General Psychopathology.* Chicago: Univ. of Chicago Press, 1963.
3. Kraepelin, E. *Dementia Praecox and Paraphrenia* (Barclay, R. M., Robertson, G. M., tran.). Edinburgh: E. S. Livingstone, 1919.
4. Othmer, E., and Othmer, S. C. *The Clinical Interview Using DSM-IV*: II. The
   Difficult Patient. Washington D.C.: American Psychiatric Press, 1994.
5. Sydenham, T. *Selected Works of Thomas Sydenham, M.D.* London: John Bales
   & Sons, Danielson, 1922.

INDEX

catecholamines, and depression,
17
cerebral arteriosclerosis, and
secondary affective disorder, 26
cerebral ventricle-to-brain ratio,
in schizophrenia, 50
charms, carrying, 142
checking rituals, 132–33, 170,
328
chest pain, in panic disorder,
86, 89, 93
childbearing rates, in schizophrenia, 58
childbirth, as precipitant of depression, 14–15
childhood conduct disorder,
203–4
children
alcoholism in, 187
Briquet's syndrome in, 118,
120
depression in, 17–18
fighting off depression for
sake of, 16
obsessive-compulsive disorder
in, 135, 142
phobic disorders in, 165
schizophrenia in, 53, 61
sociopathic, 256, 258–59,
261–63, 265–67
Chinese restaurant syndrome,
97
chippers (controlled heroin
users), 232
chloral hydrate, 206, 234
chlordiazepoxide (Librium), for
alcoholism, 238
chlorimipramine, for obsessive-
compulsive disorder, 146–
48
chlorpromazine, for mania, 31

chromosome 6, in affective disorders, 24
chromosome 11, in childhood
depression, 17
chronic alcohol hallucinosis,
201
chronic illness, diagnosing, 331
chronicity, of secondary affective disorders, 12
chronology of illness, 315
"clang" associations, in mania,
322
cleaning rituals, 133
cleanliness, inattentiveness to,
281
clonidine, for opioid
withdrawal, 229
clozapine, for schizophrenia, 66
cocaine, 222–23, 225–26, 240–
42, 323–24
codeine, 227
cognitive function
brain syndrome and, 274,
280, 318
schizophrenia and, 50
cognitive impairment of depression, 280
cognitive rehearsal, for
obsessive-compulsive disorder, 146
cognitive therapy
for panic disorder, 99
for primary affective disorder,
27
combative behavior, and brain
syndrome, 277, 279
compulsions, 95, 127, 133,
135–36, 145, 219
computerized tomography (CT)
in alcoholism, 199
in dementia, 285–86
in schizophrenia, 50

antisocial personality and,
329
psychiatric interview and, 314
schizophrenia and, 53, 57–58
sociopathy and, 259, 263, 265
seasonal affective disorder
(SAD), criteria for, 29
season of birth, in schizophrenia, 46
secondary affective disorder, 6,
9, 12
cerebral arteriosclerosis and,
26
depression and, 25
secondary depression
alcoholism and, 11
brain syndrome and, 287
secondary mania, 12
sedation, and amitriptyline, 30
sedative-hypnotics, 223–36
sedatives, brain syndrome, 289
seizures
alcoholism and, 207
lithium and, 32
selective serotonin-uptake inhibitors (SSRIs), development of, 28–29
self-harm, and depression, 8, 12
self-injury, and brain syndrome
and, 289
self-reproach, feelings of in depression, 13
serial sevens tests, 319, 326
Sernylan, 244
serotonin, in depression, 29
serotonin reuptake inhibitors
(SSRIs), 147
sex
agoraphobia, 168
Briquet's syndrome and, 114
diagnosing sexual problems,
329

loss of interest in, 13
obsessive-compulsive disorder
and, 131
panic disorder and, 94
sociopathy and, 259–60
short-term memory, and depression, 22
sidewalk cracks, stepping on,
133
signs, definition of *viii–xii*
simple phobia, 155, 165–66,
168–69
situational reaction, as term,
xii
sleep
affective disorders and, 7
alcoholism and, 189
childhood depression and, 17
depression and, 17–18, 327
imipramine and, 30
panic disorder and, 85, 88
schizophrenia and, 50
slow-wave, depression and,
17
smothering sensation, in panic
disorder, 85–86
social history
interviewing for, 314
review of, 331
social skills training, for
primary affective disorder,
27
social striving, and primary
affective disorder, 11
social unacceptability, of
depression, 15
social avoidance
in childhood depression, 17
in obsessive-compulsive disorder, 136
in panic disorder, 87
in schizophrenia, 53–54